Cytopathology of parasitic disease

Centro Médico Docente La Trinidad (CMDLT) is a non-profit making association which seeks to improve health care and medical education in Venezuela through research and the development of methods that can be applied nationally to improve quality at low cost. The association promotes and organizes lectures, courses and other scientific activities for the education of students and graduates in the medical sciences and ancillary professions. It also sets out to establish and administer clinics, hospitals and other centres which provide opportunities for the study of medicine and for progress in medical science. CMDLT aims to stimulate scientific research in various medical disciplines, so creating and helping to maintain research centres of a high scientific standard. CMDLT is grateful to the following institutions who collaborated with it locally to make this symposium possible: AsoVAC (Venezuelan Association for the Advancement of Science); the British Council; the Central University of Venezuela; CONICIT (National Council for Scientific and Technological Research); the José María Vargas Foundation; the José Francisco Torrealba Research Centre; the Ministry of Science and Technology; the Polar Foundation; and the Venezuelan Association of Weizmann Institute's Friends.

The Ciba Foundation is an international scientific and educational charity. It was established in 1947 by the Swiss chemical and pharmaceutical company of CIBA Limited—now CIBA-GEIGY Limited. The Foundation operates independently in London under English trust law. The Ciba Foundation exists to promote international cooperation in biological, medical and chemical research. It organizes about eight international multidisciplinary symposia each year on topics that seem ready for discussion by a small group of research workers. The papers and discussions are published in the Ciba Foundation symposium series. The Foundation also holds many shorter meetings (not published), organized by the Foundation itself or by outside scientific organizations. The staff always welcome suggestions for future meetings. The Foundation's house at 41 Portland Place, London, W1N 4BN, provides facilities for these meetings. Its library, open seven days a week to any graduate in science or medicine, provides information on scientific meetings throughout the world and answers general enquiries on biomedical and chemical subjects. Scientists from any part of the world may stay in the house during working visits to London. The Ciba Foundation occasionally organizes a symposium (such as this one) outside the UK, on a topic that is particularly relevant to the host country.

Cytopathology of parasitic disease

Ciba Foundation symposium 99

Organized by the Ciba Foundation, London, UK, in partnership with the Centro Médico Docente La Trinidad, Caracas, Venezuela

1983

Pitman

ISBN 0 272 79731 6

Published in September 1983 by Pitman Books Ltd, 128 Long Acre, London WC2E 9AN.
Distributed in North America by CIBA Pharmaceutical Company (Medical Education Division), Post Office Box 12832, Newark, NJ 07101, USA

Suggested series entry for library catalogues:
Ciba Foundation symposia

Ciba Foundation symposium 99
viii + xxx pages, xx figures, xx tables

British Library cataloguing in publication data:

Cytopathology of parasitic disease.—Ciba Foundation symposium; 99
1. Parasitic diseases—Congresses 2. Pathology, Cellular—Congresses
I. Ciba Foundation II. Centro Médico Docente La Trinidad III. Series
616.9′607 RC119

Text set in 10/12 pt Linotron 202 Times, printed and bound in Great Britain at The Pitman Press, Bath

Contents

Symposium on: Cytopathology of parasitic disease, held at the Centro Médico Docente La Trinidad, Caracas, Venezuela, 22-24 November 1982

Editors: David Evered (Organizer) and Geralyn M. Collins

Local organizers: Pablo A. Pulido M. and Romano Piras

This symposium was originally suggested by Pablo A. Pulido M.

Participants

Z. A. ANDRADE Gonçalo Moniz Research Center, Fundação Oswaldo Cruz Federal University of Bahia Faculty of Medicine, Rua Valdemar Falcão, 121-Brotas, Salvador, BA-40.000, Bahia, Brazil

J. L. AVILA Laboratorio de Bioquimica, Instituto Nacional de Dermatología, Apartado 4043, Caracas 1010-A, Venezuela

A. E. BUTTERWORTH Department of Pathology, University of Cambridge, Tennis Court Road, Cambridge CB2 1QP, UK

K.-P. CHANG Parasitology Laboratory, The Rockefeller University, 1230 York Avenue, New York, NY 10021, USA, *Now at:* Department of Microbiology, UHS/Chicago Medical School, 3333 Green Bay Road, North Chicago, Illinois 60064, USA

D. W. FAWCETT International Laboratory for Research in Animal Diseases, PO Box 30709, Nairobi, Kenya

W. E. GUTTERIDGE Department of Biochemical Parasitology, Wellcome Research Laboratories, Langley Court, Beckenham, Kent BR3 3BS, UK

A. G. HERNÁNDEZ Facultad de Ciencias, Universidad Central de Venezuela, Apartado 47069, Los Chaguaramos, Caracas 1041, Venezuela

L. HUDSON Department of Immunology, Jenner Wing, St George's Hospital Medical School, London SW17 0RE, UK

S. J. KLEBANOFF Allergy and Infectious Diseases, Department of Medicine, Rm-16, University of Washington School of Medicine, Seattle, Washington 98195, USA

A. MARTINEZ-PALOMO Departamento de Biología Celular, Centro Investigaciones Avanzados del Instituto Politecnico Nacional, Apartado 14–740, Mexico City 14, Mexico

D. MIRELMAN Department of Biophysics, Weizmann Institute of Science, Rehovot 76100, Israel

N. NOGUEIRA Laboratory of Cellular Physiology and Immunology, The Rockefeller University, 1230 York Avenue, New York, NY 10021, USA

R. S. NUSSENZWEIG Division of Parasitology, Department of Microbiology, New York University Medical Center, 550 First Avenue, New York, NY 10016, USA

J. A. O'DALY Laboratorio de Inmunobiología, Instituto Venezolano de Investigaciones Científicas, Apartado 1827, Caracas 1010-A, Venezuela

M. E. A. PEREIRA Department of Medicine, Division of Geographic Medicine, Tufts University School of Medicine, 136 Harrison Avenue, Boston, Massachusetts 02111, USA

H. A. PÉREZ Laboratorio de Inmunoparasitología, Centro de Microbiología y Biologí Celular, Instituto Venezolano de Investigaciones Científicas, Apartado 1827, Caracas 1010-A, Venezuela

E. R. PFEFFERKORN Department of Microbiology, Dartmouth Medical School, Hanover, New Hampshire 03756, USA

R. PIRAS Unidad de Investigaciones, Centro Médico Docente La Trinidad, Apartado 80474, Caracas 1080-A, Venezuela

P. A. PULIDO M. Centro Médico Docente La Trinidad, Apartado 80474, Caracas 1080-A, Venezuela

S. SHARMA Department of Immunology and Infectious Diseases, Research Institute, Palo Alto Medical Foundation, 860 Bryant Street, Palo Alto, California 94301, USA

A. SHER Immunology and Cell Biology Section, Laboratory of Parasitic Diseases, National Institute of Allergy & Infectious Diseases, National Institutes of Health, Bethesda, Maryland 20205, USA

J. URBINA Departamento de Biología Celular, Escuela de Biología, Facultad de Ciencias, Universidad Central de Venezuela, Apartado 21201, Los Chaguaramos, Caracas 1020, Venezuela

K. S. WARREN (*Chairman*) Health Sciences, The Rockefeller Foundation, 1133 Avenue of the Americas, New York, NY 10036, USA

D. J. WYLER Division of Geographic Medicine, Department of Medicine, Tufts University School of Medicine, 136 Harrison Avenue, Boston, Massachusetts 02111, USA

Chairman's introduction

K. S. WARREN

Health Sciences, The Rockefeller Foundation, 1133 Avenue of the Americas, New York, NY 10036, USA

The cytopathology of parasitic disease is an exceedingly important subject today because the field has really gained momentum in the past 10 years, and our knowledge about host–parasite interaction at the chemical and immunological level is increasing rapidly. Most of the people here have played a major part in the development of this work. I have previously had the pleasure of attending another Ciba Foundation meeting, in London—Parasites in the immunized host: mechanisms of survival (Ciba Found Symp 25). The discussion at that meeting almost predicted one of the major areas of parasite cytopathology today—i.e. how the parasite evades the host's responses. I hope that this meeting will be as influential on future research as that one has been. This is the second Ciba Foundation meeting held in Venezuela, the first one being in 1973, on Trypanosomiasis and leishmaniasis, with special reference to Chagas' disease (Ciba Found Symp 20). Participants here come from Europe, USA, Venezuela, Brazil, Kenya, Mexico and Israel. Thus, both the site of the meeting and the countries of those attending it attest to the truly international nature of the Ciba Foundation. It is a great honour for me to be invited to chair this meeting, and I welcome the opportunity that it provides for cooperation between the Centro Médico Docente La Trinidad and the Ciba Foundation.

1983 Cytopathology of parasitic disease. Pitman Books, London (Ciba Foundation symposium 99), p 1

Interactions between *Entamoeba histolytica*, bacteria and intestinal cells

DAVID MIRELMAN, CARMELA FEINGOLD, ADA WEXLER and RIVKA BRACHA

Department of Biophysics and Unit for Molecular Biology of Parasitic Diseases, Weizmann Institute of Science, Rehovot 76100, Israel

Abstract Axenically grown pathogenic and non-pathogenic isolates of *Entamoeba histolytica* have been shown to adhere to mammalian epithelial cells and bacteria by virtue of carbohydrate-binding proteins present on their cell surfaces. The interaction of amoeba isolates of low pathogenicity with a variety of gram-negative bacteria, mainly *Escherichia coli* strains which are readily ingested by the amoebae after relatively short periods, significantly increased the ability of the trophozoites to: (a) destroy and ingest intestinal epithelial cells; (b) secrete a cytopathic substance which morphologically affects a variety of tissue-cultured cells; and (c) cause hepatic abscesses in hamsters. Addition of carbohydrates that inhibit the lectin-mediated attachment of bacteria to amoebae prevented the enhancement of virulence. Interaction of the amoebae with bacteria that were heat-inactivated, glutaraldehyde-fixed or disrupted by sonication, as well as with bacteria precoated with antibodies or concanavalin A, did not lead to an increase in virulence. Moreover, short prior treatments of the bacteria with inhibitors of protein synthesis, but not with cell-wall synthesis inhibitors, also prevented the stimulation. The results indicate that interactions of amoebae with certain bacteria may be responsible for the increase in amoebic virulence.

1983 Cytopathology of parasitic disease. Pitman Books, London (Ciba Foundation symposium 99), p 2-30

The study of microbial interrelationships as an aspect of microbial pathogenicity is an obscure area of microbiology which has lent itself to only limited scientific investigation. It is generally recognized that the virulence of *Entamoeba histolytica* is related in part to association of the amoebae with suitable bacterial species. Early observations by Westphal (1937), Phillips & Gorstein (1966), Wittner & Rosenbaum (1970) and others have demonstrated that association of bacteria with amoebae augments the virulence of the amoebae as determined by their ability to cause lesions when inoculated into animals. Furthermore, since amoebic symptoms sometimes seem to disappear from the intestine after treatment with bactericidal but non-amoebicidal drugs such as β-lactams and sulpha-derivatives, this suggests that amoebic pathogenicity may depend on some factor(s) inherent in the interaction of amoebae with certain microorganisms.

Attachment to and ingestion of bacteria by trophozoites of *E. histolytica*

The development of *in vitro* axenic cultivation methods for *E. histolytica* by Diamond (1968) and Diamond et al (1978) has made it possible to obtain amoebic inocula free from all other microorganisms with which *E. histolytica* is usually associated in the intestine, and has facilitated the study of its interactions with bacteria.

Since surfaces of trophozoites of *E. histolytica* have been shown to contain concanavalin A receptors (Trissl et al 1977), it was logical to assume that the adherence to them by bacteria that possess mannose-binding lectins (Ofek et al 1977) would be similar to that observed for macrophages (Bar-Shavit et al 1977, 1980). Amoebae were found to be very selective in their interaction with bacteria. The attachment to the amoebae of organisms that possess organelles with mannose-binding properties, such as *Escherichia coli* 7343 or *E. coli* serotype 075, depended on time and concentration of the organisms. The average number of bacteria that attached per trophozoite at high multiplicity (1:1000) was between 40 and 100. The adherence of *E. coli* 7343 was found to be markedly inhibited by the presence of α-methylmannoside (α-MM) (Fig. 1). Precoating of the mannose receptors of the amoebae by concanavalin A also markedly blocked the attachment of *E. coli* cells (Fig. 1). Attachment of bacteria to the amoebae was mostly irreversible, and later addition of α-MM did not remove the bacteria. Only when low temperatures (5 °C) or glutaraldehyde-fixed amoebae were used—conditions that prevent ingestion—could removal of the attached bacteria by α-MM be achieved. These results implied that, after initial interaction, the amoebae began internalizing the bacteria. Further evidence for this was obtained from electron microscopic examination of thin sections (Fig. 2) as well as from the observation that phagocytized bacteria became very sensitive to solubilization by Triton X-100 (0.2%), whereas bacteria that remained attached to the surface (in incubations done in the cold) were not sensitive to the detergent (Bracha et al 1982).

Trophozoites of *E. histolytica* were found to shun bacteria that did not have a capacity to bind to mannose-containing surfaces. The only types of non-mannose binding bacteria that were found attached to trophozoites were *E. coli*, serotype 055, and *Salmonella*, serotype 050. The attachment of these bacteria was sensitive to galactose and *N*-acetylgalactosamine, as well as to a lipopolysaccharide preparation from *E. coli* 055, but was insensitive to α-MM

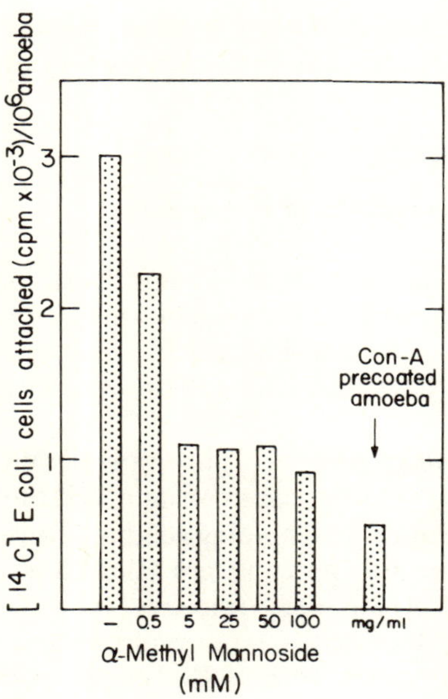

FIG. 1. Effect of increasing concentrations of α-methylmannoside and precoating of trophozoites with concanavalin A (Con-A) on the adherence of *E. coli* 7343 to amoebae. The reaction was carried out for 15 min at 37 °C. cpm, counts per minute

(Table 1). The attachment and ingestion of *E. coli* 055 was not inhibited by mannose-binding bacteria (*E. coli* 7343), but no adherence occurred with glutaraldehyde-fixed amoebae, or in the cold (5 °C). However, in contrast to *E. coli* 7343, no major differences were observed when heat-inactivated *E. coli* 055 (100 °C, 15 min) were used. Furthermore, periodate treatment of bacteria markedly affected their ability to bind to amoebae. These findings indicate that for *E. coli* 055 the interaction is mediated by an amoebic lectin (Kobiler & Mirelman 1980, Ravdin & Guerrant 1981) which recognizes a distinct carbohydrate on the bacterial lipopolysaccharide.

Other types of bacteria such as *Shigellae* species or gram-positives like *Staphylococcus aureus* and *Micrococcus luteus*, which do not have surface lectins, did not attach or interact with amoebae. On the other hand, bacteria opsonized with specific rabbit immune serum were readily attached to and ingested by the trophozoite. In contrast to peritoneal macrophages (Koide et al 1977), the attachment to the amoebae was not mediated by Fc receptors because *Shigella* precoated only with Fab′ dimers of anti-*Shigella* immunoglobulin were similarly attached (Bracha et al 1982). Adherence of opsonized *Shigella* was blocked by carbohydrates similarly to the inhibition of *E. coli* 055

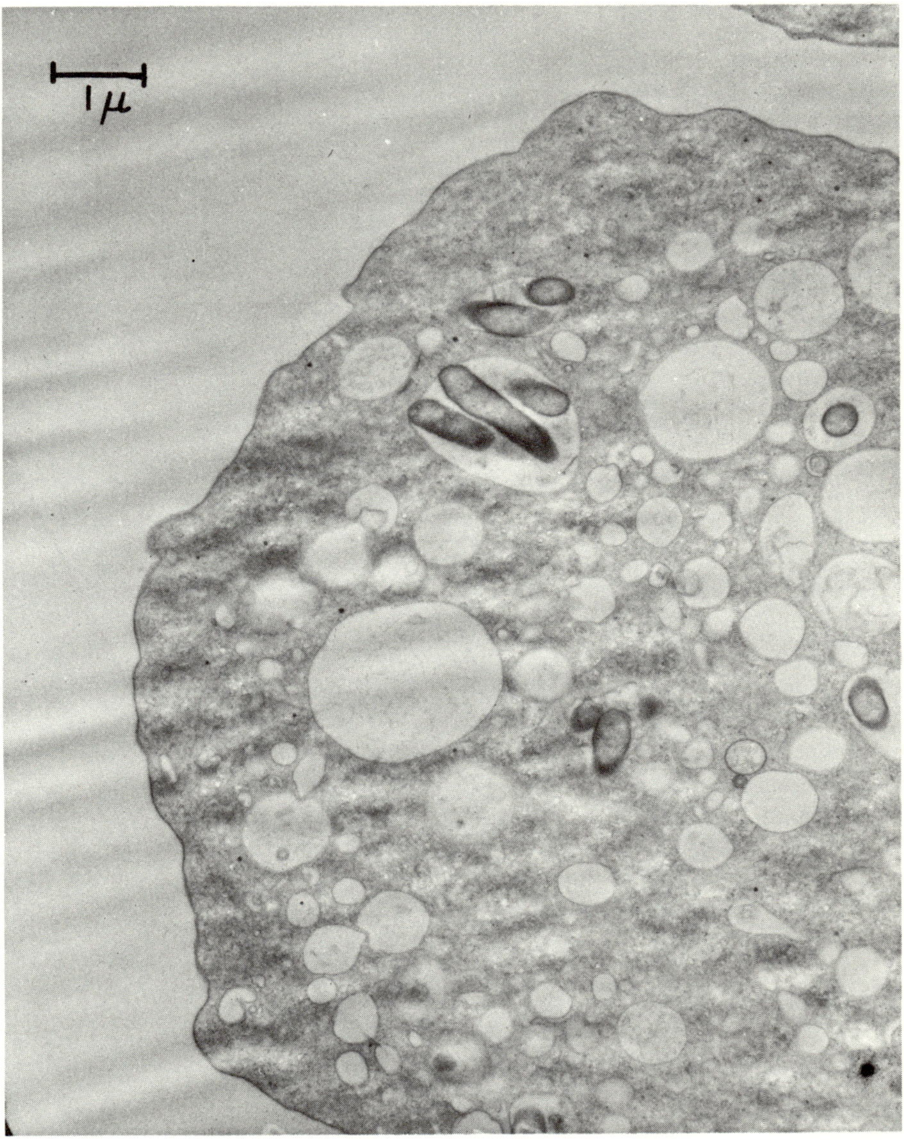

FIG. 2. Electron micrograph of thin section of an amoeba that interacted for 30 min at 37 °C with *E. coli* 7343. Bacteria were found almost exclusively inside vacuoles.

TABLE 1 Adherence of *E. coli* serotype 055[b] to trophozoites of *E. histolytica*

Variable Additions	*Attachment[a] %*
None	100
Galactose 10 mg/ml	41
α-methylmannoside 10 mg/ml	106
$GlcNAc_{2-3}$ 2 mg/ml	80
Lactose 10 mg/ml	43
GalNAc 10 mg/ml	42
Lipopolysaccharide (*E. coli* 055) (4 mg/ml)	48
Lipopolysaccharide (*E. coli* 7343) (4 mg/ml)	115
E. coli 7343 (2.5×10^8)	83
E. coli 7343 + α-MM	89
Heparin mg/ml	94
Asialofetuin mg/ml	54
Pretreatments of bacteria	
γ-irradiation (500 krad)	110
Glutaraldehyde fixation	94
Heat inactivation	89
Periodate oxidation (25 mM, 10 min)	52
Glutaraldehyde-fixed amoebae	<5

[a]The number of bacteria that adhered to each trophozoite was usually between 25–50. [b]Very similar results were obtained with *Salmonella greenside* 050 instead of *E. coli* 055. A ratio of 1000 ^{14}C-labelled bacteria per amoeba was used.

(Table 1), indicating that in these cases, too, the amoebic lectin mediated the binding to carbohydrates likely to be on the immunoglobulins that coated the bacterial surface (Niedermeier et al 1971) (Fig. 3).

In summary, our studies have shown that *E. histolytica* trophozoites that inhabit the colon have a variety of options by which to attach and ingest bacteria. Our main efforts are now directed towards understanding how such interactions might affect the pathogenicity of the amoebae.

Interactions between trophozoites and epithelial cells

The initial step in the amoebic infectious process is the attachment of the parasite to, and its proliferation on, mucosal surfaces of the caecum and colon (Chevez et al 1976). In many cases this is followed by invasion and penetration of the amoebae through the intestinal wall, leading to secondary but more serious infections such as abscesses of the liver, brain and lung (Martinez-Palomo 1982).

Carbohydrate-binding proteins on its cell surface mediate the adherence of *E. histolytica* to mammalian cell surfaces. Depending on the source of target

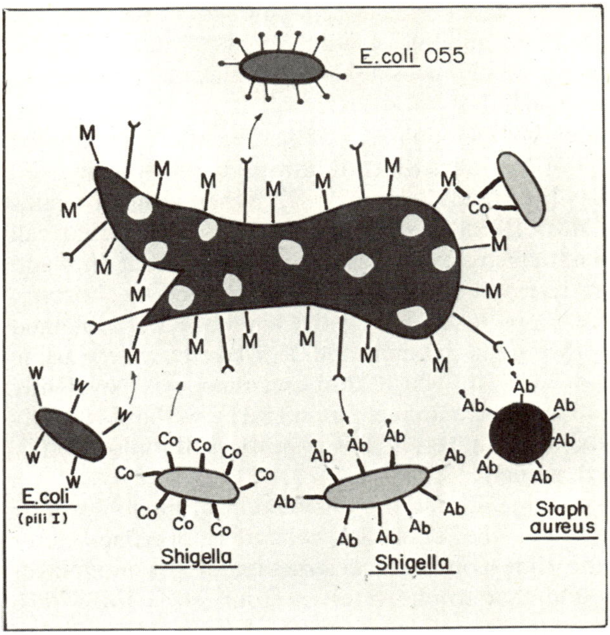

FIG. 3. Summary of various possibilities for attachment of different bacteria to the amoeba trophozoites. M, mannose-containing receptors on the amoeba surface; ——<, a carbohydrate-binding (lectin) activity; W, surface pili, on *E. coli*, which have mannose-binding properties; Co, concanavalin A bound to receptors on the bacteria; Ab, antibodies; and ——●, *N*-acetylgalactosamine or galactose moieties on bacterial surfaces or on opsonins.

cells and conditions of the assay, two mechanisms of adherence have been detected. Adherence of amoebae to a human intestinal cell line (Henle 407), to baby hamster kidney (BHK) cells (Kobiler & Mirelman 1980) and to erythrocytes (Orozco et al 1982) was specifically inhibited by oligosaccharides of *N*-acetylglucosamine $(GlcNAc)_{3-4}$, or by purified bacterial peptidoglycan preparations, as well as by precoating of the mammalian cells with wheat-germ agglutinin. Adherence of amoebae to Chinese hamster ovary (CHO) cells (Ravdin & Guerrant 1981), as well as to *E. coli* serotype 055 (see above), was inhibited by *N*-acetylgalactosamine (GalNAc) and galactose.

No significant differences in the adherence capability of various isolates of *E. histolytica* were detected (Kobiler & Mirelman 1980). The inhibitory potency of GlcNAc- or GalNAc-containing molecules implies that the mammalian cell receptor may be a surface component, probably a glycoprotein, with structures that contain such carbohydrate moieties (Yamashita et al 1978, Mizuochi et al 1978). Another potent inhibitor of trophozoite attachment to mammalian cells was a clear preparation of rabbit colonic mucus that contained considerable amounts of amino sugars (Katz et al 1982). The inhibitory action of the intestinal mucosal secretions may be important in the development of the amoebic intestinal disease.

Incubation of trophozoites with monolayers of tissue-cultured epithelial cells leads to the formation of filopodia which infiltrate the mammalian cell and form stable connections (Martinez-Palomo 1982). When virulent strains of *E. histolytica* such as HM1:IMSS are incubated with an epithelial cell monolayer, the cells begin to detach themselves from their adjacent ones and to round up; some of them lyse and others are ingested by the trophozoite. Evidence that epithelial cells are taken up by the amoebae was obtained by electron microscopy (Martinez-Palomo 1982). Moreover, by using monolayers of mammalian cells, to which fluorescamine was covalently bound before the incubation with the amobae (strain HM1), we have recently observed that after incubation the trophozoites become fluorescent (C. Feingold et al, unpublished results).

We developed an assay for quantifying the destruction of monolayers by staining, with methylene blue, the epithelial cells that remained after incubation. We studied the time course of destruction of the monolayer (5×10^5 cells/well) and found that trophozoites of strain HM1:IMSS destroyed considerably more epithelial cells than those of strain HK-9 in the same conditions (Table 2). An increased number of trophozoites per well markedly increased the rate of monolayer destruction. Inhibition of monolayer destruction was observed with a number of carbohydrates such as galactose and lactose (>85% at 10 mg/ml) as well as with serum (1%) and rabbit colonic mucus (7 mg/ml) (Katz et al 1982).

TABLE 2 Destruction of tissue-cultured monolayers by *Entamoeba histolytica* trophozoites

E. histolytica strain	*Interaction with bacteria*	*Destruction of monolayer (%)*	
		(Expt 1)	*(Expt 2)*
HM1 : IMSS	None	31 ± 1	80 ± 3
HM1 : IMSS	*E. coli* 7343	64 ± 3	–
HM1 : IMSS	*E. coli* 055	–	84 ± 6
HK-9	None	12 ± 1	19 ± 3
HK-9	*E. coli* 7343	65 ± 3	–
HK-9	*E. coli* 055	–	49 ± 1

Interaction was achieved by suspending trophozoites (4×10^5 in 0.2 ml Eagle's minimal media) in wells (0.5 cm diameter) containing a confluent monolayer of baby hamster kidney cells (5×10^5) for 60 min at 37 °C. An overnight growth of *E. coli* cells was incubated with trophozoites at a multiplicity of 1000 : 1 for 15 min at 37 °C, before their addition to the wells, and then further incubated for 60 min. Destruction of monolayers was measured by methylene blue staining of the mammalian cells that remained in the wells after the interaction. –, not measured.

Augmentation of *E. histolytica* virulence on association with bacteria

The reassociation of axenically grown amoebae with an undefined *E. coli* strain was found to restore virulence, as shown by an increase in hepatic abscess formation in the hamster model (Wittner & Rosenbaum 1970). Moreover, monoxenic strains maintained together with the protozoan flagellate *Crithidia fasciculata* or with a mixed species of *Proteus*, *Klebsiella* and *E. coli* had a significantly higher ability to form hepatic abscesses in hamsters (Bos & Hage 1975). The duration of restored virulence was relatively short, and removal of the bacteria reduced the amoebic virulence. On the other hand, passage of axenically grown amoebae through a liver and reisolation from the liver augmented their virulence, and this could be maintained in axenic media for several months (Bos & Hage 1975).

The assay for monolayer destruction was used to evaluate the effect of bacteria on the virulence of amoeba strains. Preincubation of trophozoites of strain HK-9 (2×10^5 cells/well) with varying amounts of *E. coli* 7343 (a bacterium with mannose-binding properties) gradually increased the rate of monolayer destruction. Maximal destruction rates were observed when the ratio between trophozoites and bacteria was 1 : 1000 (Fig. 4), although a 20% increase in the rate of destruction could be seen even at 1 : 10 ratios. Addition

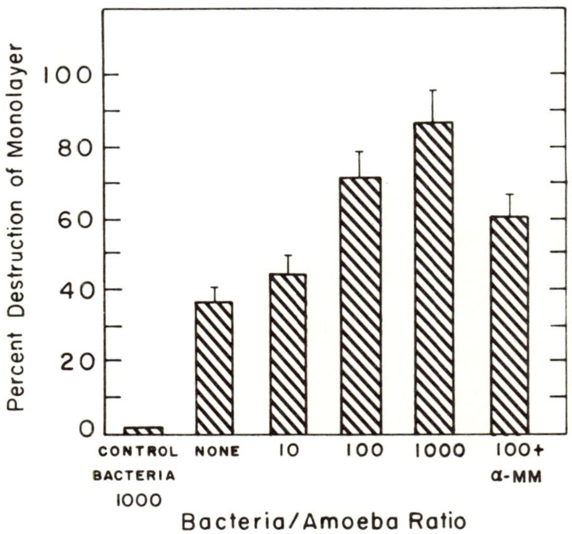

FIG. 4. Interaction of amoebae with bacteria, and augmentation of amoebic virulence. Destruction of tissue-culture monolayer by trophozoites of *E. histolytica* (strain HK-9) after interaction with cells of *E. coli* 7343 at different multiplicities. α-MM = α-methylmannoside (1%).

of α-MM (1%) to a bacteria–amoebae mixture (at 1 : 100 ratio) to provide conditions that inhibit by approximately 90% the attachment of bacteria to the amoebae, inhibited the increase in virulence (Fig. 4). Longer periods of trophozoite preincubation with bacteria did not markedly increase further the amoebic virulence. When strains HM1 : IMSS and HK-9 were compared after interaction with bacteria, the virulence increased in both, but was proportionately higher for strain HK-9 (Table 2).

Increased amoebic virulence was observed after interaction not only with *E. coli* 7343 but also with other *E. coli* strains that possessed mannose-binding activity (Table 3), as well as with strain *E. coli* 055. Mannose-binding *E. coli* strains that were cured for plasmids or were known not to contain plasmids (strains CR63 or CA274, Table 3) augmented the amoebic virulence, but *Shigella* strains and bacterial cells such as *E. coli* 09 : $K(29)^+$: H^+ that did not adhere to the amoebae did not increase the virulence. Moreover, the opsonization of *Shigella flexneri*, which we had previously shown to facilitate their ingestion by the trophozoite, did not augment the virulence of HK-9 strains (Table 3).

TABLE 3 Bacterial strains that augment amoebic virulence

Strain	*Adherence to amoebae*	*Specificity of adherence*	*Augmentation of virulence*
E. coli 055	3+	Gal,GalNAc	3+
E. coli 075	3+	Man	3+
E. coli 7343	3+	Man	3+
E. coli CR63 (no plasmids)	2+	Man	2+
E. coli CA274 (no plasmids)	2+	Man	3+
E. coli 09 : $K^{-}29$: H^{-}	0	–	0
E. coli 09 : $K^{+}29$: H^{+}	0	–	0
Serratia marcescens	3+	Man	3+
Shigella flexneri	0	–	0
Shigella flexneri (ops)	3+	Gal,GalNAc	0
Staphylococcus aureus	0	–	0
Staphylococcus aureus (ops)	3+	Gal,GalNAc	0

For experimental conditions, and the results of a marked (3+) augmentation with *E. histolytica* strain HK-9, see Table 2. —, no adherence observed.
Gal, galactose; GalNAc, *N*-acetylgalactosamine; Man, mannose.

For virulence to be stimulated, the bacteria had to be intact. Sonicates of bacteria or heat-inactivated *E. coli* 7343 did not augment the virulence (Table 4). On the other hand, bacteria exposed to 500 krad from a cobalt X-ray source (after which no capability to form colonies remained) could still enhance the virulence. Bacteria whose growth was blocked by short (1 h)

TABLE 4 Effect of pretreatments of bacteria on their ability to increase amoebic virulence

Pretreatment	*Augmentation*
None (log or stationary phase)	3+
Glutaraldehyde fixation	0
Heat-inactivation (15 min, 100 °C)	0
Sonication	0
γ-irradiation (99.9%, LD 2×10^4 rad)	3+
γ-irradiation (100%, LD 10^5 rad)	2+
γ-irradiation (100%, LD 5×10^5 rad)	1+
Growth with inhibitors of cell-wall synthesis	
(bicozamycin 200 μg/ml, 2 h)	3+
(cephalexin 8 μg/ml, 1 h)	3+
Growth with inhibitor of protein synthesis	
(amikacin 100 μg/ml, 2 h)	0

For experimental conditions, and results of marked (3+) augmentation with *E. histolytica* strain HK-9, see Table 2. The experiments were done with both *E. coli* 7343 and *E. coli* 055.
LD, lethal dose.

pretreatments with β-lactams or bicozamycin were capable of stimulating virulence, but amikacin-treated bacteria were not. Furthermore, the presence of galactose (1%) markedly inhibited all monolayer destruction.

In spite of their striking lytic ability, trophozoites of *E. histolytica* do not seem to penetrate the intact intestinal mucosa easily. In experimental *in vivo* and *in vitro* models, in which the interaction between trophozoites and the caecal mucosa of the guinea-pig was analysed, the initial penetration of amoebae was limited to the interglandular regions (Takeuchi & Phillips 1975, Mora Galindo et al 1978). These areas are usually where dying cells are continuously being sloughed off. In experiments done in our laboratory, interaction of trophozoites of strain HM1 : IMSS with guinea-pig colon sections (from the transverse region) did not damage the mucosal lining. On the other hand, trophozoites that had been reassociated with *E. coli* serotype 075 displayed a remarkable ability to penetrate and damage the mucosal lining (Fig. 5). Needless to say, incubations with the bacteria alone had no effect whatsoever. The sites of penetration again appeared to be in the interglandular zones. No damage to the mucosal lining was observed, however, when incubations were done in the presence of galactose (1%). Furthermore, there was very little damage to the mucosa when bacteria-stimulated trophozoites were incubated with sections of ascending colon.

Cytopathic effects of cell-free extracts of *E. histolytica*

Early attempts to demonstrate a trophozoite cell-free toxin were unsuccessful, apparently because of the use of serum in the culture medium (Bos 1979,

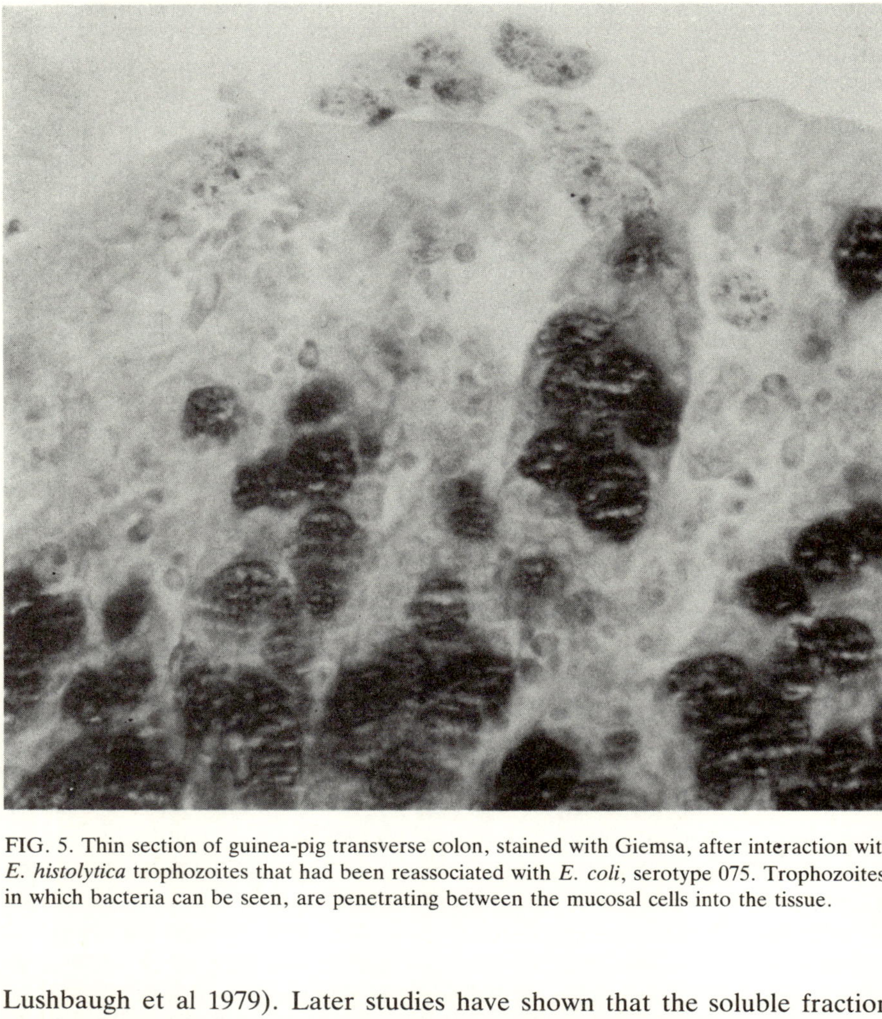

FIG. 5. Thin section of guinea-pig transverse colon, stained with Giemsa, after interaction with *E. histolytica* trophozoites that had been reassociated with *E. coli*, serotype 075. Trophozoites, in which bacteria can be seen, are penetrating between the mucosal cells into the tissue.

Lushbaugh et al 1979). Later studies have shown that the soluble fraction obtained from homogenates of pathogenic strains of amoebae possesses a substance that is toxic for a variety of mammalian cells (Lushbaugh et al 1979, 1981, Bos 1979, Ravdin & Guerrant 1981). The most commonly observed effect is the rounding up and detachment of tissue-cultured cells (Fig. 6). Some investigators have reported that amoeba homogenates can cause secretion of fluids similar to bacterial toxins in rabbit ileal loops (Lushbaugh et al 1979). This effect was demonstrated most notably in rabbits treated with indomethacin before the intraintestinal administration of the amoeba homogenate (Uedzulu et al 1982). The exact nature and mechanism of action

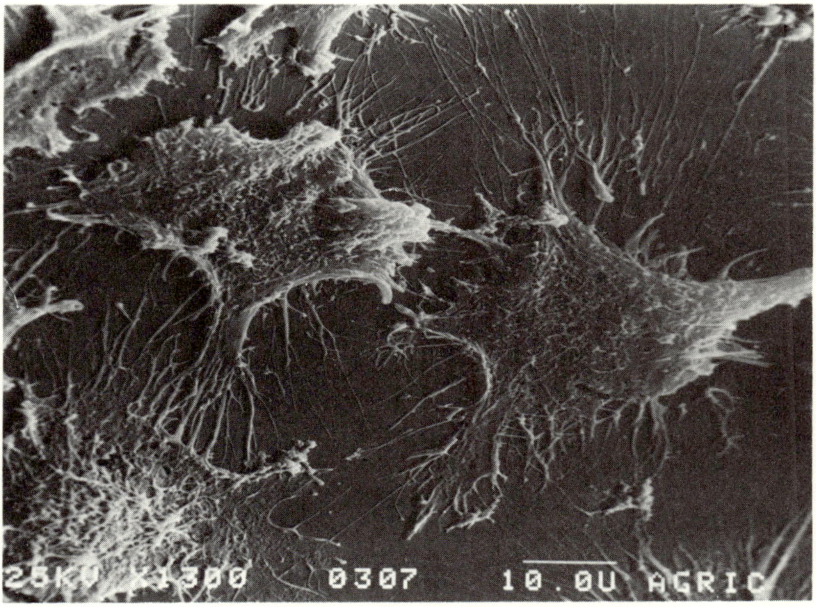

FIG. 6. Scanning electron micrograph of tissue-cultured human intestinal cells (Henle 407) after a short period of incubation with the soluble fraction of homogenates of *E. histolytica* trophozoites (strain HM1 : IMSS).

of the amoebic toxic substance is not yet completely clear, and may be the additive result of a number of biological activities. Amoebae, and particularly the pathogenic strains, have numerous proteolytic activities including collagenases (Muñoz et al 1982, Gadasi & Kessler 1983), phospholipases (J. I. Ravdin & R. L. Guerrant in Abstracts of the 22nd interscience conference on antimicrobial agents and chemotherapy, p 30, 1982, Miami) and a pore-forming ionophore type of material (Rosenberg et al 1982), all of which may affect host cells, and the intestinal mucosa in particular.

Using the above-mentioned assay system based on the detachment of tissue-cultured BHK cells, we have recently found that a soluble toxic substance, which was not a product of amoebic lysis, was slowly released by intact trophozoites that were incubated in maintenance media (Gillin & Diamond 1980) (Fig. 7). The secretion of the cytotoxic activity was inhibited when cytochalasin B was added to the incubation mixtures (C. Feingold et al, unpublished observations). The cytopathic effect on monolayers of mammalian tissue-cultured cells was inhibited by several serum factors including fetuin (Mattern et al 1980, Kobiler et al 1981) α-macroglobulin and α-1-

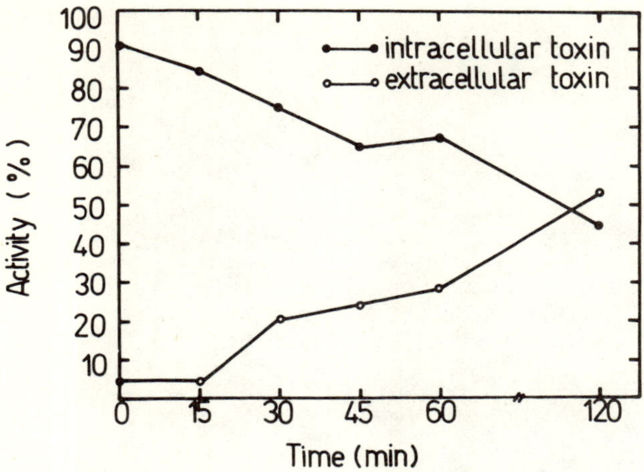

FIG. 7. Time-dependent release of cytopathic activity, by trophozoites of strain HM1 : IMSS, on incubation at 37 °C in saline that contained minimal media without serum. After incubation, the trophozoites were sedimented and the cytopathic activity released into the medium, as well as that remaining in the cells, was determined by their effect on baby hamster kidney cells.

TABLE 5 Inhibitors of the cytopathic activity of cell-free extracts of *E. histolytica*

Inhibitors	*Concentration added (mg/ml)*	*Destruction of tissue-culture monolayer (%)*
None	–	>95
Fetuin	2	17
Fetuin	25	<5
Asialofetuin	1	72
Thyroglobulin	2.5	28
Mucin	2.5	<5
Sialic acid	10	15
Sialic acid	4	35
Concanavalin A	1	40
Wheat-germ agglutinin	1	20
Soybean agglutinin	1	>95
Peanut agglutinin	1	>95

The tissue-cultured cells (baby hamster kidney) were preincubated with the lectins before being exposed to the cell-free extract (from 10^6 amoebae/well) The glycoproteins were added to the amoebic extract. The cell-free extract was obtained by freeze–thaw disruption of trophozoites of *E. histolytica* strain HM1 : IMSS.

antiprotease (Lushbaugh et al 1981). We have recently found that the cytopathic effect could also be inhibited by sialic acid-containing compounds (Table 5) and by precoating of the cells with wheat-germ agglutinin (1 mg/ml) but not by soybean or peanut lectin, which indicates that sialic acid may act as a recognition site on the mammalian cell surface.

Since homogenates of non-pathogenic strains such as HK-9 and NIH : 200 had very small amounts of the toxic substance (Bos 1979), it was interesting to see whether these cell-free cytopathic activities would increase after pre-interaction of the HK-9 trophozoites with bacteria. Interaction between *E. histolytica* strains HK-9 or HM1 : IMSS and *E. coli* 7343 or 055 at a ratio of 1 : 1000, for 1 h before homogenization, produced a remarkable increase in the cytopathic activity of the amoebae (Fig. 8). The increase was greater for

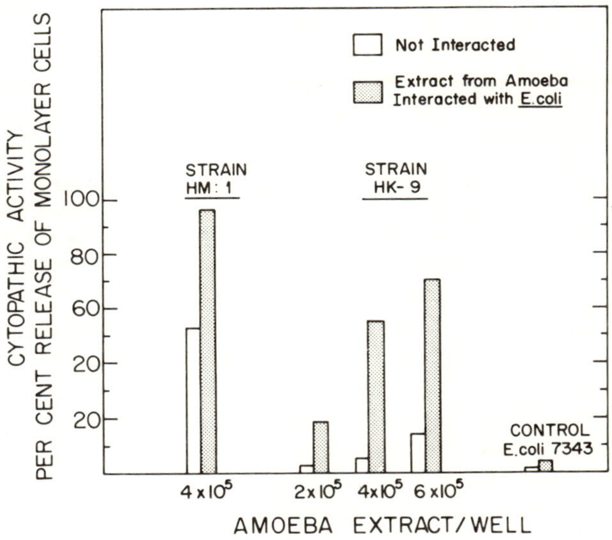

FIG. 8. Cytopathic activity of homogenates of *E. histolytica*, strains HK-9 and HM1 : IMSS, on baby hamster kidney cells before and after interaction with *E. coli* 7343.

strain HK-9 than for strain HM1 : IMSS. No increase was observed when homogenates of amoebae and bacteria were used or when sonicates of both bacteria and amoebae were used. Neither was there an increase in virulence when we used bacteria that did not adhere to the amoebae, such as *Shigella* (see above), or heat-inactivated or glutaraldehyde-fixed bacteria (Table 4).

Concluding remarks

One of the fundamental aspects of studying amoebiasis is to elucidate the factors that determine virulence of the parasite and its conversion sometimes from a harmless commensal to an aggressive invader. It is generally accepted that a balanced host–parasite equilibrium facilitates the commensal relationship and that alterations in this balance may convert it to a virulent state. Disruption of the balance may be due to changes in either the host or parasite. Among a variety of possible host factors, consideration has been given to geographical location, race, sex, age, nutritional and immunological condition, diet, local climate and previous history of medication. Very little is known, however, about how such factors specifically alter the host. The parasite can also be affected apparently by many factors. Numerous strains with different pathogenicities have been isolated, and studies in several laboratories have begun to shed light on these differences as well as on the conditions that modify the degree of virulence in different strains.

Our results clearly indicate that specific mechanisms of carbohydrate recognition are critical for the interaction of trophozoites with both mammalian and bacterial cells. Moreover, our studies support the notion that association of axenically grown trophozoites with certain types of bacteria augments their virulence. The molecular mechanism behind the increased amoebic virulence is not yet clear. Transfer of bacterial genetic information is not likely to be the cause since the augmentation is quite rapid and plasmids are apparently not essential. Furthermore, inhibitors of protein or DNA-synthesis do not inhibit the augmentation. More appealing is the idea that bacterial ingestion supplies the trophozoite with a key nutrient ingredient (for example, iron) or an enzymic activity that liberates a cryptic virulent potential. It is tempting to speculate that most trophozoites have the potential for virulence and that certain conditions may trigger its expression.

The wider implications about the role of bacteria in the establishment of *E. histolytica* colonies and in the subsequent invasion of the colonic mucosa are far from being understood. On the one hand, certain bacteria that are not recognized or taken up by the amoebae may hinder the direct contact and attachment of the trophozoite to the apical surface of the intestinal epithelial cell (Martinez-Palomo 1982). On the other hand, bacterial strains that readily adhere to and are ingested by the amoebae may serve both as focal points of attachment to the intestinal mucosa and as triggers for enhanced trophozoite virulence. The nature of the intestinal microbial flora may thus have considerable importance for the pathogenicity of the amoebae and for the aetiology of the disease.

Acknowledgement

Our studies were supported by a grant from the Rockefeller Foundation. (Bicozamycin was obtained from Dr Kradolfer, Ciba-Geigy, Basel.)

REFERENCES

Bar-Shavit Z, Ofek I, Goldman R, Mirelman D, Sharon N 1977 Mannose residues on phagocytes as receptors for the attachment of *Escherichia coli* and *Salmonella typhi*. Biochem Biophys Res Commun 78:455-460

Bar-Shavit Z, Goldman R, Ofek I, Sharon N, Mirelman D 1980 Mannose-binding activity of *Escherichia coli*: a determinant of attachment and ingestion of the bacteria by macrophages. Infect Immun 29:417-424

Bos HJ 1979 *Entamoeba histolytica* cytopathogenicity of intact amebae and cell-free extracts: isolation and characterization of an intracellular toxin. Exp Parasitol 47:369-377

Bos HJ, Hage AJ 1975 Virulence of bacteria-associated, *Crithidia*-associated, and axenic *Entamoeba histolytica*: experimental hamster liver infections with strains from patients and carriers. Z Parasitenkd 47:79-89

Bracha R, Kobiler D, Mirelman D 1982 Attachment and ingestion of bacteria by trophozoites of *Entamoeba histolytica*. Infect Immun 36:396-406

Chevez A, Sepulveda B, Segura M, Corona D, Diaz J 1976 Initial phases of pathogenic activity of *E. histolytica* in colon and liver of hamsters. In: Sepulveda B, Diamond LS (eds) Proc 6th Int Seminar Amebiasis, 1976. Instituto Mexicano del Seguro Social, Mexico City, p 418-517

Diamond LS 1968 Techniques of axenic cultivation of *Entamoeba histolytica* Schaudinn, 1903 and *E. histolytica*-like amebae. J Parasitol 54:1047-1056

Diamond LS, Harlow DR, Cunnick CC 1978 A new medium for the axenic cultivation of *Entamoeba histolytica* and other *Entamoeba*. Trans R Soc Trop Med Hyg 72:431-432

Gadasi H, Kessler E 1983 Correlation between virulence and collagenolytic activity in *Entamoeba histolytica*. Infect Immun 39:528-531

Gillin FD, Diamond LA 1980 Attachment and short-term maintenance of motility and viability of *Entamoeba histolytica* in a defined medium. J Protozool 27:220-225

Katz S, Izhar M, Ashkenazi S, Halperin Z, Mirelman D 1982 Isolated colonic loop in rabbit. An *in vivo* system for studying intestinal mucus. Digestion 24:99-104

Kobiler D, Mirelman D 1980 A lectin activity in *Entamoeba histolytica* trophozoites. Infect Immun 29:221-225

Kobiler D, Mirelman D, Mattern CFT 1981 Lectin and toxin-like activities of *E. histolytica*: comparison of properties. Am J Trop Med Hyg 30:955-959

Koide N, Nose M, Muramatsu T 1977 Recognition of IgG by Fc receptor complement: effects of glycosidase digestion. Biochem Biophys Res Commun 75:838-844

Lushbaugh WB, Kairalla AB, Cantey JR, Hofbauer AF, Pittman FE 1979 Isolation of a cytotoxin–enterotoxin from *Entamoeba histolytica*. J Infect Dis 139:9-17

Lushbaugh WB, Kairalla AB, Hofbauer AF, Arnaud P, Cantey JR, Pittman FE 1981 Inhibition of *Entamoeba histolytica* cytotoxin by alpha-1-antiprotease and alpha-2-macroglobulin. Am J Trop Med Hyg 30:575-585

Martinez-Palomo A 1982 The biology of *Entamoeba histolytica*. John Wiley, Chichester (Trop Med Res Studies Ser) see: Parasite factors of virulence, p 95-117

Mattern CFT, Reister DB, Natovitz PC 1980 *Entamoeba histolytica* 'toxin' fetuin neutralizable and lectin-like. Am J Trop Med Hyg 29:26-30

Mizuochi T, Yonemasu K, Yamashita K, Kobata A 1978 The asparagine-linked sugar chains of subcomponent $C1^{17}$ of the first component of human complement. J Biol Chem 253: 7404-7409

Mora Galindo J, Martinez-Palomo A, Chavez B 1978 Interaccion entre *Entamoeba histolytica* y el epitelio cecal del cobayo. Arch Invest Med 9 (Suppl 1):261-274

Muñoz ML, Calderón J, Rojkind M 1982 The collagenase of *Entamoeba histolytica*. J Exp Med 155:42-51

Niedermeier W, Kirkland T, Acton RT, Bennet JC 1971 The carbohydrate composition of immunoglobulin G. Biochim Biophys Acta 237:442-449

Orozco E, Guarneros G, Martinez-Palomo A 1982 Clonas de *E. histolytica* deficientes en fagocitosis presentan deficiencia en virulencia. Arch Invest Med 13 (Suppl 3):137-143

Ofek I, Mirelman D, Sharon N 1977 Adherence of *Escherichia coli* to human mucosal cells mediated by mannose receptors. Nature (Lond) 265:623-625

Phillips BP, Gorstein F 1966 Effects of different species of bacteria on the pathology of enteric amebiasis in monocontaminated guinea-pigs. Am J Trop Med Hyg 15:863-868

Ravdin JI, Guerrant RL 1981 Role of adherence in cytopathogenic mechanisms of *Entamoeba histolytica*. J Clin Invest 68:1305-1313

Ravdin JI, Croft BY, Guerrant RL 1980 Cytopathogenic mechanisms of *Entamoeba histolytica*. J Exp Med 152:377-390

Rosenberg IM, Gitler C, Lynch EC 1982 An ion channel forming protein produced by *Entamoeba histolytica*. EMBO J 1:801-805

Takeuchi A, Phillips BP 1975 Electron microscope studies of experimental *Entamoeba histolytica* infection in the guinea-pig. I:Penetration of the intestinal epithelium by trophozoites. Am J Trop Med Hyg 24:34-48

Trissl D, Martinez-Palomo A, Arguello C, de la Torre M, de la Hoz R 1977 Surface properties related to concanavalin A-induced agglutination. A comparative study of several *Entamoeba* strains. J Exp Med 145:652-665

Uedzulu IA, Leitch GJ, Bailey GB 1982 Use of indomethacin to demonstrate enterotoxic activity in extracts of *Entamoeba histolytica* trophozoites. Infect Immun 36:795-801

Westphal A 1937 Betrachtungen und experimentelle untersuchungen zur virulenz der *Entamoeba histolytica* beim menschen. Arch Schiffs Trophenhyg 41:262-279

Wittner M, Rosenbaum RM 1970 Role of bacteria in modifying virulence of *Entamoeba histolytica*. Am J Trop Med Hyg 19:755-761

Yamashita K, Tachibana Y, Kobata A 1978 The structures of the galactose containing sugar chains of ovalbumin. J Biol Chem 253:3862-3869

DISCUSSION

Piras: Are you not worried about fixing the mammalian tissue-cultured cells with glutaraldehyde, which can make some surface components unavailable for other interactions?

Mirelman: I agree that glutaraldehyde fixation is not an ideal method, but we find so many difficulties in trying to dissociate the step of amoebic adherence from the step of tissue-cultured cell destruction that we have to resort to this type of technique. Using various controls we found that the mechanism of amoebic adherence that was sensitive to carbohydrates was unchanged when we used as target cells the glutaraldehyde-fixed monolayers.

Piras: What happens when you use low temperatures?

Mirelman: Amoebae will 'round up' at low temperatures or in the presence of cytochalasin B, and under these conditions they will not bind to mammalian cells or inert surfaces. The amoebae have to be at an optimum temperature to form the filaments and filopodia needed for adherence.

Nussenzweig: You mentioned that you can inhibit the first phase of interaction by addition of sugars. But once the amoebae have adhered to the cells, can you inhibit the second phase i.e. pathogenicity?

Mirelman: It is almost impossible to reverse the first stage. As I mentioned, if α-methylmannoside is added after amoebae have adhered to bacteria, one cannot remove the bacteria from the amoebae, except at low temperature, in which case ingestion of the bacteria does not occur. It seems, therefore, that the initial recognition is mediated by a carbohydrate recognition mechanism but this step is rapidly followed by a stronger but, as yet, unclear attachment mechanism.

Chang: Have you followed the fate of the bacteria within the amoebae? Protozoa very often ingest intracellular bacteria. In some cases (e.g. in the work of Jeon & Jeon 1976) one can even establish intracellular symbiosis by feeding *Amoeba proteus* with bacteria. Another point is in relation to the *kappa* particle in *Paramecium* (Preer et al 1974). There appears to be some kind of bacteriophage which helps the bacteria or kappa particles to release a toxin that kills sensitive *Paramecium* without the particles. Does this connect with your work?

Mirelman: This is a very interesting question. A relevant example comes from recent findings on *Legionella* bacteria. Their natural reservoir appears to be in water-borne amoebae which hold the *Legionella* and give rise to the associated bacterial disease when the amoebae are inhaled in damp or closed quarters (air-conditioning water reservoirs). Ten minutes after the bacteria are inside the *Entamoeba histolytica* trophozoite, they are extremely sensitive to detergents, unlike most bacteria, and their outer membrane ceases to function as a protective barrier so they are dissolved. After two hours, thin sections of amoeba trophozoites under electron microscopy show that the bacteria are partially digested. Most bacteria under these conditions have no survival potential inside the amoebae. The possibility of using a potentially toxic substance from the bacteria to enhance the virulence of the amoebae has not escaped our notice. In Canada, Dr De Voe is finding that when *Neisseria meningitidis* (De Voe 1976) are ingested by macrophages, the macrophages cannot digest the endotoxin of the *Neisseria*. This endotoxin is released by the macrophages and can cause the toxic symptoms just as if it were the bacterium itself. It is possible that the amoebae cannot digest some bacterial toxins, e.g. lipopolysaccharide, for which no degrading enzymes have been found. We often use bacteria that are completely non-toxic—i.e. the K-12 derivatives that have no endotoxins and no exotoxins, and yet are capable of augmenting amoebic virulence. However, it is possible that in some cases the effects may be compounded, and the bacteria may also contribute some intrinsic toxic effect.

Hudson: I am reminded by your results of macrophage activation. What is the morphology of activation of *amoebae*, if you indeed accept that this is an activation process; and have you tried any of the classical activators that immunologists use?

Mirelman: We could not demonstrate any activation of amoebae by any of the classical soluble compounds that activate macrophages. As for the morphology, we can see that amoebae which have ingested bacteria are very much more motile than those that have not. We don't understand the connection. We have not looked at other morphological aspects, and we should do this. I agree with you however that there may be some common aspects between the activated state of the macrophage and the amoeba. Many studies are being done to try to understand macrophage activation in biochemical terms but, as far as I am aware, there are no definite answers yet.

Warren: Zanvil Cohn's group (Aley et al 1980) have done some interesting work on the connection between the macrophage and the amoeba.

Klebanoff: One of the consequences of activation of macrophages is, of course, the increased ability of the cells to respond to a stimulus with a respiratory burst. Is there any comparable response in amoebae?

Mirelman: Amoebae are anaerobic and in this respect appear not to have systems similar to those in the macrophage (Martinez-Palomo 1982). We have tried to detect oxygen bursts in the amoebae but have failed so far.

O'Daly: Have you studied with your model the system that secretes immunoglobulin A (IgA)? IgA is built on the lamina propria and is secreted throughout epithelial cells. It is very richly concentrated in epithelial cell granules, in the glycocalyx and also in mucus. Secretory IgA has a lot of carbohydrate in the Fc portion of the alpha chain and in the secretory component. Can the natural molecule be used by the amoebae, and does it function in the adherence process, leading to infection?

Mirelman: The natural defences of the body's mucosal surfaces consist of secretions that include mucus and secretory IgA. These gel-like materials are rich in carbohydrates and consequently provide endless possibilities for competition as receptors for the attachment mechanisms of pathogens. The mucus components coat the mammalian epithelial cells and protect them by preventing pathogens from adhering to them. Thus, even if the amoeba is extremely pathogenic and has many bacterial activators, if the host has a healthy production of mucus and secretory IgA the amoeba will find it difficult to harm the intestinal mucosa. On the other hand, as I mentioned in my paper, secretion of mucus components depends very much on the host and can be impaired in a variety of ways. Such an impairment would then render the host intestine susceptible to amoeba. Uedzulu et al (1982) made animals susceptible to amoebiasis by injecting them with indomethacin, which is a very effective blocker of prostaglandin synthesis (Smith et al 1981). In this case the secretion of the mucus is partially blocked, so it becomes less efficient in inhibiting amoebic damage. Most patients with amoebiasis come from undernourished backgrounds, and it is well known that secretion of mucus and IgA in undernourished children is very different from that in normal people. Immunosuppressive drugs or radiation are also known to cause a lot of intestinal problems, and this is probably due to the lack of the surface defence that is provided normally by these secretions.

Nogueira: Can you show the appearance of collagenase activity in the previously non-virulent amoebae? What do you think is the mechanism by which bacterial ingestion enhances amoebic virulence?

Mirelman: As I mentioned, Gadasi & Kessler (1983) and Muñoz et al (1982a) have shown a correlation between collagenase activity and virulence of trophozoites. We have also recently found that collagenase is one of the activities that increases following ingestion of bacteria, *provided that* the bacteria are taken up as intact particles. It is possible that the ingested bacteria supplies an enzyme (such as a nuclease or proteolytic activity) that cleaves and de-regulates an intrinsic activity in the amoeba. When the amoeba digests the bacterium the enzyme would then be released and, in turn, would activate the amoeba. A second possibility is that the bacterium provides a key ingredient or nutrient—perhaps an iron- or sulphur-containing material that the amoeba requires—and becomes activated by it.

Sher: Activated macrophages, and also amoebae (Orozco et al 1981), show an increased ability to phagocytose red blood cells and other particles. Has your group demonstrated such an effect after *E. histolytica* has ingested bacteria?

Mirelman: We have tested for this effect, and we don't see a significant increase in erythrocyte phagocytosis. An amoeba such as HK-9 has a poor erythrophagocytic activity. If, after it has ingested bacteria, it is presented with red blood cells we do not observe the level of erythrocyte phagocytosis that is demonstrated by the HM1:IMSS strain. Perhaps the HK-9 strain has used all its available energy for phagocytosis of the bacteria so that less is left for taking up the red blood cells.

Piras: You said that the amoeba has a lectin that interacts with *N*-acetylglucosamine (GlcNAc). What is the role of this lectin?

Mirelman: The initial lectin that we discovered in amoeba had a specificity for oligosaccharides of GlcNAc. The amoeba has chitin in its cyst coat (Arroyo-Begovich et al 1980, Avron et al 1982). During the encystation process the amoeba assembles this chitin coat. Since chitin is a polymer of GlcNAc, the lectin that we have discovered may have a role in assembling this chitin coat. I think the GlcNAc-specific lectin may also be important for attachments to certain types of cells (erythrocytes), whereas the second lectin, which is very loosely bound to the amoeba and is specific for *N*-acetylgalactosamine (GalNAc) and galactose, mediates attachment to epithelial cells.

Butterworth: Do the non-pathogenic isolates have receptors only for the GlcNAc and do the pathogenic isolates have receptors only for GalNAc? Do they differ in their adherence to cells?

Mirelman: No. All the different types of amoebae have the same efficiency of adherence. To test for this kind of adherence one has to fix the monolayer cells so that the amoebae will not destroy them as soon as they touch them. We must differentiate between the step of adherence and the step of ingestion and destruction of the cells. If we fix the monolayers with glutaraldehyde, and put radio-labelled amoebae onto them and watch for their adherence capability, we find that all strains of amoebae tested have the lectin and the ability to adhere, and their attachment can be blocked by carbohydrate-containing compounds. So the various amoeba strains do not differ too much in adherence, but in their ability to destroy the monolayers (Kobiler & Mirelman 1981).

Warren: Are the amoebae that exhibit no increase in erythrocyte phagocytosis still able to phagocytose other particles, such as bacteria?

Mirelman: We have tested for the ingestion of the tissue-cultured cells. As I mentioned, we label the tissue-cultured cells with fluorescamine, and then watch for the amoebae to become fluorescent as they ingest the labelled cells. The fluorescent-labelled cells are taken up more by the amoebae that have already interacted with bacteria. The phagocytosis and ingestion by the amoebae of mammalian tissue-cultured cells appears to increase, although that of red blood cells does not.

Warren: Have you demonstrated any increase in destructive factors such as the newly described pore-forming protein produced by amoeba (Lynch et al 1982)?

Mirelman: Non-pathogenic amoebae have very little soluble toxic substance but after they have ingested bacteria they have much more of this substance, which is probably a mixture of several factors—proteolytic enzymic activity, such as collagenase, as well as the amoeba pore-forming material. The latter is now being studied by Carlos Gitler in our institute, who has found that an amoebic protein will form holes in artificial membranes, thus changing the electric potential that the membrane holds. According to Dr Gitler, this is one of the killing effects on target cells. Dr Gitler and I are now trying to see if the amoeba pore-forming material was present, but was mostly not apparent, in these non-pathogenic amoebae until after interaction with the bacteria.

Hudson: How does the amoeba protect its own membrane from this pore-forming toxin?

Mirelman: The toxic substance is probably present in the amoebic vacuoles. The amoeba membrane is extremely fluid and is constantly internalizing, unlike bacterial cell wall, which is stable and defined. During amoeba membrane internalization, the content of vacuoles may be released outside, and it fails to interact with the amoeba membrane probably because the membrane has a different composition from that of bacteria or mammalian cells. The amoeba membrane contains a lipopeptidophosphoglycan (Isibasi et al 1982). The theory of how the amoeba bilayer membrane is built is very different from that for other eukaryotic cells.

Hernández: You said earlier that inhibitors of protein synthesis stop the process of activation. Have you tested any of the glycosylation inhibitors like tunicamycin? Secondly, you said that lysis is associated with the rounding up of the cells, and that Dr Gitler has found the pores in the cell surface of the target mammalian cells. Surely it is likely that the amoeba is secreting something that digests the cell coat, causes rounding up of the cells and later induces pore formation?

Mirelman: Tunicamycin blocks synthesis of the cell-wall coat of the bacteria and is similar to cephalexin, but it doesn't affect the amoeba at all; these glycosylations don't cause any amoebic damage. As to the second question, according to Carlos Gitler, once the amoeba adheres to the target cell it injects this pore-forming material and other enzymes which help it in rounding up and in breaking the cytoskeleton of the target cells. When the amoeba has made the cells round up it can more readily engulf them.

Warren: Dick Guerrant's group have done cinemicrographs of amoebae and cells which show that when a cell and an amoeba come together, a little bump appears on the surface of the amoeba and it appears to punch the cell, which then immediately rounds up (Ravdin et al 1980).

Hernández: It is possible that induced movement of the mammalian cell coat may cause the rounding up, with the consequent destruction of the cytoskeleton.

Butterworth: I have a follow-up question about whether it is the amoeba or the ingested bacterium that is responsible for the augmentation of toxicity. You say that you can block this augmentation by inhibitors of protein synthesis. If you use irreversible inhibitors of protein synthesis to pretreat either the bacterium or the amoeba, which pretreatment prevents the augmentation of toxicity?

Mirelman: The protein-synthesis inhibitor has to be added to the bacteria culture before the bacteria are harvested and supplied to the amoebae. Such treated bacteria do not augment virulence. The protein synthesis inhibitors don't affect the amoebae and when added at the time of the interaction between bacteria and amoebae they do not prevent the ensuing augmentation of virulence.

Butterworth: This suggests that augmentation of toxicity is a property of the bacterium and not the amoeba.

Mirelman: Yes. That is correct.

Gutteridge: Do your observations have any implications for chemotherapeutic strategy? Is there a case for saying, when considering the chemotherapy of amoebic dysentery, that one has an alternative to an approach involving a direct action on the parasite (as seen with drugs such as metronidazole)? This would involve killing the bacteria that markedly enhance the degree of virulence of the parasite, or limiting their virulence by manipulating the diet of the patient.

Mirelman: There is a lot of circumstantial evidence that many antibiotics which are strictly antibacterial—the tetracyclines or even the β-lactams—have some beneficial effect on amoebiasis. Bicyclomycin has no anti-amoebic activity but is effective against most of the enterobacteria that the amoebae can ingest. Thus, by eliminating the bacterial flora that activate the amoebae, the antibiotic may sometimes be effective against amoebiasis. In invasive amoebiasis, with a liver abscess, there is little chance of any effect. Bicyclomycin will be useful only for the intestinal dysenteric stage. Drugs that stimulate secretions, however, e.g. prostaglandin activators, may increase the resistance of the host to invasion, and may also affect the virulence. The interactions that we are observing offer many possibilities for interference with amoebic virulence and may help in alleviating the disease.

Gutteridge: Is this an alleviation or a true irradication of the problem? In other words, are such drugs alternatives to those with a direct action on the parasite?

Mirelman: They are probably not drastic enough to eliminate the problem completely. A basal level of virulence will remain. With antibiotic therapy one usually sees resistant flora that are not eliminated. For example, by using metronidazole one will eliminate a lot of the commensal anaerobic flora, thus opening up the way for the development of a resistant flora. One will definitely not obtain a 'sterile' colon using only antibiotics. On the other hand, it would be interesting to test the flora of the amoebiasis patients because some bacteria, which we don't know about, may be capable of enhancing virulence even more than those that we are studying at present. In collaboration with Dr Martinez-Palomo we will try to study some of these 'super-activating' bacteria.

Warren: Faeces from people in certain parts of Mexico and South Africa may contain virulent organisms. In some parts of the world *E. histolytica* is highly virulent e.g. in the Natal area of South Africa and in parts of Mexico. In other parts of the world where *E. histolytica* is commonly carried one sees very little evidence of disease.

Mirelman: I have started to collaborate with Dr P. Sargeaunt from the London School of Tropical Medicine who collects amoebae from patients and grows them polyxenically, together with the flora from the same patients, to see whether the zymodene patterns of amoeba are affected by the type of bacteria that they interact with. We hope that this study may produce some answers to this interesting question.

Warren: Another unique parasite interaction is the formation of the cyst. I believe you have a new approach to preventing formation of cysts in amoebiasis, which would therefore prevent transmission of the disease.

Mirelman: As I mentioned before, the cysts contain chitin microfibrils as part of their cell coat which protects the amoebae from the hostile environmental conditions once they are outside the body. A number of chitin-synthesis inhibitors has been developed. They are usually analogues of UDP-*N*-acetylglucosamine, which is the precursor of chitin synthesis. These analogues are good inhibitors of fungal chitin synthesis, and are being used as antifungal drugs in agriculture. Since chitin is not present in mammals, these chitin synthesis inhibitors have very low toxicity. We recently tested the effect of chitin synthesis inhibitors on the encystation process of *Entamoeba*. We also developed a method to separate the different encystation stages, using gradients of Percoll, and found that we can block over 90% of cyst formation as well as chitin synthesis with these materials. Our rationale for using these drugs is that they may be useful for preventing transmission of the disease: if the amoeba cannot form a cyst then it will not be resistant to the environment, and the motile trophozoite will die once it comes out from the body. One of the frustrating things about this approach is that we cannot yet test this theory in any animal, as no animal will reproducibly produce cysts of *Entamoeba*, but in cultures we get nice results. We also have now developed a new system for chitin biosynthesis in the pre-cyst forms, and it is blocked by the drugs. However, we would like to test whether the drugs are effective in blocking cyst formation also in humans. We know that the drugs are not toxic, but considerably more information about their pharmacology is needed before we can test them in humans.

Warren: Are these drugs being used for fungus diseases in humans?

Mirelman: Fungal diseases that affect humans are mostly candidiasis and aspergillosis, which are not sensitive to the drugs, so they have not been used in humans. The fungal wall seems not to allow the drug to penetrate through. All the patents on these drugs are for their use as agricultural fungicides. Becker & Naider (1977) have found that yeasts have a peculiar transport system that specifically incorporates tripeptides. By modifying these drugs and binding them to a tripeptide they can, however, get the drug taken up by the *Candida*, where it will then inhibit chitin synthesis and hence will block cell-wall synthesis. The *Candida* then becomes very sensitive to detergents. This is one way of detecting whether or not the skeletal chitin is being synthesized by the fungi. These studies may eventually lead to development of a drug for humans.

Warren: In a place like Mexico, where carriers of amoebae are common, one can see the effect on the protozoan infection when antifungal treatment is indicated.

Butterworth: There are other problems. One would not be treating the disease itself, in infected patients, but would be using the drug solely as a measure for preventing subsequent transmission.

Mirelman: Yes, it is true that the afflicted person may not benefit from such a drug. However, we think it may also be used in combination with the standard use of metronidazole. When one treats with metronidazole, some of the amoebae trophozoites curiously escape the drug by forming cysts. A drug combined with metronidazole could actually block this escape route into cysts.

Cell biology of amoebiasis

Martinez-Palomo: I have some comments about the contribution of bacteria to the virulence of *E. histolytica*. In the liver form of the disease the amoebae are unrelated to bacteria, and practically all cases of liver necrosis are sterile in this sense. On the other hand, invasive amoebiasis in the gut requires the presence of bacteria.

We have been studying the structural basis of the cytopathic effect of *E. histolytica* in epithelial cells without bacteria. It is difficult to understand how a protozoon parasite that is not much larger than a liver cell can induce the damage that is seen in focal sterile necrosis of the liver. Of the several models that we have used the one that has worked best is a culture of epithelial MDCK (Madin-Darby canine kidney) cells. These cells establish a monolayer a few hours after seeding. If we use the Nomarsky technique we can identify clearly the formation of domes, which reflect the fact that these cells are transporting water. The cells therefore lift from the substrate at some regions where there is active transport of water, and so this cultured epithelium behaves much as a real epithelium would. If we add amoebae, after 30 min to 1 h of interaction, we observe tremendous damage to the cell culture; the culture will be almost entirely wiped out if we use a strain of high virulence, such as HM1 in a 1:1 ratio. Scanning electron microscopy (see Fig. 1) shows an interaction between the trophozoites and the upper surface of the epithelial cell cultures. The first structural damage that we can identify is the opening of the intercellular junctions, with passage of electron-dense tracers from the upper surface of the epithelial culture to the lateral spaces and the basal surface of the cells. (Normally the tracer is stopped from penetrating into the lateral space.)

We can quantitate the opening of intercellular spaces by measuring the transmural resistance in cultured epithelium that is mounted on collagen and nylon discs. We see a very sharp drop of resistance during the first five minutes, indicating early interaction between *E. histolytica* and the artificial epithelium. The lytic effect of trophozoites on cultured epithelial cells is revealed, by scanning electron microscopy, to be a surface modification of the cells. This is a focal effect, and only the cells that are directly in contact with the trophozoite show the damage. The trophozoites have a mechanical effect of lifting the cell from its substrate. Once the target cell is damaged, portions of the cytoplasm

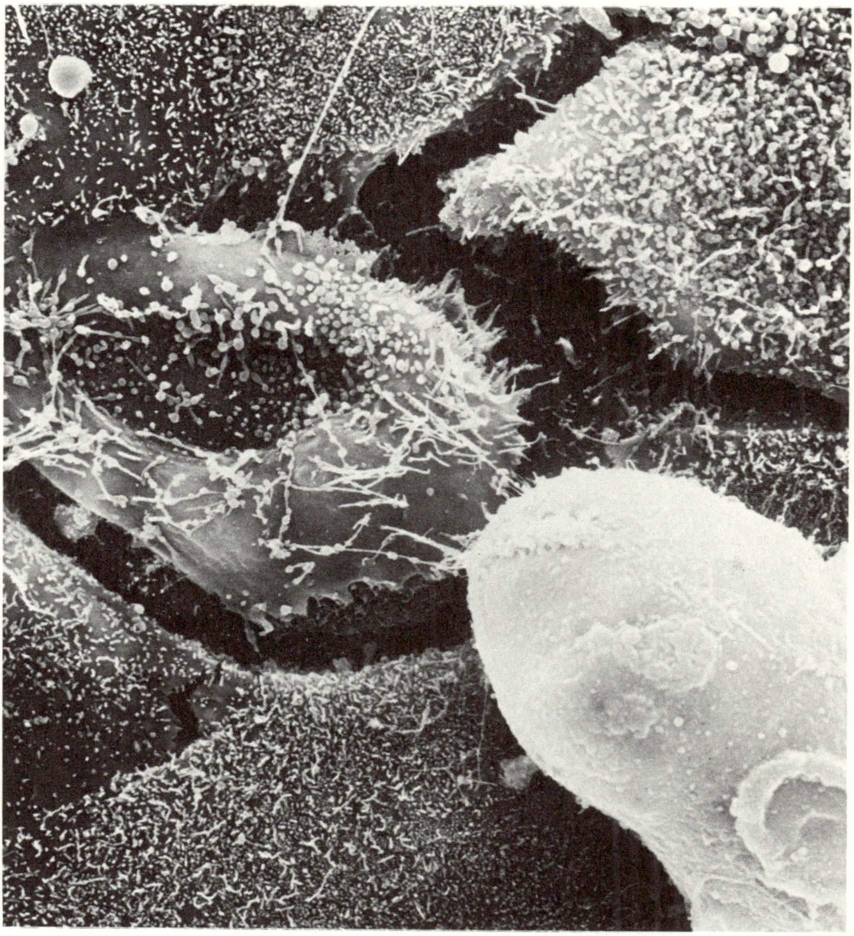

FIG. 1. (*Martinez-Palomo*) Scanning electron micrograph of epithelial cells in contact with a trophozoite of *E. histolytica* (lower right). Early damage appears as retraction of neighbour cells and structural modification of surface microvilli. Magnification, × 1000.

can be pinched off by the amoeba. The damaged cell is then phagocytized by the amoeba (see Fig. 2). The result of this interaction is the intracellular degradation of the engulfed cell. The basic morphological sequence is therefore adhesion, lysis, mechanical effects, phagocytosis and intracellular degradation. We have seen these effects in epithelial cells both in this cell line and in primary cultures of liver cells. The gut is very different. David Mirelman's results are very important because we know little about why amoebiasis may be

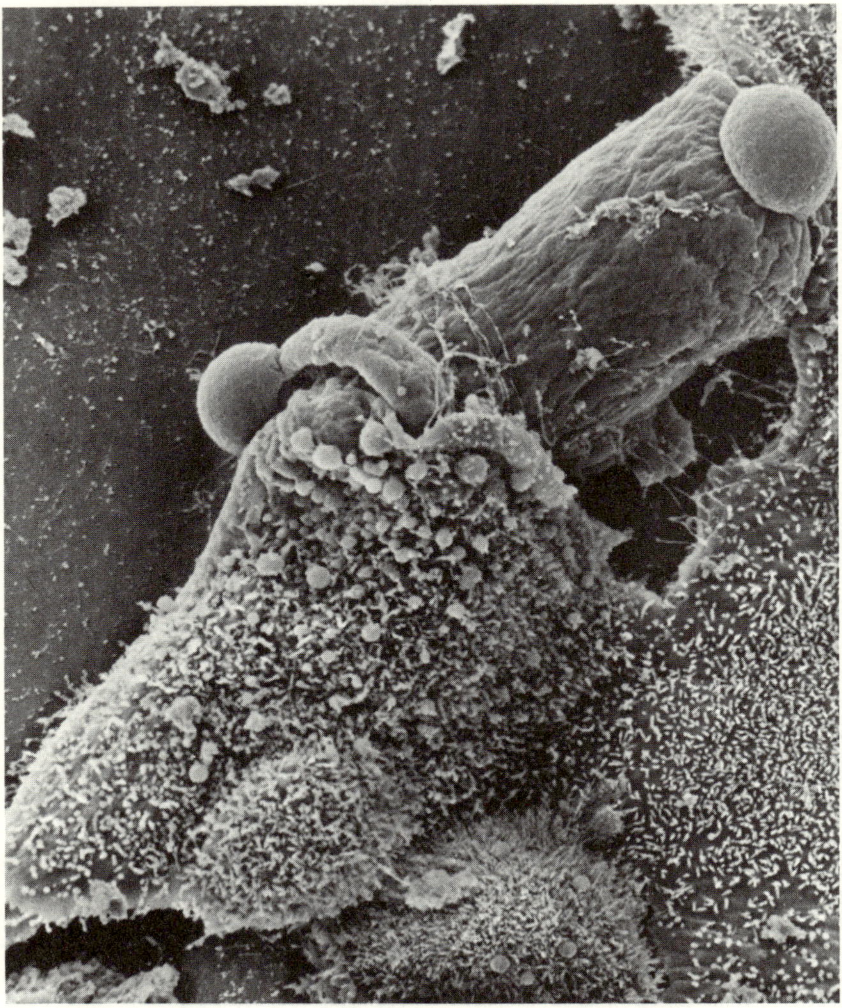

FIG. 2. (*Martinez-Palomo*) A trophozoite of *E. histolytica* (upper right) engulfing a damaged epithelial cell (lower left). Scanning electron micrograph. Magnification, × 1100.

restricted to a commensal phase, or may transform into an invasive phase, in the gut. In collaboration with Dr L.S. Diamond we have shown that axenic strains of *E. histolytica* were capable of inducing ulceration of the caecum in newborn guinea-pigs, but *only* when we worked in Mexico. We attempted the same experiments at NIH in Maryland, using the same strain of amoebae, the same type of guinea-pig and the same food (i.e. maternal milk). We failed miserably: not a single animal had ulcers. When we repeated the work back in Mexico we had the same results as before: we observed the ulcers. This means that something else, in addition to the parasite, the host and the food, is influential, and this may be the presence of bacteria, as Dr Mirelman has described. What exactly are these bacteria modifying in the amoeba? We have had the impression for a number of years that bacteria may in some way activate trophozoites of *E. histolytica* as in the activation of macrophages. This interaction may result in activation of adhesion, lysis and the mechanical activity of the parasite on phagocytosis or degradation, and this provides a direction for future work. We must establish the factors that can enhance or produce this activation of trophozoites that work with human flora. Dr Mirelman's group and our own may be able to establish collaborative work on the isolation of different bacteria from humans who have commensal or invasive amoebiasis, to test the bacterial effects on amoebae in culture.

Pulido: In the activation of trophozoites, have you tried any of the experiments that David Mirelman has done with bacteria and dietary factors?

Martinez-Palomo: All we can do is to study in the laboratory certain physiological parameters of amoebae. At present we are investigating whether there is some sort of activation in terms of phagocytosis and liberation of collagenase, which our group has shown is produced by *E. histolytica* (Muñoz et al 1982b). We don't have an answer yet.

REFERENCES

Aley SB, Scott WA, Cohn ZA 1980 Plasma membrane of *Entamoeba histolytica*. J Exp Med 152:391-404

Arroyo-Begovich A, Cabarez-Trejo A, Ruiz-Herrera J 1980 Identification of the structural component in the cyst wall of *Entamoeba invadens*. J Parasitol 66:735-741

Avron B, Deutsch RM, Mirelman D 1982 Chitin synthesis inhibitors prevent cyst formation by *Entamoeba* trophozoites. Biochem Biophys Res Commun 108:815-821

Becker JM, Naider F 1977 Peptide transport in yeast: uptake of radioactive trimethionine in *Saccharomyces cerevisiae*. Arch Biochem Biophys 178:245-255

De Voe IW 1976 Egestion of degraded meningococci by polymorphonuclear leukocytes. J Bacteriol 125:258-266

Gadasi H, Kessler E 1983 Correlation between virulence and collagenolytic activity in *Entamoeba histolytica*. Infect Immun 39:528-531

Isibasi A, Cruz MS, Ramirez A, Kumate J 1982 Localizacion en los trofozoitos de *Entamoeba histolytica* de una lipopeptidofosfoglicana extraida por fenol-agua de la cepa HK-9. Arch Invest Med 13:57-62

Jeon KW, Jeon MS 1976 Endosymbiosis in amoebae: recently established endosymbionts have become required cytoplasmic components. J Cell Physiol 89:337-347

Kobiler D, Mirelman D 1981 Adhesion of *Entamoeba histolytica* trophozoites to monolayers of human cells. J Infect Dis 144:539-546

Lynch EC, Rosenberg IM, Gitler C 1982 An ion-channel forming protein produced by *Entamoeba histolytica*. EMBO J 1:801-804

Martinez-Palomo A 1982 The biology of *Entamoeba histolytica*. John Wiley, Chichester (Trop Med Res Studies Ser) see: Parasite factors of virulence, p 95-117

Muñoz ML, Calderón J, Rojkind M 1982a Presencia de actividad colagenolitica en trofozoitos de *Entamoeba histolytica*. Arch Invest Med 13 (Suppl 3):191-202

Muñoz ML, Calderón J, Rojkind M 1982b The collagenase of *Entamoeba histolytica*. J Exp Med 155:42-51

Orozco E, Guarneros G, Martinez-Palomo A 1981 Aislamiento de una clona de *E. histolytica* deficiente en fagocitosis. Correlacion de la facocytosis en la virulenci. In: Proc IX Seminar on amebiasis. Instituto Mexicana del Segura Social, Mexico City

Preer JR Jr, Preer LB, Juran A 1974 Kappa and other endosymbionts in *Paramecium aurelia*. Bacteriol Rev 38:113-163

Ravdin JI, Croft BY, Guerrant RL 1980 Cytopathogenic mechanisms of *Entamoeba histolytica*. J Exp Med 152:377-390

Smith PL, Blumberg JB, Stoff JS, Field M 1981 Antisecretory effects of indomethacin on rabbit-ileal mucosa *in vitro*. Gastroenterology 80:356-365

Uedzulu IA, Leitch GJ, Bailey GB 1982 Use of indomethacin to demonstrate enterotoxic activity in extracts of *Entamoeba histolytica* trophozoites. Infect Immun 36:795-801

Trypanosoma cruzi–fibroblastic cell interactions necessary for cellular invasion

R. PIRAS, M. M. PIRAS and D. HENRÍQUEZ

Unidad de Investigaciones, Centro Médico Docente La Trinidad, Apartado 80474, Caracas 1080-A, Venezuela

Abstract Detailed knowledge of the mechanism by which vertebrate cells are invaded by the haemoflagellated parasite *Trypanosoma cruzi* is of paramount importance for understanding one of the early events in the life cycle of this obligatory intracellular parasite. The ability to infect vertebrate fibroblastic cells was found to be only partially expressed in trypomastigotes that were recently liberated from cell cultures. These trypomastigotes could increase by several fold their capability for adhesion and infection by a time-dependent *in vitro* process. This activation phenomenon was used to study how certain inhibitors of macromolecular biosynthesis (actinomycin D, puromycin, tunicamycin), proteases, protease inhibitors, and a combination of them, acted on adhesion and infection. The effect of exposing the parasites and, independently, the host fibroblasts to various lectins and carbohydrates was also investigated. Most of these treatments either inhibited or stimulated adhesion and infection. Exposure of fibroblastic cells to trypsin and to drugs altering the cytoskeleton impaired their susceptibility to infection. Tunicamycin blocked the recovery of infection, but not of adhesion, in trypsinized cells. The results obtained have been interpreted as indicating that the process of fibroblast infection by *T. cruzi* trypomastigotes occurs through two distinct and independent steps (adhesion and penetration), mediated by components of both the parasite and the host cell. The parasite components seem to be: (a) a lectin-like protein involved in adhesion; (b) an activating inducible system, probably of proteolytic nature, which enhances parasite adhesion; and (c) a tunicamycin-sensitive glycoprotein, related to penetration only. As for the fibroblastic cell components, these are postulated to be two glycoproteins (one insensitive and the other sensitive to tunicamycin), which are involved in the steps of parasite attachment and penetration, respectively.

1983 Cytopathology of parasitic disease. Pitman Books, London (Ciba Foundation symposium 99), p 31-51

Our knowledge of various aspects of the morphology, life cycle, differentiation, biochemical composition, metabolism and immunology of the haemoflagellated parasite *Trypanosoma cruzi* has improved substantially during the last few years (Brener 1979, 1980, Gutteridge 1981). Nevertheless, several important basic aspects of the relationship between this parasite and its host cells remain obscure. Among these aspects, the mechanism controlling the parasite's capacity to penetrate cells is of paramount importance. Because *T. cruzi* is an obligatory intracellular parasite, an adequate knowledge of the cell-invasion process might facilitate the formulation of strategies for blocking this early stage of the biological cycle of the parasite.

Since one of the first events in parasite interiorization into a host cell is the interaction between the two plasma membranes, it is reasonable to assume that certain cell-surface components of both *T. cruzi* and the host cell are involved in interiorization. This membrane interaction is unlikely to be either highly specific, like that described for some viruses and bacteria (Markwell & Paulson 1980, Ofek et al 1977), or non-specific. In fact, although *T. cruzi* can invade a variety of hosts, it displays a certain degree of tissue tropism *in vivo* (Melo & Brener 1978). Infections show no cell specificity *in vitro*, but the extent of cell invasion varies with the *T. cruzi* strain and the cell type used. The parasitic form and the cell type are important, as indicated by the fact that both the epimastigote and the trypomastigote forms are interiorized by 'professional' phagocytic cells but only the trypomastigotes can invade 'non-professional' phagocytes, such as fibroblasts. Moreover, even for a given cell line and parasitic form (e.g., Vero fibroblasts and cell culture-derived trypomastigotes) variable infections can be obtained, depending on the inoculum used (Piras et al 1980a). These observations point out that although a highly specific interaction is unnecessary for infection to occur, certain requirements must be met to allow *T. cruzi* to invade cells. In this paper we shall summarize our findings about these requirements and about some of the components involved in the interaction between *T. cruzi* trypomastigotes and vertebrate fibroblastic cells. More detailed accounts of some of these results have been published (Piras et al 1980b, Henríquez et al 1981b, Piras et al 1982a, b).

Definitions and assay systems

Trypomastigotes of *T. cruzi* (EP strain) derived from infected Vero-cell monolayers were used routinely. The parasites were grown, isolated and purified as already described (Piras et al 1982a), and we shall refer to them here as CCT (cell-culture-derived trypomastigotes).

We shall be using the terms 'adhesion' and 'attachment' synonymously. We have studied this process by causing parasites to interact with monolayers of fibroblastic cells (Vero cells, unless otherwise stated) at 0 °C for 2 h, followed by extensive washings to remove the free parasites, and staining; the 'adhesion index' expresses the average number of extracellular parasites bound per cell. 'Infection', 'invasion' and 'interiorization' will also be used as synonyms; these terms include two distinct and consecutive steps: adhesion and penetration. The latter has not been measured directly, but it has been assumed that a decrease in infection that was not concurrent with a decrease in adhesion indicated an alteration in the penetration step *per se*. Infection was studied in a similar way to adhesion, but incubations were done at 37 °C; the 'infection index' expresses the average number of intracellular parasites found per cell. These procedures have been reported in detail (Henríquez et al 1981b, Piras et al 1982a).

Results and discussion

Role of the parasite

The presence of amastigote forms in the trypomastigote preparations derived from cell cultures has not received much attention, probably because it has been assumed that they arose as a small contamination from the premature disruption of cells which contained parasites that had not yet differentiated into trypomastigotes. We consistently observed, in our preliminary studies, that trypomastigotes obtained as soon as they first burst out from infected monolayers of Vero cells contained few amastigotes and that their ability to invade fresh Vero cells was very poor. Trypomastigotes that were not collected and were used immediately after bursting had a variable, but usually high, invasive capability and amastigote content (Piras et al 1980a). Incubation of fresh CCT in a cell-free medium has demonstrated that the ability of the parasites to invade fibroblasts did indeed increase 5- to 15-fold with time (Fig. 1). Concomitantly, the adhesion of *T. cruzi* to Vero cells increased, and the morphology of the CCT changed profoundly. Thus, the typical trypomastigote, originally present in recently isolated preparations, began to transform first into intermediate forms and then to round forms. Since the total number of parasites remained constant during incubation (20–26 h), the decrease in trypomastigotes was accounted for by the increase in the round forms. We have referred to these round parasites as 'spheromastigotes' or 'amastigote-like forms', since they are similar, but not identical to true intracellular amastigotes (Piras et al 1982a). The main differences are the kinetoplast ultrastructure, the lack of DNA synthesis in the spheromastigotes, and the very efficient ability of the spheromastigotes to infect cells. The changes in infectivity and, to a lesser extent, of morphology were observed also with two other isolates (BEC and MEN). Moreover, they were independent of the cell line used for producing the CCT (Vero, BHK-21, HEP-2), as well as of the target cell used to determine their invasive capability (Vero, MA-103, chick embryonic muscle cells, normal human macrophages). Hence,

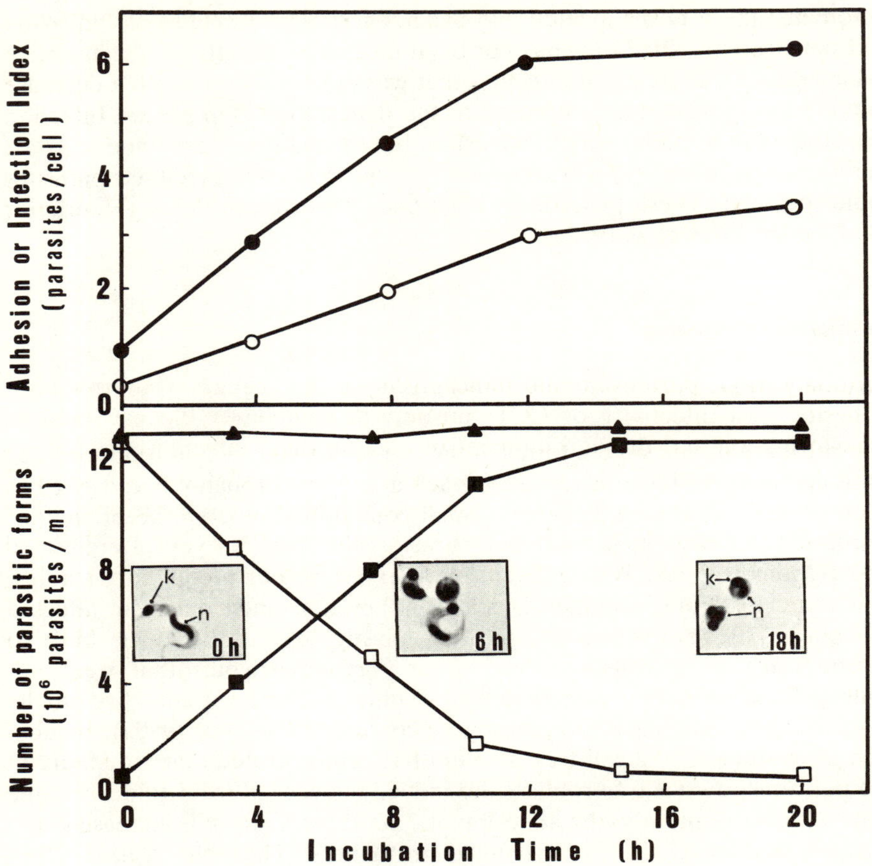

FIG. 1. The effect on adhesion, infectivity and morphology of *T. cruzi* after extracellular incubation of trypomastigotes that were recently liberated from Vero cells. Aliquots of incubated parasites were used to measure adhesion (open circles), infection (filled circles), total parasite content (filled triangles), and trypomastigote (open squares) and spheromastigote (filled squares) forms. The inserts are photomicrographs of stained parasites incubated for the periods shown: k, kinetoplast; n, nucleus. Adapted from Piras et al (1982a).

this *in vitro* enhancement of infectivity seems to be quite general, suggesting that trypomastigotes liberated from the infected cell cultures can express only part of their total invasive capacity. This phenomenon can be detected and studied as long as recently released trypomastigotes and short incubation periods are used for the determination of adhesion and infection.

Regardless of whether this extracellular 'maturation' has an *in vivo* significance, the demonstrated increase in adhesion and infection *in vitro* might be used as a tool in studies directed: (a) to identify the trypomastigote components responsible for the invasive process; and (b) to understand the mechanism of the host–parasite relationship at the membrane level. Particle engulfment into both professional and non-professional phagocytes has been shown to consist of an adhesion and interiorization step (Silverstein et al 1977). In *T. cruzi*, only recently has it been possible to measure adhesion as a separate phase from infection, a process that includes both adhesion *and* penetration (Henríquez et al 1981a, Piras et al 1982a, Andrews & Colli 1982). Determining how these parameters are affected by inhibitors of RNA, protein and glycoprotein biosynthesis has allowed us to clarify whether the enhancement of infectivity was due to an activation or to a *de novo* synthesis of *T. cruzi* macromolecules (Piras et al 1982b). Fig. 2 summarizes the effect of actinomycin D, puromycin and tunicamycin on the changes of morphology, adhesion and infectivity of CCT: puromycin completely blocked parasite transformation and the development of adhesion and infectivity; cycloheximide had a similar effect; but chloramphenicol was ineffective (not shown). Actinomycin D and tunicamycin completely inhibited the development of infectivity, without blocking adhesion and transformation. The blockage by puromycin of the development of parasite adhesion and the suppression by actinomycin and tunicamycin of infectivity (in the absence of inhibition of adhesion) indicate that during parasite maturation a *de novo* synthesis of the macromolecules involved in both adhesion and penetration is necessary, and that these two steps are independent. Moreover, the tunicamycin effect also suggests that a parasite glycoprotein(s) with N-glycosidic-linked oligosaccharides is involved in the penetration step of *T. cruzi* into fibroblasts. Morphological transformation requires protein biosynthesis but is independent of the development of infectivity, which can be abolished without altering transformation. Hence, during extracellular parasite maturation the following processes seem to be taking place: (a) translation of pre-existing RNA with the information for parasite adhesion and, eventually, for transformation; and (b) transcription of the RNA and biosynthesis of the corresponding glycoprotein(s) necessary for penetration.

Using exogenous modifications of the surface membrane of CCT, we have attempted to obtain additional information about the parasite components involved in infection. These modifications included CCT interaction with lectin and carbohydrates (Piras et al 1980b) as well as alterations by periodate and trypsin (Henríquez et al 1981a). Some of the results obtained with trypsin are summarized in Fig. 3. The treatment of fresh CCT with trypsin stimulated adhesion by 4- to 6-fold but this enhancement became less evident, and eventually disappeared, when parasites already partially or totally activated were used. High trypsin concentrations also precluded us from observing the stimulation (not shown). When CCT were incubated extracellularly in the

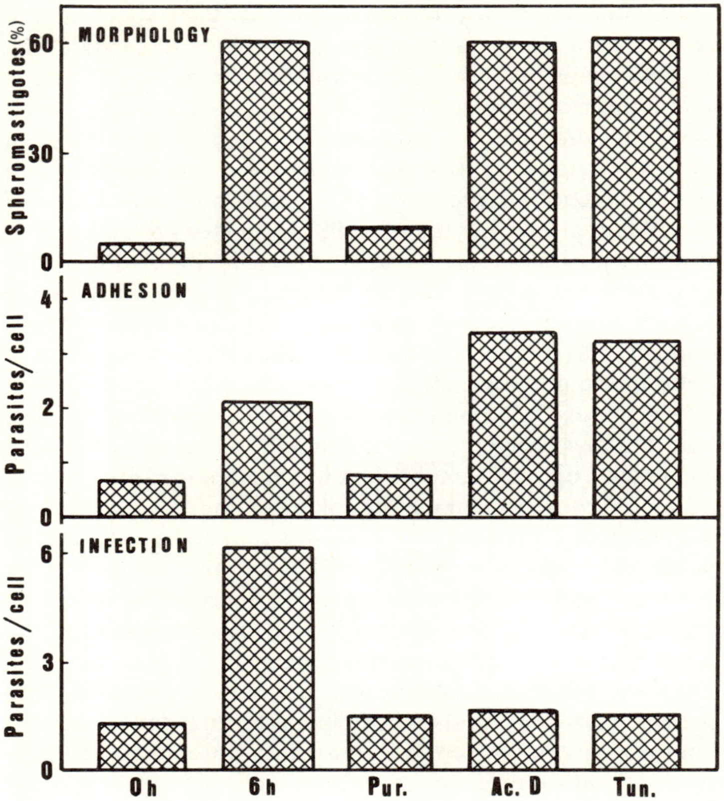

FIG. 2. The effect of puromycin, actinomycin D and tunicamycin on the changes in morphology, adhesion and infection induced by extracellular incubation of *T. cruzi* trypomastigotes. Parasites were incubated for 6 h either alone or in the presence of 5 μg/ml puromycin (Pur.), 8 ng/ml actinomycin D (Ac.D) or 30 ng/ml tunicamycin (Tun.), washed, and used for the measurements indicated.

presence of protease inhibitors (phenylmethylsulphonylfluoride, aprotinin, antipain, pepstatin, chymostatin and trypsin inhibitors) the development of adhesion was blocked. However, trypsinization caused the parasites to reacquire an adhesion capability similar to that of controls. A similar result was observed when puromycin was included during the activation period. Trypsinization of parasites activated in the presence of tunicamycin (which were already very adherent by themselves; see also Fig. 2) stimulated adhesion only very slightly. Thus, a similar and high adhesion value (the upper part of the empty bars in Fig. 3) was obtained both by a 24 h extracellular incubation and by trypsinization of the other types of parasites

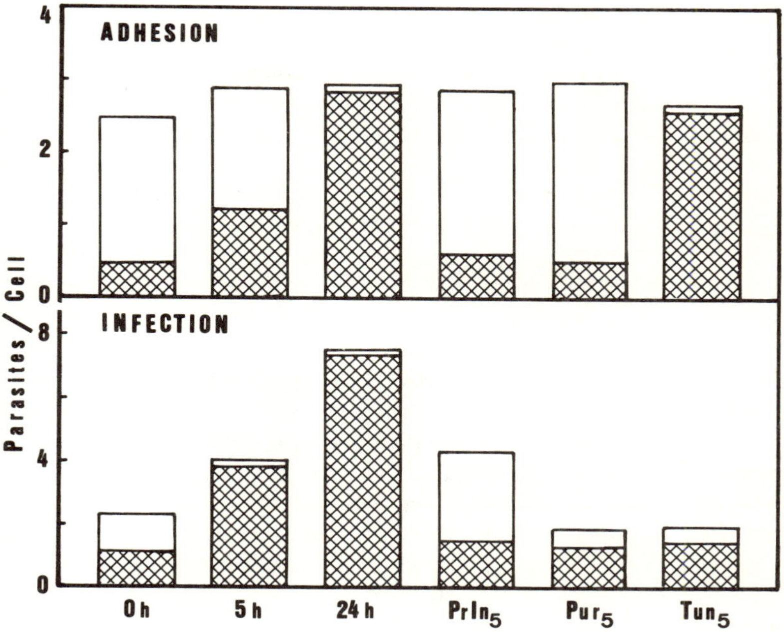

FIG. 3. The effect of trypsinization of *T. cruzi* trypomastigotes activated in the absence and presence of protease inhibitors, puromycin and tunicamycin. Trypomastigotes were incubated alone for 5 and 24 h, or for 5 h in the presence of either a mixture of 15 μg/ml aprotinin, leupeptin and antipain (PrIn), or 5 μg/ml puromycin (Pur) or 50 ng/ml tunicamycin (Tun); the parasites were then washed and used directly (cross-hatched bars) or after trypsinization (empty bars) to determine adhesion and infection.

studied. This suggests that the adhesion capability was already present in fresh CCT and that puromycin blocked the biosynthesis of an enzyme responsible for activating pre-existing molecules. The effect of exogenous proteases and protease inhibitors makes it tempting to speculate that this endogenous activity is an inducible protease of the parasite. We have recently detected a protease activity in intact CCT, which is apparently located in the external surface membrane of the trypomastigotes (Recover & Piras 1982). As for the infectivity, trypsin stimulation occurred only with fresh CCT, and trypsinization of parasites pretreated with protease inhibitors, puromycin and tunicamycin restored the infectivity to the proper control levels only in protease-treated parasites. These results again point to the independence of the adhesion and penetration steps, as well as to the fact that the glycoprotein(s) necessary for penetration are probably synthesized *de novo* during the maturation period.

Using cell-culture-derived trypomastigotes Andrews & Colli (1982) have recently observed that exposure of these parasites to high levels of fetal calf serum inhibited their adhesion and infectivity, and that trypsinization restored these processes. No effect of trypsin was found if the trypomastigotes were not pretreated with fetal calf serum. They have interpreted these results as indicating that a serum factor binds to trypomastigotes and impairs adhesion and infection. However, in our system we have not found any inhibitory effect of serum on adhesion and infection. In fact, CCT were optimally activated during extracellular incubation with media that contained fetal calf serum and, during assays, their infectivity was best expressed with such media. Moreover, the trypsin-induced activation of adhesion and infection could be obtained even with CCT liberated from cells grown in serum-free medium. Differences in parasite strains and in isolation conditions, together with the high trypsin concentration and the length of assay used could be the reasons why a stimulatory effect of trypsin was not observed on the parasites *per se*. Trypsinization of blood-form trypomastigotes substantially stimulates their uptake by macrophages (Nogueira et al 1980, Kipnis et al 1981). Reincubation of trypsinized parasites restored the low uptake that was characteristic of untreated blood trypomastigotes, and cycloheximide blocked this recovery. This effect of trypsin has been interpreted as due to the removal of a surface glycoprotein (relative molecular mass, M_r, 90 000) of the parasites, which acted as an antiphagocytic factor (Nogueira et al 1980, 1981). Since we did not observe any decrease of CCT adhesion and infectivity on reincubation of trypsinized CCT for up to 6–8 h, the mechanism of activation of CCT, and their interaction with fibroblasts, is unlikely to be identical to that between blood trypomastigotes and macrophages.

We have examined the pattern of surface-membrane proteins in fresh CCT and in parasites activated either by prolonged incubation or by trypsin (Fig. 4). Iodination with [^{125}I]iodogen of recently isolated CCT, followed by sodium dodecyl sulphate–polyacrylamide gel electrophoresis showed several bands tightly clustered in the region of 60 000 to 110 000 M_r. This pattern is complex, with prominent bands of M_r approximately 105 K, 95 K, 86 K and 68 K, coinciding, in general, with that reported recently by Zingales et al (1982). Since it is not known yet whether the membrane components involved in adhesion and penetration are immunogenic and, if glycosylated, of what specificity they are, we have preferred as a first approach not to sort out any special class of molecules *a priori* by immunoprecipitation or by lectin chromatography. CCT activation for 20 h brought about the disappearance and the decrease of the 105 K and 95 K bands, respectively, and the intensification of the 68 K species. Trypsinization of fresh CCT resulted in a pattern similar to that observed for the 20 h-activated parasites. The persistence of the 86 K species in the highly infective parasites would be consistent with the suggestion that an 85 K protein might be related to infection

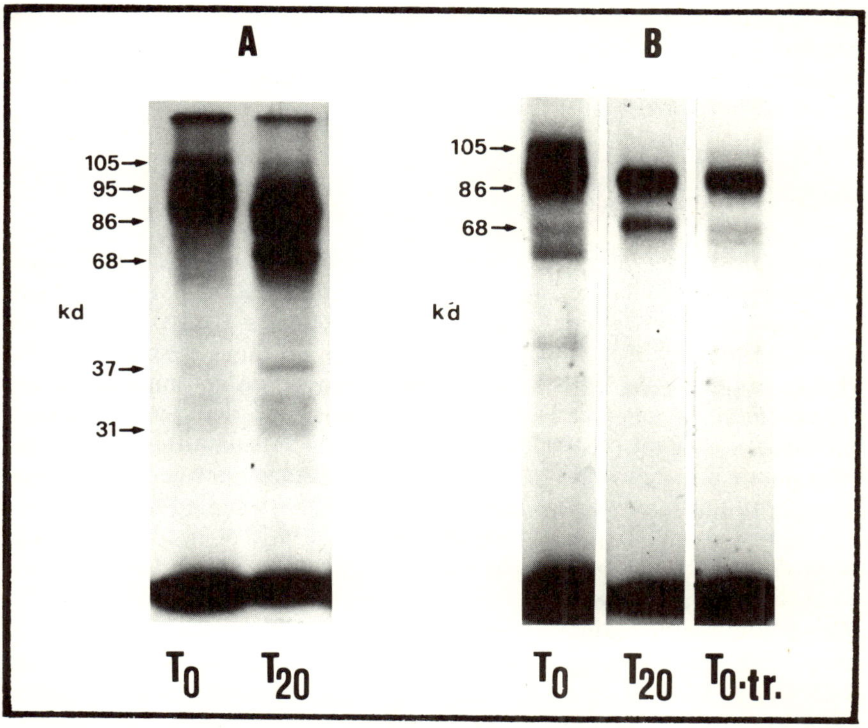

FIG. 4. Autoradiographies of *T. cruzi* surface-membrane proteins labelled with [^{125}I]iodogen. T_0, recently isolated cell-cultured trypomastigotes (CCT); T_{20}, CCT incubated for 20 h; $T_{0.tr}$, T_0 parasites that were trypsinized and then radioiodinated.

(Zingales et al 1982). Moreover, removal of the high M_r bands is concomitant with (but may be not causally related to) the increase in adhesion and infectivity; Nogueira et al (1981) have reported that trypsin activation of blood trypomastigotes removes an immunogenic 90 K glycoprotein.

Several possible interpretations can be advanced to explain the CCT activation process and its relationship to infection of fibroblasts. Among these would be that the parasite component necessary for adhesion is present in recently liberated CCT mainly as an inactive precursor, which is then activated during the maturation process by an inducible endogenous membrane protease. A slight variation of this interpretation would be that the component is active and preformed, but masked or unavailable, and that activation brings about a membrane rearrangement that unmasks the component. A relatively different possibility would be that parasites are released from infected fibroblasts coated with a *host* component, which is then removed extracellularly to increase adhesion. As already discussed, the possibilities that this inhibitory factor could be of parasite origin, as for blood trypomastigotes, or that it was a serum factor picked up from the incubation medium are not consistent with our results.

*Fibroblasts–*T. cruzi *interactions*

To determine if the interaction between fibroblasts and CCT takes place through a specific ligand–receptor mechanism mediated by glycoproteins in one cell and the corresponding lectin-like molecules in the other, we have explored the effects of lectins and carbohydrates on this system (Piras et al 1980b, Henríquez et al 1981b). This type of recognition and interaction has been identified between viruses, bacteria, yeasts, etc. and vertebrate cells (e.g. Markwell & Paulson 1980, Ofek et al 1977). Parasites are no exception, and the interaction is thought to take place, for instance, between *Leishmania donovani* promastigotes and hamster macrophages (Chang 1981), *Plasmodium falciparum* and human erythrocytes (Perkins 1981, Weiss et al 1981) and between *Entamoeba histolytica* and intestinal epithelial cells and erythrocytes (Kobiler & Mirelman 1980).

The carbohydrate residues available for interactions on the cell surface of *T. cruzi* have been investigated in detail by means of lectin binding (Araujo et al 1980) and lectin-induced agglutination of parasites (Pereira et al 1980). In spite of some apparent discrepancies between these two reports, some common features are evident. Thus, all parasite forms seem to have the following sugar residues accessible for interaction with the corresponding lectins: galactose, mannose and/or glucose, *N*-acetylglucosamine, *N*-acetylgalactosamine and probably sialic acid; fucose does not seem to be available, according to these workers. If these parasitic carbohydrate residues were to act as ligands in the cell–parasite attachment, it would be expected that treatment of the CCT and the host cell with the proper lectins and sugars, respectively, should impair parasite adhesion to host cells. The results we have obtained first on infection (Piras et al 1980b), and now also on adhesion, show that rather than an inhibition, a 2- to 3-fold stimulation of both adhesion and infection was brought about by parasite exposure to concanavalin A, wheat-germ agglutinin and phytohaemagglutinin (Table 1). Neither adhesion nor infection were altered by *Ulex europeus* lectin (as expected by the lack of available fucosyl residues in the parasite, as already discussed) or by ricin I agglutinin (for which galactosyl residues were supposed to be accessible). Moreover, when Vero cells were pretreated with various monosaccharides and then infected with CCT, adhesion and infectivity were not altered (Table 1). Hence, the existence of specific CCT 'ligands' interacting with 'lectin-like'

TABLE 1 The effect on adhesion and infection of treating cell-culture trypomastigotes (CCT) with lectins and Vero cells with carbohydrate residues

Conditions[a]	*Adhesion* (%)	*Infection* (%)
CCT treatment		
None	*100*	*100*
Concanavalin A	275	252
Wheat-germ agglutinin	210	189
Phytohaemagglutinin	220	251
Ricin I lectin	75	79
Ulex europeus lectin	95	107
Vero cell treatment		
None	*100*	*100*
D-Mannose	98	105
D-Galactose	120	95
L-Fucose	100	101
N-Acetyl-D-glucosamine	90	95
N-Acetyl-D-galactosamine	110	100

[a]CCT were treated with 10 μg/ml lectin for 30 min at 24 °C in a serum-free medium, washed, and then used to determine adhesion and infection under standard conditions. Vero cells were pretreated similarly, but with 50 mM carbohydrate.

molecules of the host cell could not be substantiated by these experiments. However, while removal of the saccharides before infection avoids the possibility of carbohydrates acting simultaneously on parasites, this might have precluded us from detecting an effect, if the binding affinity of the saccharides for the cell sites were low. In addition, the stimulation of adhesion found when parasites are treated with certain lectins could be due to the formation by the multivalent lectins of new, artificial binding sites, which could then bridge to glycoproteins of the counterpart cell. This non-specific process might be masking the 'legitimate' lectin effect; the monovalent derivative of concanavalin A—succinyl-concanavalin A—should be useful to test this point.

Another possibility for a ligand–receptor interaction involving carbohydrate moieties would be that these ligands were on the host cell, and the lectin-like molecules on the CCT. We have already established (Piras et al 1980b) that CCT treated with mannose, α-methylmannoside, mannan, *N*-acetylglucosamine and *N*-acetylgalactosamine had a decreased infectivity, while parasites exposed to other sugars were unaffected. Table 2 summarizes these results and compares them with those on adhesion. Mannosyl, *N*-acetylglucosaminyl and *N*-acetylgalactosaminyl residues seem to affect CCT mainly at the adhesion step. The effect of mannan is especially noteworthy because of the low initial concentration used and the fact that is a high M_r polysaccharide that probably does not permeate into the parasite. Since these

TABLE 2 The effect on adhesion and infection of treating CCT with carbohydrates and Vero cells with lectins

Conditions[a]	*Adhesion* (%)	*Infection* (%)
CCT treatment		
None	*100*	*100*
D-Mannose	55	41
α-D-Methylmannoside	40	24
Mannan	48	20
L-Fucose	87	95
D-Galactose	116	100
N-Acetyl-D-glucosamine	55	32
N-Acetyl-D-galactosamine	48	28
Vero cell treatment		
None	*100*	*100*
Concanavalin A	340	30
Wheat-germ agglutinin	45	40
Phytohaemagglutinin	45	29
Ricin I lectin	82	27
Ulex europeus lectin	90	105

[a]Conditions were similar to those of Table 1, except that parasites and cells were treated with carbohydrate and lectin, respectively.

inhibitory effects were seen with only some of the carbohydrate residues, and after removing excess unbound saccharides, it is likely that they reflect the existence of lectin-like protein(s) in the *T. cruzi* cell surface. Recently, Crane & Dvorak (1982) have also found evidence that *N*-acetylglucosamine blocks infection of vertebrate cells by *T. cruzi*. However, they found that mannose (and to a lesser extent *N*-acetylgalactosamine) was not effective. Whether these differences are due to *T. cruzi* strains or to other experimental variables remains to be determined. To test if these lectin-like proteins of the parasite have a counterpart in host cells, we treated the host cells, before infection, with lectins. We had already reported (Henríquez et al 1981b) that such treatment inhibits the infection process. These results are summarized in Table 2, together with those on adhesion. Of the three lectins we tested and expected to inhibit adhesion (concanavalin A, wheat-germ agglutinin and phytohaemagglutinin), the last two did so while concanavalin A, in contrast, actually stimulated adhesion. Ricin I and *Ulex europeus* lectins, which we anticipated would be inactive, did not affect adhesion. Thus, with the exception of the concanavalin A stimulation of adhesion, the results obtained both with carbohydrates and lectins seem to be consistent with the presence of carbohydrate ligands in the host cell and with the corresponding lectin-like molecules in the CCT. Studies with lectins and sugars can provide information only on interactions between glycoproteins or glycolipids and their counterparts; however, other types of interaction might also be occurring. In fact, we never observed a total inhibition of adhesion and infection with lectin-treated cells or with sugar-treated parasites. Thus, while most of the data so far obtained favour the hypothesis that a specific ligand–receptor mechanism is involved in the attachment phase of CCT to fibroblasts, further and independent evidence is desirable to substantiate this point firmly. The possibility that other mechanisms might also be acting, either alone or in conjunction with the previous one, cannot yet be dismissed.

Role of the host cell

The surface membrane of host fibroblasts does not seem to play a simple, passive part in the infective process. This is indicated by the differences in infectivity observed when fibroblasts were subjected to various treatments (Piras et al 1980b, Henríquez et al 1981b). Thus, we found reduced infectivity: (a) when non-confluent cells were used instead of confluent cells; (b) when we used fibroblasts exposed to drugs that disrupt the cell cytoskeleton; and (c) when fibroblasts treated with periodate or trypsin were used. Recently, Dvorak & Crane (1981) found that HeLa cells in the S phase of the growth cycle are more suceptible to infection by *T. cruzi* than cells in the other phases. Any of the above conditions and procedures brings about important changes in the composition and distribution of numerous surface-membrane components. Some of them may play a specific and prominent part in the steps of adhesion and penetration and it is therefore important to identify them.

Trypsin-treated Vero cells are less susceptible to infection by CCT than control cells (Piras et al 1980b, Henríquez et al 1981b). Similarly, host-cell trypsinization has been reported to impair the uptake of *T. cruzi* by macrophages (Nogueira & Cohn 1976), the binding of *L. donovani* promastigotes to macrophages (Chang 1981) and the invasion of erythrocytes by *P. falciparum* merozoites (Perkins 1981). We have now examined whether tunicamycin influences the return of trypsinized Vero cells to 'normal' adhesion and infection by CCT (Table 3). The decreased susceptibility to parasite adhesion and infection of these cells was restored completely within 4–5 h of incubation after trypsinization. When tunicamycin was present during the recovery period, infection was not re-established, despite the fact that adhesion returned to normal values. Tunicamycin did not affect adhesion and infection of untreated cells under the conditions used. Neither did it inhibit amino acid incorporation into proteins, but it did suppress the stimulated mannose incorporation that occurs after cell trypsinization (not shown). These results confirm earlier observations on lectin- and periodate-

TABLE 3 The effect of tunicamycin on the recovery of *T. cruzi* adhesion and infectivity of trypsin-treated Vero cells

Treatment[a]	*Adhesion*	*Infection*
	(*Parasites/cell*)	
None	0.8	1.5
Trypsin	0.1	0.5
Trypsin + (5 h incubation)	0.7	1.4
None + (tunicamycin + 5 h incubation)	0.8	1.4
Trypsin + (tunicamycin + 5 h incubation)	0.7	0.5

[a]Vero cells were first either trypsinized (1.2 mg/ml for 10 min at 24 °C) or not, and then incubated for 5 h either alone or in the presence of 100 ng/ml tunicamycin; adhesion and infection were then measured.

treated cells, indicating that adhesion and infection could respond independently in host fibroblasts (Henríquez et al 1981b). Moreover, they also suggest that a tunicamycin-sensitive glycoprotein(s) of the host cell is involved in the penetration step of the parasites into the cells. The adhesion results could suggest that the glycosylated ligand postulated as a cell receptor for the parasite is a tunicamycin-insensitive glycoprotein rather than, for example, a glycolipid. This would be consistent also with the observation that cycloheximide blocked the recovery of adhesion and infection of trypsinized cells (not shown). However, we cannot yet discard the notion that trypsin could have acted indirectly, that is, by producing a general disorganization of the cell membrane, which rendered the cell receptor unavailable or non-functional.

Conclusions

Cell-culture-derived trypomastigotes of *T. cruzi* invade fibroblastic cells through two distinct, independent steps: adhesion and penetration. Surface-membrane components of both the parasite and the host fibroblasts need to interact for infection to occur. The parasite components involved seem to be: (a) a lectin-like protein related to adhesion, (b) an activating system, probably proteolytic, which enhances parasite adhesion through activating or unmasking pre-existing inactive or masked molecules, or through removing an inhibitory factor originating in the host cell, and (c) a tunicamycin-sensitive glycoprotein related to penetration only. Two host-cell glycoproteins are also postulated to be involved: one in the attachment and the other in the penetration phase. The isolation and characterization of these components should help to establish their real involvement and the mechanism by which cell-cultured trypomastigotes invade fibroblastic cells.

Acknowledgements

The able technical assistance of Stefania Negri is greatly acknowledged, as well as the continuous support and interest of Dr Pablo A. Pulido. This work was financed in part by funds from CONICIT of Venezuela (Project S1-1303), the UNDP/World Bank/WHO Special Programme for Research and Training in Tropical Diseases, the Fundación José María Vargas, and the Centro Médico Docente La Trinidad.

REFERENCES

Andrews NW, Colli W 1982 Adhesion and interiorization of *Trypanosoma cruzi* in mammalian cells. J Protozool 29:264-269

Araujo FG, Handman E, Remington JS 1980 Binding of lectins to the cell surface of *Trypanosoma cruzi*. J Protozool 27:397-400

Brener Z 1979 O parasito: relaçoes hospedeiro-parasito. In: Brener Z, Andrade Z (eds) *Trypanosoma cruzi* e doença de Chagas. Guanabara Kogan, Rio de Janeiro, p 1-41

Brener Z 1980 Immunity to *Trypanosoma cruzi*. Adv Parasitol 18:247-291

Chang KP 1981 *Leishmania donovani*–macrophage binding mediated by surface glycoproteins/antigens: characterization *in vitro* by a radioisotopic assay. Mol Biochem Parasitol 4:67-76

Crane MSJ, Dvorak JA 1982 Influence of monosaccharides on the infection of vertebrate cells by *Trypanosoma cruzi* and *Toxoplasma gondii*. Mol Biochem Parasitol 5:333-341

Dvorak J, Crane MSJ 1981 Vertebrate cell cycle modulates infection by protozoan parasites. Science (Wash DC) 214:1034-1036

Gutteridge WE 1981 *Trypanosoma cruzi*: recent biochemical advances. Trans R Soc Trop Med Hyg 75:484-492

Henríquez D, Piras R, Piras MM 1981a Surface membrane interactions of *Trypanosoma cruzi* and Vero cells: dissociation of the adhesion and penetration steps. J Cell Biol 91:108a

Henríquez D, Piras R, Piras MM 1981b The effect of surface membrane modifications of fibroblastic cells on the entry process of *Trypanosoma cruzi* trypomastigotes. Mol Biochem Parasitol 2:359-366

Kipnis TL, David JR, Alper CA, Sher A, Da Silva WD 1981 Enzymatic treatment transforms trypomastigotes of *Trypanosoma cruzi* into activators of alternative complement pathway and potentiates their uptake by macrophages. Proc Natl Acad Sci USA 78:602-605

Kobiler D, Mirelman D 1980 Lectin activity in *Entamoeba histolytica* trophozoites. Infect Immun 29:221-225

Markwell MAK, Paulson JC 1980 Sendai virus utilizes specific sialyloligosaccharides as host cell receptor determinants. Proc Natl Acad Sci USA 77:5693-5697

Melo RC, Brener Z 1978 Tissue tropism of different *Trypanosoma cruzi* strains. J Parasitol 64:475-482

Nogueira N, Cohn Z 1976 *Trypanosoma cruzi*: mechanism of entry and intracellular fate in mammalian cells. J Exp Med 143:1402-1420

Nogueira N, Chaplan S, Cohn Z 1980 *Trypanosoma cruzi*: factors modifying ingestion and fate of blood form trypomastigotes. J Exp Med 152:447-451

Nogueira N, Chaplan S, Tydings JD, Unkeless JC, Cohn Z 1981 *Trypanosoma cruzi*: surface antigens of blood culture forms. J Exp Med 153:629-639

Ofek I, Mirelman D, Sharon N 1977 Adherence of *Escherichia coli* to human mucosal cells mediated by mannose receptors. Nature (Lond) 265:623-625

Pereira MEA, Loures MA, Villalta F, Andrade AFB 1980 Lectin receptors as markers for *Trypanosoma cruzi*. Developmental stages and a study of the interaction of wheat germ agglutinin with sialic acid residues on epimastigote cells. J Exp Med 152:1375-1392

Perkins M 1981 Inhibitory effects of erythrocyte membrane proteins on the *in vitro* invasion of the human malarial parasite (*Plasmodium falciparum*) into its host cell. J Cell Biol 90: 563-567

Piras MM, Henríquez D, Negri S, Piras R 1980a Transformación *in vitro* de tripomastigotes de *Trypanosoma cruzi* en amastigotes extracelulares: cambios en la infectividad y efecto de la inhibición de la síntesis de proteínas. Acta Cient Venez 31(Supl 1):197

Piras R, Henríquez D, Piras MM 1980b Studies on host–parasite interactions: role of fibroblastic cell surface functions and *Trypanosoma cruzi* forms in the infective process. In: Van den Bossche H (ed) The host–invader interplay. Elsevier/North-Holland, Amsterdam, p 131-134

Piras MM, Piras R, Henríquez D 1982a Changes in morphology and infectivity of cell culture-derived trypomastigotes of *Trypanosoma cruzi*. Mol Biochem Parasitol 6:67-81

Piras R, Piras MM, Henríquez D 1982b The effect of inhibitors of macromolecular biosynthesis on the *in vitro* infectivity and morphology of *Trypanosoma cruzi* trypomastigotes. Mol Biochem Parasitol 6:83-92

Recover P, Piras R 1982 Actividad proteásica de tripomastigotes enteros de *Trypanosoma cruzi* frente a ^{125}I-caseína. Acta Cient Venez 33(supl 1):441

Silverstein SC, Steinman R, Cohn Z 1977 Endocytosis. Annu Rev Biochem 46:669-722

Weiss MM, Openheim JD, Vanderberg JP 1981 *Plasmodium falciparum*: assay *in vitro* for inhibitors of merozoite penetration of erythrocytes. Exp Parasitol 51:400-407

Zingales B, Andrews NW, Kuwajima VY, Colli W 1982 Cell surface antigens of *Trypanosoma cruzi*: possible correlation with the interiorization process in mammalian cells. Mol Biochem Parasitol 6:111-124

DISCUSSION

Hudson: How does the proteolytic activator system that you have described relate to the enzymic cleavage of antibody molecules described by Harvey Eisen: is it the same thing?

Piras: We don't think that the activation system relates specifically to antibodies that coat the parasite because one can obtain the same increase in adhesion with trypomastigotes obtained from cells cultured in serum-free medium and then activated and assayed in serum-free medium.

Hudson: Is the proteolytic activity of a sufficiently wide spectrum to degrade antibody molecules?

Piras: It might be, since it is inhibited by different types of protease inhibitor.

Nogueira: Your results fit well with those that I shall be describing (see p 52-73). You mentioned that the activation of infection is seen in the presence of serum. If you leave the trypomastigotes for 6-20 h in the absence of serum, do you obtain the same results?

Piras: Morphological transformation and the development of adhesion are exactly the same in the absence or presence of serum. Serum seems in some way to be stabilizing, and even stimulating, the system, in that the invasive activity is larger when serum is present.

O'Daly: We have been working for the last four years on the problem of obtaining antigens from *Trypanosoma cruzi*. We have found, in *T. cruzi*, *Leishmania mexicana* and *Leishmania donovani*, a tremendous amount of proteolytic enzymes at pHs ranging from 2.5 to pH 8 (O'Daly et al 1983). These enzymes can break down not only labelled substrates but also endogenous proteins from these parasites. We have been able to inhibit this proteolytic enzyme activity and we have also localized the enzymes by electron microscopy, with the method of silver proteinate. In both *T. cruzi* and the *Leishmania* species we have found a laminar structure that is exocytosed from the epimastigotes into the culture medium, and on this structure we can identify a proteolytic enzyme directly. We can see the enzyme also in electron-dense bodies, in the cytoplasm, in the kinetoplast and in the nuclei. This high loading of the parasites with proteolytic enzymes makes isolation of antigens very difficult. I wonder if this wide range of proteolytic activity is producing fragments from a variety of molecules. This could explain many of the parasite's proposed biological effects.

Piras: We have been trying to establish whether there is proteolytic activity in intact trypomastigotes (Recover & Piras 1982). Here we are not considering activity within the cell, which we know is full of proteases. To detect this ecto-activity we need to use a high specific activity—^{125}I-labelled casein. The protease activity of the intact trypomastigotes represents less than 0.5% of the activity that one can measure in total parasite extracts. In experiments with haemoglobin bound to Sepharose we find this activity, which is not free in the supernatant. Therefore a small part of the total protease activity seems to be located in the external membrane of the trypomastigotes. However, because this activity is inhibited by various protease inhibitors, we are dealing either with more than one enzyme or with a non-specific enzyme.

Gutteridge: Do you have any evidence that trypomastigotes, as they are released initially *in vivo*, are required to undergo a period of maturation? Is there any way that you can test for this?

Piras: No. We have not tried any *in vivo* work yet. What you are proposing would be very difficult to test because one would need to follow up a trypomastigote that is liberated from a tissue in the animal and see whether infection eventually increases with time.

Gutteridge: I am curious about this because although many strains of *T. cruzi* have a dichotomy of trypomastigote structure between the 'slender' and 'broad' (or 'stout') form, *in vivo* one sees only rarely structures similar to what you have called spheromastigotes.

Piras: We do not know whether this phenomenon that we have observed *in vitro* has any significance *in vivo*. Nevertheless, there are some early reports from Brazilian workers (De Morais Rego 1956, Pereira Da Silva 1959) that amastigote forms of *T. cruzi* were found in circulating blood of mice. If these forms do exist *in vivo*, and if they are so infective, the chance of seeing them in the peripheral blood would be low, because as they became more adhesive and more infective they would rapidly infect new cells.

Mirelman: I have a question and a suggestion. Have you tested any of the proteolytic digests by collecting them and seeing whether they are inhibitory? Moreover, a number of cell lines have been developed that are resistant, for example, to ricin toxin or to wheatgerm agglutinin attached to ricin. Perhaps these cell lines with modified surface receptors would be helpful for distinguishing between adherence and invasive processes.

Piras: I agree; we haven't done it but it would be useful to use a resistant line to test their response.

Nussenzweig: I am interested in the *in vivo* relevance of the protease you identified on the surface of *T. cruzi*. Have you examined non-pathogenic trypanosomes such as *Trypanosoma lewisi* to see if they show the same kind of activation?

Piras: Not yet.

Sharma: You mentioned that in trypomastigotes in culture there is translation and transcription of mRNA. How do the trypomastigotes get the signal for that *in vitro*, and what significance could this have *in vivo* ?

Piras: We really do not know.

Sharma: With ^{125}I-labelling you found that a protein of relative molecular mass (M_r 125 000 was missing, and that a protein of M_r 90 000 had been reduced. Are those proteins found once again when the amastigotes are transformed to trypomastigotes inside the cell before they are released?

Piras: We have not done this kind of experiment. The transformation to which you refer occurs *within* the cell, whereas we are studying the trypomastigote once it is *outside* the cell. We haven't labelled intracellular amastigotes to see whether their pattern would be similar to the spheromastigotes obtained by extracellular incubation of trypomastigotes *in vitro*.

Sharma: Do you know what percentage of the membrane protein is the glycoprotein that is necessary for infection?

Piras: We have no idea because we have not yet isolated a specific glycoprotein. We are simply inferring that it exists, on the basis of the effect of tunicamycin on the development of infectivity.

Wyler: Perhaps you are seeing an effect of a sub-population. If you take the next generation of parasites—that is, the cells that have been infective, and do the same kinds of experiments—do you see the same effects?

Piras: We do. We find that activated parasites that have not gone into cells on a first infection can infect new cells to a similar extent on a second infection. So we are seeing a property not just of a sub-population but of the whole population.

Wyler: If you use parasites that have *entered* the cells and are then retrieved, do you observe the same effect?

Piras: Cells that are infected by either the trypomastigotes or by the activated trypomastigotes would behave similarly, except that the period necessary for transformation into amastigotes that multiply and give rise to new trypomastigotes is shorter if one uses the more infective trypomastigotes or spheromastigotes.

Nogueira: I have a comment following up Dr Sharma's question. We have found that the major surface antigens of *T. cruzi* are developmentally expressed. The insect stages of *T. cruzi* (epimastigotes and metacyclic trypomastigotes) possess a 75 K glycoprotein, which is absent in the mammalian stages of the organism (blood-form trypomastigotes and amastigotes). These, in turn, possess a 90 K glycoprotein not usually seen in the insect stages. That is, when a metacyclic enters a cell it displays the 75 K glycoprotein on the surface. When it is transformed intracellularly into an amastigote form it will lose the 75 K glycoprotein and start expressing the 90 K glycoprotein. This is the same antigen that will be found in the surface when the amastigotes develop into trypomastigotes and leave the host cells. Preliminary experiments in our laboratory suggest that under certain conditions of culture medium and temperature one can induce, in the absence of cells, expression of developmentally specific antigens. This could explain some of the observations described by Dr Piras. We are now investigating the genetic and molecular regulators of the expression of these antigens.

Piras: If our incubated trypomastigotes are shifted to a lower temperature (28 °C) then they will transform into epimastigotes. But if we leave them at 37 °C, after two or three days they will begin to die out.

Chang: You mentioned that intracellular amastigotes don't seem to enter into the fibroblast. Do they adhere to the cells?

Piras: The intracellular amastigotes are obtained by gentle disruption of cells that are full of replicating amastigotes, and isolation of the parasites on a gradient of metrizamide. These were not infective. We don't know whether they attached to fibroblasts or not because at that time our system for measuring adhesion was still being developed. We have not re-checked that. Epimastigotes in our hands attach only very poorly. We have tried to trypsinize the epimastigotes, to see if they would acquire an adhesion and infection similar to that of the trypomastigotes, but this did not change these parameters.

Nogueira: I wish to follow up the subject of the amastigotes. I have found that amastigotes are highly infective and that they possess on the surface the same 90 K glycoprotein as trypomastigotes. I should point out, however, that we obtain them in a different way. You have obtained amastigotes by disrupting the host cells, while we looked at amastigotes released spontaneously into the medium from infected muscle cells. We achieve this by maintaining the infected cells in fetal calf serum rather than in horse serum. Under these conditions, very few organisms differentiate intracellularly into trypomastigotes. When the cells rupture one can obtain pure populations of amastigotes.

Gutteridge: A number of years ago, when isolating amastigotes from infected animals, we looked at their infectivity. We found exactly the same results that Dr Piras described for his tissue culture work: no infectivity (Gutteridge et al 1978). We also know there is a surface difference, at least in charge, between the amastigotes and the trypomastigotes. When we poured a mixture of morphological forms through cellulose columns, the amastigotes always stuck to the columns but the trypomastigotes, if present, passed through (Gutteridge et al 1978).

Wyler: With *Leishmania* species the situation may be a little different. Amastigotes from foot-pads of mice that have all been infected simultaneously, but are harvested at different times after infection, differ in their ability to attach to human monocytes *in vitro* (D.J. Wyler, unpublished observations). Amastigotes harvested from mice early in infection attach to monocytes less readily than those obtained from mice later in infection. Perhaps this represents alteration in some surface property of the parasite within the host. In contrast, if amastigotes are permitted to incubate at 37 °C *in vitro* they progressively lose their attachment ability.

Hernández: With *Leishmania* species being different from *T. cruzi* in these respects I wonder if the trypomastigotes, when treated with tunicamycin, change in shape?

Piras: No. Under phase-contrast optical microscopy the morphology is similar regardless of whether they have been incubated with tunicamycin or not.

Hernández: We found that treatment with tunicamycin increased adhesion, as you found, but also it increased the penetration into macrophages. But in *Leishmania* species there are probably bigger changes than in *T. cruzi* in form and structure. For example, the leishmanial cell coat disappears completely. The binding of concanavalin A to this tunicamycin-treated parasite also increases; so, this could fit with increasing adhesion.

Warren: Are Dr Wyler and Dr Hernández both talking about the same species?

Wyler: This is a critical issue. We work with *Leishmania tropica major* (or *L. major*, as some prefer to call it). Of course, the whole issue of taxonomy in leishmaniasis is a nightmare at present. Criteria for defining species have not been widely accepted. Does one use isoenzyme patterns or kinetoplast DNA hybridization, for example? And what is a species when one is talking about an asexual parasite, after all?

Hernández: And we are working with *Leishmania braziliensis* and/or *L. mexicana*.

Nogueira: Investigators working with any species of *Leishmania* agree that *Leishmania* all multiply within parasitophorous vacuoles. When *Leishmania* amastigotes are released, they come out with the host membrane still around them. After some time under *in vitro* conditions, the host membrane may be shed. Couldn't this phenomenon explain the differences in infectivity that you have described, Dr Wyler?

Wyler: Our experience suggests that the vacuolar membrane is shed within an hour. By electron microscopy we are unable to detect host membrane surrounding our amastigotes by the time we do attachment studies. I wonder, though, whether this membrane surrounds the amastigote *in vivo*, as it attaches to a macrophage that it is about to infect.

Chang: I have worked on both *L. donovani* and *L. mexicana*. *L. donovani* amastigotes often have host membranes around them, but this is not true of *L. mexicana*. So if one uses *L. donovani* there is a complication when one does the binding mentioned by Dr Nogueira.

Piras: When we measure binding of a [^{125}I]-labelled concanavalin A on fresh and on incubated trypomastigotes, there is no significant difference.

Nogueira: They are free in cytoplasts and don't come out with any host membrane around them.

REFERENCES

De Morais Rego SF 1956 Sobre o encontro de formas tissulares do *Trypanosoma cruzi* Chagas 1909 no sangre circulante do camundongo branco (*Mus musculus*). Folia Clin Biol 26:17-46

Gutteridge WE, Cover B, Gaborak M 1978 Isolation of blood and intracellular forms of *Trypanosoma cruzi* from infected rats and other rodents and preliminary studies of their metabolism. Parasitology 76:159-176

O'Daly JA, Serrano LE, Rodríguez MB 1983 Free aminoacid pool and proteolytic enzymes in *Trypanosoma cruzi*. Int J Parasitol, in press

Pereira Da Silva LH 1959 Observaçoes sobre o ciclo evolutivo do *Trypanosoma cruzi*. Rev Inst Med Trop Sao Paulo 1:99-118

Recover P, Piras R 1982 Actividad proteásica de tripomastigotes enteros de *Trypanosoma cruzi* frente a ^{125}I-caseína. Acta Cient Venez 33 (Supl 1):441

Host and parasite factors affecting the invasion of mononuclear phagocytes by *Trypanosoma cruzi*

N. NOGUEIRA

Laboratory of Cellular Physiology and Immunology, The Rockefeller University, 1230 York Avenue, New York, NY 10021, USA

Abstract Epimastigotes and trypomastigotes of *Trypanosoma cruzi* enter mouse and human macrophages by phagocytosis. Organisms are initially found in a parasitophorous vacuole, and fusion with lysosomes promptly ensues. Epimastigotes are rapidly killed and digested in phagolysosomes. Trypomastigotes, however, soon escape the confines of the vacuolar system and reach the cytoplasm, where they replicate. Metacyclic trypomastigotes are quickly taken up by mouse and human macrophages. In contrast, blood-form trypomastigotes are resistant to interiorization by mononuclear phagocytes. This effect can be overcome, without affecting parasite survival, by opsonization of the parasites with immunoglobulin G (IgG)-class antibodies or by removal of trypomastigote surface peptides with trypsin. The major surface glycoprotein (relative molecular mass 90 000) of the mammalian stages of *T. cruzi* has been implicated in this antiphagocytic effect. This surface glycoprotein seems to have glycosidase activity, and the antiphagocytic effect may be mediated via the removal of sugar residues necessary for parasite internalization by macrophages. This enzyme activity may explain other evasion mechanisms displayed by *T. cruzi* bloodstream forms. These include antibody-mediated complement lysis and Fc-receptor-mediated phagocytosis. Trypomastigotes are, however, promptly killed in mouse and human macrophages activated by either *in vivo* infection or *in vitro* treatment with sensitized, antigen-stimulated, T-cell products. Increased production of reactive oxygen intermediates by activated cells has been implicated as the mechanism of intracellular killing in mononuclear phagocytes. Opsonization by IgG-class antibodies enhances uptake of the parasites but does not affect their fate in normal mononuclear phagocytes. In contrast, it enhances their killing by activated macrophages, suggesting that antibodies may have a major protective role only in the presence of concomitant cell-mediated immunity.

1983 Cytopathology of parasitic disease. Pitman Books, London (Ciba Foundation symposium 99) p 52-73

One of the principal functions of 'professional' phagocytic cells (neutrophils, eosinophils and mononuclear phagocytes) is to ingest and destroy micro-organisms. Mononuclear phagocytes, however, may also provide a favourable environment for the survival and multiplication of a variety of intracellular pathogens, including obligate intracellular parasites, such as *Trypanosoma cruzi*.

Our studies of the interactions between *T. cruzi* and mouse or human macrophages have shown that these cells initially support the growth of the organisms but, on sensitization of the host, will become efficient killers of the phagocytized parasites. In this review I shall discuss some of the data on the mechanisms of uptake, survival and replication or death of *T. cruzi* in mononuclear phagocytes. I shall also discuss some of the characteristics evolved by the different developmental stages of the parasite to cope with the host's immune system.

Uptake and fate in normal macrophages

Insect stages

Macrophage interiorization of epimastigotes and metacyclic trypomastigotes of *T. cruzi*, obtained from acellular cultures, takes place by a phagocytic process, mediated by receptor-like peptides on the macrophage surface. Trypsin and chymotrypsin treatment of the macrophage surface abolishes the uptake of *T. cruzi* by mouse peritoneal macrophages (Nogueira & Cohn 1976). The uptake is mediated by non-specific receptors and does not involve C_3 or Fc receptors. Interiorization of the organisms is inhibited by cytochalasin B.

Once the organisms are inside the parasitophorous vacuole they fuse with lysosomes, to form phagolysosomes. Epimastigotes are killed rapidly and digested within these cellular organelles, while metacyclic trypomastigotes escape from the phagolysosome and multiply in the host-cell cytoplasm. The mechanisms by which the phagolysosome membrane is lysed are not clear, but they may be related to enzymic activity of the *T. cruzi* surface glycoproteins, as discussed at the end of this paper.

Opsonization of metacyclic trypomastigotes with specific immune serum increases their uptake without affecting their intracellular fate (Fig. 1).

Mammalian stages

T. cruzi is able to replicate in practically any cell type in the mammalian host; only the macrophage is potentially microbicidal for the parasites. Therefore, avoiding phagocytosis by the macrophage can be an advantageous evasion mechanism. Indeed, the blood-form trypomastigotes (BFTs) of *T. cruzi*

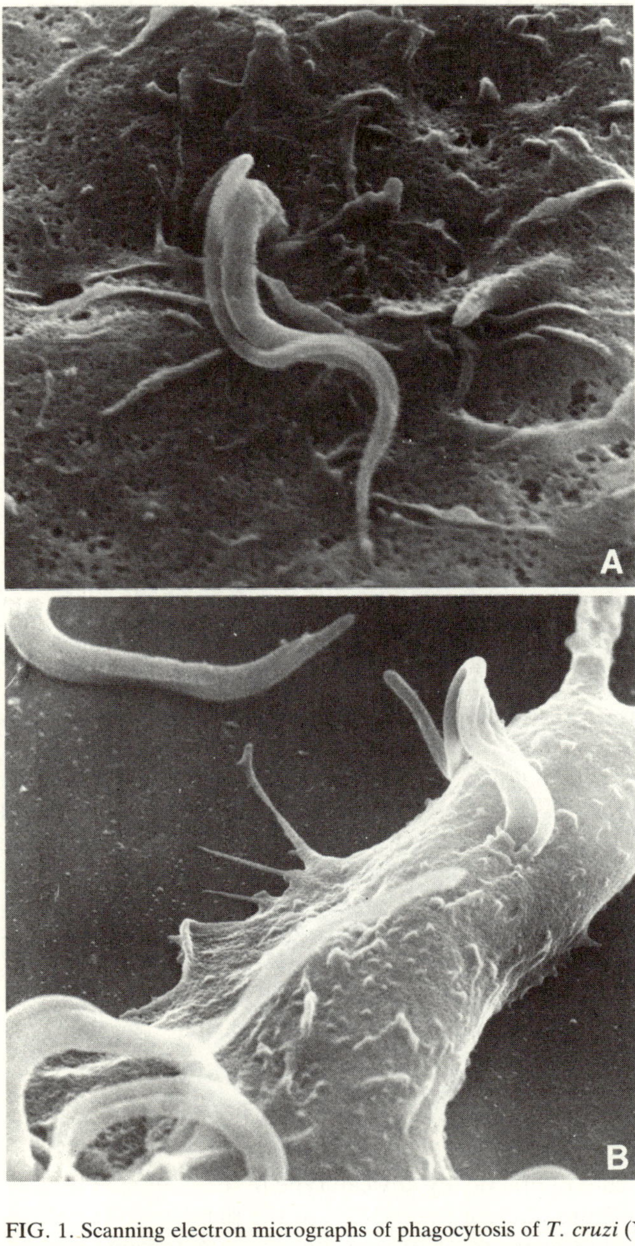

FIG. 1. Scanning electron micrographs of phagocytosis of *T. cruzi* (Y strain) trypomastigotes by mouse peritoneal macrophages. A, the trypomastigote has already burrowed into the macrophage; B, the organism is enveloped by projections of the macrophage membrane.

possess on their surface an anti-phagocytic factor that dramatically reduces their uptake by mouse or human macrophages (Nogueira et al 1980, M. Reesink & N. Nogueira, unpublished results); this is also true of tissue-culture trypomastigotes (TCTs) obtained from infected rat embryonic myoblasts (N. Nogueira, unpublished observations).

TCTs and BFTs can, however, be rendered susceptible to phagocytosis in two ways: first, by opsonization with hyperimmune serum; and, second, by proteolysis with trypsin. These two treatments appear to enhance ingestion by separate mechanisms. Hyperimmune serum works through specific immunoglobulin G (IgG)-class antibodies, opsonizing the organisms in a classical fashion, and resulting in binding and interiorization mediated by the Fc receptor (Nogueira et al 1980). Therefore, a monoclonal antibody (2.4G2) directed against this receptor (Unkeless 1979) blocks any opsonizing effect. Trypsin, on the other hand, removes an antiphagocytic factor and promotes infection via a non-Fc-mediated mechanism. Trypsin and specific IgG have an additive effect in enhancement of parasite uptake (Table 1).

TABLE 1 Effect of hyperimmune serum and trypsin on the uptake and fate of BFT[a] by mouse peritoneal macrophages

Macrophage treatment with anti-Fc antibody	*Treatment of parasites*		*Parasites per 100 macrophages at 3 h*	*Parasites per 100 macrophages at 72 h*	*Infected macrophages at 72 h (%)*
	Trypsin	*Serum*			
None	–	–	Undetectable	15	1
2.4G2	–	–	Undetectable	4.5	0.5
None	–	+	35	230	20
2.4G2	–	+	Undetectable	7	1.5
None	+	–	18	130	9
2.4G2	+	–	14	102	8
None	+	+	58	344	38
2.4G2	+	+	17	97	9.5

[a]CL strain of blood-form trypomastigotes of *T. cruzi*. (Courtesy of J Exp Med.)

The antiphagocytic factor was found not only in the reportedly myotropic CL strain of *T. cruzi* but also in the Y strain, which is considered to parasitize the macrophages preferentially (Alcantara & Brener 1978). Once taken up by macrophages *in vitro*, BFTs and TCTs behave identically to metacyclic trypomastigotes in their uptake, subcellular localization and fate within normal and activated macrophages, as discussed below.

Activation and intracellular killing in mouse and human mononuclear phagocytes

Mechanism of macrophage activation

Infection and boosting of mice with live BCG or *T. cruzi*, but not injection with thioglycollate broth or protease peptone (Nogueira et al 1977a), results in peritoneal macrophages being capable of destroying trypomastigotes of *T. cruzi* (i.e. *in vivo* activation).

The mechanisms underlying macrophage activation in this system were clarified under *in vitro* conditions (Nogueira et al 1977b, Nogueira & Cohn 1978). Normal, resident peritoneal macrophages were induced *in vitro* to display microbicidal activity against *T. cruzi* trypomastigotes by exposure to products from antigen-stimulated, sensitized T-cell populations (i.e. *in vitro* activation). The requirements for induction of optimal microbicidal activity *in vitro* were the presence of an antigen-specific T-cell product (lymphokine) and the constant exposure of macrophages to, and daily renewal of, the T-cell mediators. Removal of the lymphokines, or failure to add fresh mediators, resulted in reversal of the microbicidal effect. Macrophage activation was found to be non-specific: that is, once activated, mouse macrophages are able to kill a variety of microorganisms.

A similar modulation has been observed for human mononuclear phagocytes *in vitro* (Nogueira et al 1982b). *T. cruzi*-induced lymphokines, derived from antigen-stimulated mononuclear cells from the peripheral blood of patients with chronic Chagas' disease, as well as BCG and concanavalin A-induced lymphokines, were shown to induce microbicidal activity against trypomastigotes of *T. cruzi*. In contrast to the murine system, in human macrophages optimal microbicidal activity could be achieved without the need for daily addition of lymphocyte factors. But, as with the murine system, induction of microbicidal activity depended on the dose of lymphokine (Fig. 2).

Mechanism of intracellular killing of T. cruzi *in mononuclear phagocytes*

A remarkable correlation was found between the conditions required for macrophages to express microbicidal activity and the conditions under which macrophages released large amounts of reactive oxygen intermediates, which had previously been implicated in the bactericidal activity of neutrophils (Nathan & Root 1977, Johnston et al 1978). Indeed, the ability of the mouse macrophages to release H_2O_2 closely parallels their level of antimicrobial function under a number of experimental conditions (Nathan et al 1979).

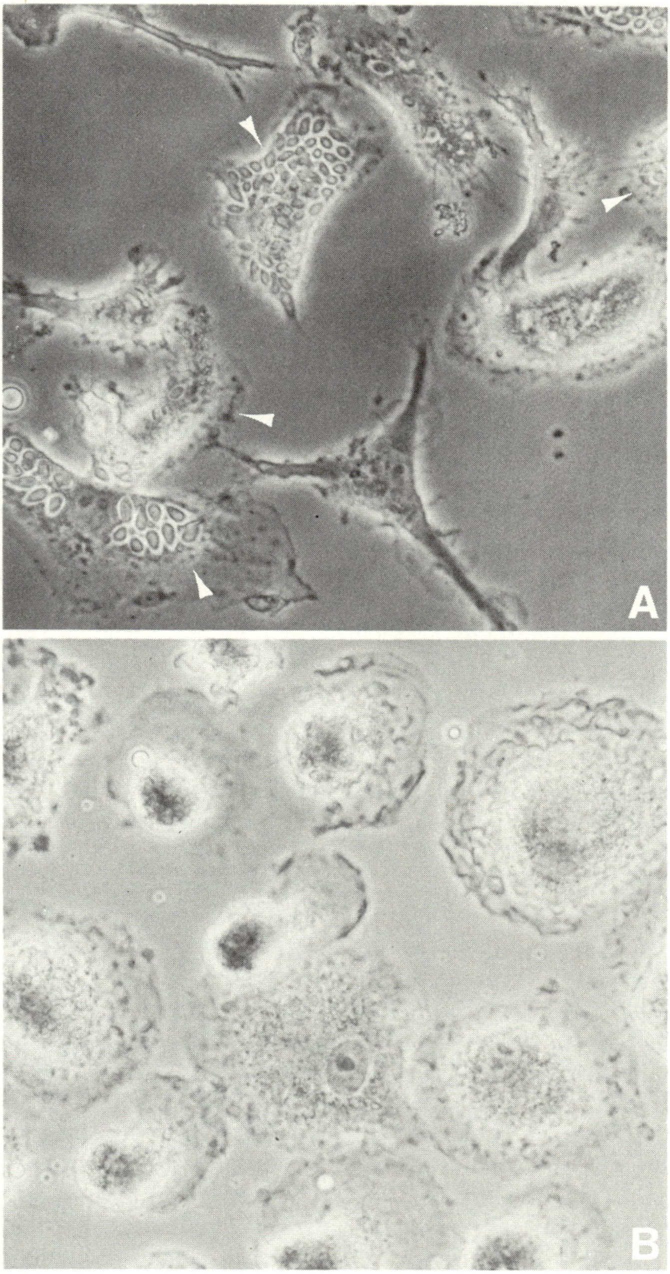

FIG. 2. Human monocyte-derived macrophages exposed to 2.5% control lymphokine (A) or 2.5% *T. cruzi*-induced lymphokine from a patient with chronic Chagas' disease (B), 72 h after infection with *T. cruzi*. Notice abundance of intracellular parasites (arrows) in samples exposed to control lymphokine, as compared to *T. cruzi*–lymphokine induced cells, where parasites are absent.

Both functions were found to follow the same time course and dose–response curve and were reversible over a similar period of time.

Similar studies with human cells revealed that supernatants from human mononuclear blood cells stimulated by mitogen or antigen also enhanced the ability of peripheral-blood monocytes or monocyte-derived macrophages to release H_2O_2 or O_2^- in response to phorbol myristate acetate or zymosan (Nagakawara et al 1982).

An investigation of the sensitivity of *T. cruzi* to H_2O_2 generated by glucose and glucose oxidase resulted in an LD_{50} of 6.5 nmol/min for epimastigotes and 9.4 nmol/min for trypomastigotes. Such concentrations of H_2O_2 could possibly be achieved within the vacuolar system, as supported by recent measurements by Tanaka et al (1982). They used glucose oxidase coupled to zymosan to measure the amount of H_2O_2 needed to kill one parasite, and estimated that this could be achieved by a flux of 2.7×10^{-7} nmol/min.

The lower resistance of epimastigotes of *T. cruzi* to H_2O_2 can explain their higher sensitivity to killing by even normal peritoneal macrophages, which produce very low levels of reactive oxygen intermediates. Epimastigotes of *T. cruzi* are reported to lack catalase and glutathione peroxidase (Boveris et al 1980). This lower level of antoxidant defences can therefore explain their exquisite susceptibility to H_2O_2.

Additional evidence for the role of H_2O_2 as a possible mediator of intracellular killing by macrophages is provided by experiments where metacyclic trypomastigotes and BFTs are rendered sensitive to intracellular killing by normal human and mouse macrophages after being coated with eosinophil peroxidase, as discussed by Dr Seymour Klebanoff (this volume; and see Nogueira et al 1982a).

Surface antigenic determinants on different developmental stages of *T. cruzi*, and their possible role in evasion mechanisms

Developmental stages of *T. cruzi* display two major surface antigens. One, a 75 000 M_r glycoprotein, is found in the insect stages of the organism, epimastigotes and metacyclic trypomastigotes. The other, a 90 000 M_r glycoprotein, is found in the mammalian stages, blood-form trypomastigotes (BFTs), tissue-culture trypomastigotes (TCTs) and amastigotes. The two glycoproteins were found, by two-dimensional tryptic and chymotryptic peptide mapping, to be unrelated and to be non-cross-reactive immunologically (Nogueira et al 1981, 1982c). The same surface-antigen profile has been found in six strains of *T. cruzi* from widely different geographic areas of Latin America.

The 90 K glycoprotein has been implicated in the antiphagocytic effect displayed by TCTs and BFTs for the following reasons.

(a) Trypsinization of the organisms abolishes the antiphagocytic effect and removes the 90 K glycoprotein. This was demonstrated in surface-iodinated as well as in biosynthetically labelled organisms (Fig. 3).

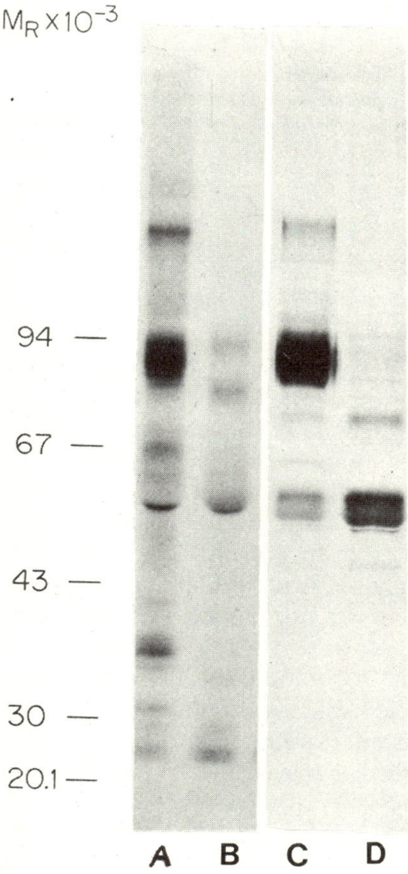

FIG. 3. Effect of trypsin treatment of blood-form trypomastigotes of *T. cruzi* on the immunoprecipitated proteins. A, Y strain-immunoprecipitation of ^{125}I-labelled whole-cell lysate with human immune IgG (patients 2). B, as in (A), but parasites trypsinized before iodination. C, CL strain, [^{35}S]methionine-labelled surface components immunoprecipitated with hyperimmune mouse serum. D, as in (C), but parasites trypsinized before incubation with hyperimmune mouse serum. (Courtesy of J Exp Med.)

(b) Within 3 h after trypsinization the 90 K component is re-expressed at the surface of the organisms, and the antiphagocytic effect is restored.

(c) Addition of 5 μg/ml of cycloheximide to the trypsinized organisms completely blocks the incorporation of [^{35}S]methionine into BFT and TCT polypeptides. This treatment therefore prevents the re-expression of the 90 K glycoprotein and also prevents the restoration of the antiphagocytic effect (Table 2).

TABLE 2 Re-expression of BFT[a] anti-phagocytic activity after trypsinization

Treatment of parasites	*Time after trypsinization (hours)*	*Intracellular parasites per 100 macrophages*	*Infected macrophages (%)*
None	–	8	1.5
Trypsin	0	63	9
Trypsin	3	25	4
Trypsin + cycloheximide	3	56	10

[a]Blood-form trypomastigotes of *T. cruzi*, Y strain. (Courtesy of J Exp Med.)

Pereira (1983) recently demonstrated a developmentally regulated neuraminidase activity in *T. cruzi*. The enzyme is expressed in BFTs and TCTs but not in epimastigotes or metacyclic trypomastigotes. We have recently demonstrated (M.E.A. Pereira & N. Nogueira, unpublished results) that this neuraminidase activity is selectively bound both by a rabbit antisera against the 90 K glycoprotein and a monoclonal antibody, 5D10.8, also directed against the 90 K glycoprotein (N. Nogueira et al, unpublished work). The enzyme activity is retained neither by normal sera (rabbit, human, mouse or fetal calf) nor by anti-75 K glycoprotein antisera nor monoclonal antibodies (N. Nogueira et al, unpublished results).

This neuraminidase activity may mediate the antiphagocytic effect of the 90 K glycoprotein, by removing sialic acid residues required for parasite interiorization by macrophages. It is also interesting to postulate that this enzyme activity is responsible for the defective role of the IgG antibodies–BFT complex in complement fixation and in Fc receptor-mediated phagocytosis of opsonized BFTs and TCTs (Nogueira et al 1980). Both these Fc-mediated functions occur in *T. cruzi* BFTs and TCTs only in the continuing presence of high concentrations of specific IgG. Removal of unbound antibody results in failure to fix complement and failure to bind the macrophage Fc receptor. Removal of sugars from the carbohydrate chains of IgG molecules has been reported to alter these Fc-mediated activities (Koide et al 1977). Variations among *T. cruzi* strains could result from differences in specific activity and/or in substrate specificity of the glycosidase activity of the 90 K glycoprotein. In collaboration with M.E.A. Pereira, we are currently analysing the validity of these postulates.

The function of the 75 K glycoprotein is still unknown, but it is tempting to speculate that it, too, may possess an enzymic activity.

Acknowledgements

I thank Professor Zanvil A. Cohn for his support and advice during the course of these studies. The scanning electron micrographs in this paper were kindly taken by Dr Gilla Kaplan. This work is supported by a Research Career Development Award in Geographic Medicine from the Rockefeller Foundation and by a grant from the Biomedical Sciences Component of the United Nations Development Program/World Bank/World Health Organization Special Program for Research and Training in Tropical Diseases.

REFERENCES

Alcantara A, Brener Z 1978 The *in vitro* interaction of *Trypanosoma cruzi* bloodstream forms and mouse peritoneal macrophages. Acta Trop 35:209-219

Boveris A, Sies H, Martino EE, DoCampo R, Turrens JF, Stoppani ADM 1980 Deficient metabolic utilization of hydrogen peroxide in *Trypanosoma cruzi*. Biochem J 188:643-648

Johnston RB, Godzik CA, Cohn ZA 1978 Increased superoxide anion production by immunologically activated and chemically elicited macrophages. J Exp Med 148:115-127

Koide N, Nose M, Muramatso T 1977 Recognition of IgG by Fc receptors and complement: effects of glycosidase digestion. Biochem Biophys Res Commun 75:838-844

Krettli AV, Carrington PW, Nussenzweig RS 1979 Membrane-bound antibodies of bloodstream *T. cruzi* in mice: strain differences in susceptibility to complement-mediated lysis. Clin Exp Immunol 3:1–8

Nakagawara A, DeSantis NM, Nogueira N, Nathan CF 1982 Lymphokines enhance the capacity of human monocytes to secrete reactive oxygen intermediates. J Clin Invest 70:1042–1049

Nathan CF, Root RK 1977 Hydrogen peroxide release from mouse peritoneal macrophages. Dependence on sequential activation and triggering. J Exp Med 146:1648-1662

Nathan CF, Nogueira N, Juangbhanich C, Ellis J, Cohn ZA 1979 Activation of macrophages *in vivo* and *in vitro*. Correlation between hydrogen peroxide release and killing of *Trypanosoma cruzi*. J Exp Med 149:1056-1068

Nogueira N, Cohn ZA 1976 *Trypanosoma cruzi*: mechanism of entry and intracellular fate in mammalian cells. J Exp Med 143:1402-1420

Nogueira N, Cohn ZA 1978 *Trypanosoma cruzi*: *in vitro* induction of macrophage microbicidal activity. J Exp Med 148:288-300

Nogueira N, Gordon S, Cohn ZA 1977a *Trypanosoma cruzi*: modification of macrophage function during infection. J Exp Med 146:157-171

Nogueira N, Gordon S, Cohn ZA 1977b *Trypanosoma cruzi*: the immunological induction of macrophage plasminogen activator requires thymus-derived lymphocytes. J Exp Med 146:172-183

Nogueira N, Chaplan S, Cohn Z 1980 *Trypanosoma cruzi*: factors modifying ingestion and fate of blood-form trypomastigotes. J Exp Med 152:447-451

Nogueira N, Chaplan S, Tydings JD, Unkeless J, Cohn Z 1981 *Trypanosoma cruzi*: surface antigens of blood and culture forms. J Exp Med 153:629-639

Nogueira NM, Klebanoff S, Cohn ZA 1982a *T. cruzi*: sensitization to macrophage killing by eosinophil peroxidase. J Immunol 128:1705-1708

Nogueira N, Chaplan S, Reesink M, Tydings J, Cohn ZA 1982b *Trypanosoma cruzi*: induction of microbicidal activity in human mononuclear phagocytes. J Immunol 128:2142-2146

Nogueira N, Unkeless J, Cohn Z 1982c Specific glycoprotein antigens on the surface of insect and mammalian stages of *Trypanosoma cruzi*. Proc Natl Acad Sci USA 79:1259-1263
Pereira MEA 1983 A developmentally regulated neuraminidase activity in *Trypanosoma cruzi*. Science (Wash DC) 219:1444-1446
Tanaka Y, Kiyotaki C, Tanowitz H, Bloom B 1982 Reconstitution of a variant macrophage cell line defective in oxygen metabolism with a H_2O_2-generating system. Proc Natl Acad Sci USA 79:2584-2588
Unkeless J 1979 Characterization of a monoclonal antibody directed against mouse macrophage and lymphocyte Fc receptors. J Exp Med 150:580-596

DISCUSSION

Warren: The new movement in parasitological research towards the use of modern chemical, immunological, and molecular biological techniques is most promising. How does your work compare with Harvey Eisen's 'fabulation' (Krettli et al 1980)?

Nogueira: Harvey Eisen's ideas about fabulation in *Trypanosoma cruzi* may well be right, but the evidence for proteolytic cleavage of antibody is still inconclusive. Two years ago, with two students in my laboratory, S. Chaplan and J. Tydings, I investigated the fate of antibody on the surface of blood-form trypomastigotes of the Y and CL strains of *T. cruzi*. We bound radiolabelled specific antibody to the organisms and looked for release of labelled antibodies and/or fragments at 4 °C and 37 °C. We were never able to demonstrate any proteolytic cleavage of the antibody molecules by sodium dodecyl sulphate–polyacrylamide gel electrophoresis. We could, however, recover antigen and antigen–antibody complexes in the medium. That is how we started looking into the release of the 90 K glycoprotein, which normally occurs even in the absence of antibody. We are now suggesting that the glycosidase activity of the 90 K glycoprotein at the surface of the trypomastigotes may alter the Fc domain of the antibody molecule, rendering it ineffective for complement or Fc receptor binding.

Sharma: You mentioned phospholipase activity in response to lysing the phagosome. Do you think that phospholipase is associated with a specific granule or is it present in the cell membrane?

Nogueira: My suggestion of a phospholipase activity is just that: a suggestion. I have no evidence that such activity exists at the surface of the organisms. The analogies between the interiorization of *T. cruzi* and that of some viruses are compelling. Virologists have shown that for influenza and paramyxoviruses an acid pH is required for activation of a fusion-promoting protein, which allows the escape of the viral nucleocapsid into the cytoplasm (Matlin et al 1981). We therefore speculated that there may be a surface phospholipase on the parasites, which could be activated by acid pH, resulting in lysis of the phagosomal membrane.

Sharma: We have some evidence that phospholipase associated with the macrophage membrane may be involved in killing *Toxoplasma*. We also have some preliminary results on the lysis of epimastigotes but not yet on trypomastigotes by phospholipase.

Nogueira: Opperdoes & Van Roy (1982) and Hambrey et al (1981) have described phospholipase A_1 activities in several *Trypanosoma* species, but without evidence for a surface localization of the enzyme.

Sher: If your hypothesis is correct—that the neuraminidase is the antiphagocytic substance—then you should be able to treat macrophages with neuraminidase to block the uptake of metacyclic trypomastigotes. Have you done that?

Nogueira: We are doing that now.

Mirelman: Which neuraminidase are you using? Its specificity may be a problem.

Nogueira: We are using *Vibrio cholerae* neuraminidase from Calbiochem, reported to be free of contaminating proteases. We are also testing an inhibitor of neuraminidase, FANA (see Meindl et al 1974), kindly supplied by Dr Peter Palese.

Sher: There is an interesting hypothesis to explain the antiphagocytic effect that Dr Nogueira has just described of trypsin on trypomastigotes. Czop et al (1978) have demonstrated the presence on the human monocyte surface of phagocytic receptors that recognize structures on particles responsible for activation of the alternative pathway of complement. Kipnis et al (1981) showed that trypsinization converts non-activating bloodstream trypomastigotes into activators of the alternative pathway and enhances their uptake by mouse macrophages. Dr Kipnis hypothesized that the latter effect was due to recognition of the trypsin-treated trypanosomes by the phagocytic receptors, demonstrated by Czop et al (1978) to recognize alternative pathway-activating substrates. Thus, the 'antiphagocytic substance' may be a parasite-produced inhibitor of the alternative pathway.

Hernández: How did you first see the link between the neuraminidase and the 90 K protein? Did you use concanavalin A–Sepharose in the purification?

Nogueira: Dr M.E.A. Pereira first described this neuraminidase as a developmentally expressed protein, only present in blood-form and tissue-culture trypomastigotes. This was the first analogy. In discussing his results with me (see also p 68-72), a few other analogies were obvious to us: first, that this neuraminidase activity bound strongly to concanavalin A–Sepharose, being impossible to elute out just with the specific competitor sugar; and secondly, that the activity was released into the supernatant of trypomastigote suspensions. Both features are true of the 90 K glycoprotein as well.

Hernández: The same thing happens with *Leishmania* species, which may explain the different results obtained in different labs. For example, many people have said that *Leishmania donovani* has sialic acid on its cell surface but we didn't find it in our strains. When we tried to purify the cell-surface components of *Leishmania* species, about 70% of the protein remained attached to concanavalin A and it was impossible to remove it.

Nogueira: We have the same result with the 65 000 surface component of *L. donovani*. We cannot elute it out from a concanavalin A–Sepharose column with α-methyl mannoside. One can show that binding is specific by preventing it in the presence of 0.25 M α-methyl mannoside but, once the component is bound, it cannot be eluted out with the sugar.

Hernández: We shall have to check for neuraminidase! I also think that we have to check for galactosidase because results with sodium borohydrate do not agree with results reported for other systems (A.G. Hernández and A. Misle, unpublished work).

Nogueira: I agree. There is no published evidence, as far as I am aware, that neuraminidase treatment *alone* of IgG molecules affects the Fc-mediated function. Koide et al (1977) reported that only endo-H treatment would result in alteration of the Fc-mediated function of the IgG molecules. It is thus possible that neuraminidase is just one glycosidase activity on this protein. Maybe it also has an endo-H activity.

O'Daly: In 1979 (O'Daly & Aso) we found that membranes from epimastigotes and promastigotes of *T. cruzi*, *Leishmania mexicana* and *L. donovani* lysed red blood cells and mammalian cells. Later, Brizuela (1981) found phospholipase in the membranes of *T. cruzi* and the *Leishmania* species. You have found this neuraminidase on the surface, and Rangel et al (1981) previously found the protease (by using antibody) on the surface of the parasite. Our electron microscopic work did not confirm that of Rangel et al (1981), although we found the protease in very limited areas in buds on the surface of epimastigotes. The protease is therefore very localized and the neuraminidase is around the parasite. This emphasizes that we must try to culture parasites in a medium with as few substances as possible, and at different temperatures, to see if the various surface components like those you have found are expressed.

Nogueira: I agree. The developmental expression of the different antigens could well explain most of the divergent published reports on interactions of the organism with cells and immune factors.

Avila: We demonstrated (Avila et al 1979a) in *T. cruzi* not only the presence of different proteolytic enzymes but also very high specific activities of neutral α-glucosidase and acid α-mannosidase. Have you tried to measure lysosomal contamination in the membrane preparations that you used in order to explain the presence of neuraminidase?

Nogueira: Dr Pereira was aware of this problem when he described the enzyme. I believe he has not looked at the supernatant for the presence of other lysosomal enzymes, but the pH optimum of this neuraminidase is 6.5. The fact that we can bind the enzyme with a monoclonal that is specific for a surface antigen provides the most important clue that we are looking at a surface component.

Avila: The optimum pH of the neuraminidase is not important because there are several neutral proteases inside lysosomes, and one must be careful about saying that this neuraminidase activity belongs to the membrane preparation.

Nogueira: I think that the monoclonal data provide the most compelling evidence that we have.

Avila: Steiger et al (1980) have demonstrated neuraminidase activity, in African trypanosomes, located in lysosomes.

Piras: In our experiments on interaction between the parasite and the lectins, concanavalin A was one of three lectins that stimulated adhesion. Since the 90 K protein or neuraminidase binds to concanavalin A it would be interesting to correlate these observations.

Nogueira: Yes. Many aspects of our data should be compared to see if it all fits together in a simple way.

Wyler: Does your monoclonal antibody inactivate the neuraminidase activity?

Nogueira: No. Neither do any of the Chagas' immune sera tested. The role of the antibody in negating the antiphagocytic effect seems to be independent of neuraminidase activity. It may be explained by interiorization mediated by the Fc receptor.

Chang: How long are the organisms exposed to lysosomal contents in phagolysosomes?

Nogueira: I don't know how long the organisms are within phagosomes or phagolysosomes before they come out into the cytoplasm. Until recently it was impossible to synchronize entry of the organisms into cells. Within two hours one can see organisms already outside the vacuole, but they might have been there for a matter of minutes, since the infection is not synchronous.

Sher: Have you ever looked at the surface of *true* metacyclic trypomastigotes, in other words bug-derived trypomastigotes, for expression of the 90 K protein?

Nogueira: No.

Klebanoff: The lysis of phagolysosomes, and the release of the organism into the cytoplasm proper, was surprising to me in the sense that the macrophages can survive this release of proteolytic and other lytic enzymes. Does this process limit the survival of macrophages in any way?

Nogueira: I suspect that it may, if all the organisms are in true phagolysosomes and the cell has been heavily infected. In contrast, one could imagine that if there are only two or three organisms to escape from phagolysosomes, the host cell could cope with the released hydrolases. However, Galloway et al (1983) have recently described that prelysosomes (endosomes) can be already acidified. So, the concept of the prelysosomes not having a proton pump, and therefore an acid pH, has to be modified. Our results, and those of others showing fusion of trypomastigote-containing vacuoles with lysosomes, are derived from qualitative, ultrastructural studies without any quantitation. It is possible that not all organisms have to go through a fusion with lysosomes in order to escape. Again, by analogy with the viral system, if an acid pH is what is needed to allow the organisms to escape into the cytoplasm, fusion with acidified endosomes may be enough to activate whatever is responsible for lysing the membrane. This would resolve the conceptual problem of 'spilled hydrolases'.

O'Daly: The dynamics of Chagas' disease may involve the parasites entering at the inoculum site and then going to the heart. Is it worth looking at the adherence and penetration process in the heart itself or in heart-cell cultures, because myocarditis is found in Chagas' disease?

Nogueira: Dr Pereira is looking at the effect of parasite interiorization and neuraminidase action in heart cells in tissue culture. I believe the results are preliminary.

Pulido: I see that you have used sera from patients in some instances. Have you continued this work and compared results on patients from different geographical areas?

Nogueira: We continue to look at different strains from different areas. (We plan to test some Venezuelan strains from Dr Avila.) This is interesting also in view of the differences in chemotherapeutic susceptibility of the different strains. All the strains that I have examined so far seem to have the same surface make-up. All the sera that I have looked at always recognize the same major components. Maybe we don't need to have qualitatively different surface components in the various strains, to explain differences in the host. The specific activity of whatever enzymes are expressed at the surface may explain the parasites' preferences for this or that tissue, justifying distinct clinical manifestations in the host. We don't really know what other functions these antigens may have.

Butterworth: You said that trypsinization and antibody are synergistic in preventing the antiphagocytic effect. This presumably has one of two implications: either that the removal of the 90 K neuraminidase then exposes underlying antigenic determinants, or that your antibodies do bind to the surface of the untrypsinized organism, but that the neuraminidase activity inhibits a subsequent interaction between the bound antibody and the cell's Fc receptors. That is testable, by checking the relative binding of antibody to the trypsinized and untrypsinized organisms, respectively.

Nogueira: Yes. Antibodies are effective both before and after trypsinization.

After trypsinization, in the presence of antibodies, the additional binding and interiorization may be mediated through other determinants that are on the surface of the parasites and not removed by protease treatment but are recognized by the polyclonal serum. In contrast, in the absence of serum, the enhancement in uptake may be due to the persistence of sialic acid which may be necessary for binding and/or interiorization. These are the molecules which would normally be removed by the trypanosome neuraminidase.

Wyler: Of obvious relevance to this discussion, Dr Butterworth, is the recent work of Henricks et al (1982) indicating that partial removal of sialic acid from the surface of polymorphonuclear leucocytes enhances their phagocytic ability. The same might be true for macrophages, thus explaining how *T. cruzi* neuraminidase might enhance infectivity.

Warren: I believe Dr Nogueira is doing some very exciting work using *T. cruzi* intracellularly to study lepromatous and tuberculoid leprosy. Perhaps she could summarize some of this for us.

Nogueira: For the last year and a half, a joint investigation by a group in our Department and scientists in Brazil has been examining aspects of cell-mediated immune function in human leprosy. We recently reported the characteristics of the cell infiltrates in cutaneous lesions of patients with lepromatous, tuberculoid and intermediate forms of leprosy (Van Voorhis et al 1982). The main finding of this study was that the T cells in the lesions of lepromatous patients are devoid of OKT4/Leu 3a-positive ('helper') cells and consist almost exclusively of OKT8/Leu 2a-positive ('suppressor') populations. In contrast, the tuberculoid infiltrates present the OKT4/Leu 3a-positive subset as the predominant T-cell type. These major differences in the T-cell subsets may influence the microbicidal activity of macrophages in the lesions.

In agreement with these data are the results we have obtained '*in vitro*' with mononuclear cells from patients. We have been investigating the possibility that the suppressor effect could be mediated through a direct action of soluble mediators generated by suppressor lymphocytes on the macrophages themselves. By using *T. cruzi* and *L. donovani* as intracellular targets, we have been able to test this hypothesis. Our results suggest that mononuclear cells from patients with the tuberculoid form of leprosy generate factors, on stimulation by the specific antigen, that activate macrophages to kill parasites, as one would expect. In contrast, peripheral blood mononuclear cells from patients with the lepromatous form of leprosy, on stimulation by the specific antigen, generate factors that inhibit the intracellular killing of the parasites by macrophages. This factor seems to be produced by suppressor T cells since its production is abrogated by treatment of the cells with OKT-8 monoclonal antibodies, which recognize a suppressor/cytotoxic subset of T cells. We suggest that there is a subpopulation of lymphocytes which, when activated, can down-regulate macrophage function directly.

Avila: Do you know if this problem has a genetic basis?

Nogueira: At this moment, no.

Pereira: Lectin has been mentioned by several people at this symposium, perhaps because it is becoming evident nowadays that sugar is involved in cell–cell interaction in general, and in host–parasite interaction in particular. Investigators in parasitology commonly use the word 'lectin-like' to describe a cell–cell interaction that is inhibited by sugar. It is difficult to define a 'lectin-like' material, in the same way that it is difficult to describe an 'enzyme-like' or an 'immunoglobulin-like' substance. Lectin is now defined as being a sugar-binding protein of non-immune origin, with multiple sugar-combining sites: any substance that does not have this property is not a lectin. Thus, when inhibition of cell–cell interaction is observed with sugars, it would be better to say that the interaction is due to a *sugar-binding protein*; it could be due to a lectin, or to a glycosidase, or to a glycosyl transferase or to a sugar kinase, and so on.

Our own work is on the neuraminidase that we found in *T. cruzi*. This enzyme is not a lectin as far as we know because, although it is a sugar-binding protein, it does not agglutinate, probably because it has only one sugar-binding site. (There is no reason why an enzyme could not be a lectin, as is the case for galactose oxidase, which agglutinates cells having galactose in the outer membrane because it has two sugar-binding sites per molecule; M.E.A. Pereira & H. Wigzell, unpublished observations.) The *T. cruzi* neuraminidase activity is developmentally regulated because it is present only in trypomastigotes—in particular in those obtained from fibroblasts and from the bloodstream of infected mice. The activity is absent from amastigotes and is found in very low amounts in epimastigotes. Indirect evidence suggests that it is present on the outer membrane of the parasite. It digests sialoglycoproteins (or sialoglycolipids) from the circulation, as well as erythrocytes, platelets and lymphocytes. The infection of mice by *T. cruzi* is thus accompanied by the consequent release of sialic acid, as is the infection of host cells *in vitro*, such as myocardial cells and fibroblasts. As Dr Nogueira has mentioned, the neuraminidase is apparently the 90 K protein, although we need to do more experiments to define that point more clearly.

Incubation of live parasites with fetuin, which is a sialoglycoprotein, causes the release of free sialic acid, which is part of the evidence that the enzyme is located on the cell surface (Fig. 1). We didn't find any enzyme activity in the supernatant of the reaction mixtures shown in Fig. 1. If we lyse the cells in water, and use either the pellet after washing (100 000 $g \times 3$) or the whole lysate, containing cytosol and particles, we find that the activity is approximately the same as with the live cells. This also suggests that most of the enzyme is on the outer membrane. The enzyme has a certain specificity, the best one being for the acute-phase protein orosomucoid (or α-l-acid glycoprotein). Some

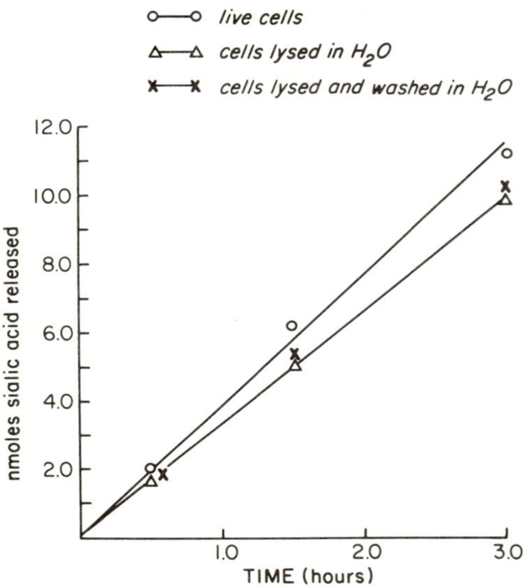

FIG. 1. (*Pereira*) Progress curve of *T. cruzi* neuraminidase. Trypomastigotes from human fibroblast cultures were used as viable cells or after lysis in distilled water. 5×10^6 trypomastigotes or the equivalent lysed in water per reaction mixture. The incubations were conducted at pH 6.5 for the lengths of time indicated, with fetuin used as substrate.

sialocompounds—ovomucoid and bovine submaxillary mucin—are not good substrates, whereas sialolactose and fetuin are relatively good. If human erythrocytes are treated with *T. cruzi*, they become strongly agglutinated by peanut lectin (Pereira 1983). In infection of mice with the Y strain of *T. cruzi* we see a parallel between the parasitaemia and the titre of peanut lectin against the erythrocytes of the infected mice. For three days before infection there were no parasites in the blood and the erythrocytes were not agglutinated with the lectin. When the parasites emerged in the bloodstream the erythrocytes became agglutinated with the lectin. The parasite thus contains a neuraminidase activity, which is developmentally regulated and acts on cells both *in vitro* and *in vivo*. Cardoso & Brener (1980) recently showed that mice infected with *T. cruzi* have a pronounced thrombocytopaenia and anaemia, which could very well be explained by the *T. cruzi* neuraminidase. The enzyme may thus be relevant to the pathogenesis of Chagas' disease.

Piras: I believe you have shown that the metacyclic trypomastigotes obtained from LIT medium have a very low sialidase activity. Will this parasite infect fibroblastic cells as well as the other ones?

Pereira: Yes. Trypomastigotes from LIT cultures will infect both fibroblasts and macrophages much better than trypomastigotes obtained from fibroblasts and from infected mice.

Sher: An alternative explanation for the results of Cardoso & Brener (1980) that you mentioned is that the removal of sialic acid from red cells makes them more susceptible to lysis by the alternative complement pathway. Have you incubated red cells with trypomastigotes to see if they become more sensitive to lysis?

Pereira: Incubation of human erythrocytes with *T. cruzi in vitro* shows two things. First, it exposes T receptors as judged by the ability of the erythrocytes to be agglutinated by normal human sera. Secondly, the erythrocytes are lysed by fresh serum but not by serum inactivated at 56 °C, presumably by activating the alternative complement pathway.

Avila: Have you tried using 4-methylumbelliferyl neuraminic acid as a substrate for this neuraminidase?

Pereira: Not yet.

Avila: How would you explain the differences in neuraminidase specific activity between parasites that originate from the bloodstream and from fibroblasts?

Pereira: I don't know.

Avila: We know that *T. cruzi* has a high pinocytic activity. Have you considered the possibility that this neuraminidase comes from the blood or from fibroblast culture media?

Pereira: It is possible; although, if we trypsinize the trypomastigotes in the conditions that Dr Nogueira used to remove the 90 K protein, we completely remove the enzyme activity, and incubation of that parasite in serum-free media at 37 °C will restore some of the enzyme activity. Although we haven't done metabolic labelling, these findings argue that the enzyme is neither absorbed nor stored inside the cell by pinocytic activity.

Mirelman: You mentioned that the 90 K protein has, in addition to sialidase, other glycosidase activities. I noticed that you find an increase in the amount of peanut agglutinin (PNA) bound. Have you incubated further to see if the PNA binding capacity goes down? That would indicate that the galactose is being digested as well. Secondly, I noticed that the colominic acid is not a substrate for the sialidase. Is it an inhibitor? If it is, perhaps it could be used for purification of this enzyme activity by affinity. You could perhaps also use *Escherichia coli* K1, which contains colominic acid as a capsule, to localize the activity of the sialidase on the surface of the parasite.

Pereira: Those are good suggestions. I will certainly look for the possibility of colominic acid as an affinity adsorbent. Free sialic acid is not released from colominic acid by *T. cruzi*, but the enzyme could bind to the polysaccharide.

Martinez-Palomo: I am interested in Dr Avila's comment about the active pinocytosis of *T. cruzi*, but as far as I know the only evidence for this is our work on freeze-fractured membranes of epimastigotes and trypomastigotes (De Souza et al 1978). Trypomastigotes do not have any pinocytic activity except for the cytostome, whereas the trypomastigotes do have many endocytic vesicles. Has anybody else studied this activity?

Avila: Yes; Bretaña & O'Daly (1976) have done this, but on epimastigotes. We also have recently demonstrated the possibility of culturing virulent *T. cruzi* epimastigotes in a minimal medium containing inorganic salts, folic acid, choline, glucose and bovine liver catalase as the only amino acid source of the culture medium. This suggests that through pinocytosis the intralysosomal digestion of this haemoprotein provides epimastigotes with all amino acids needed for active multiplication (Avila et al 1979b, 1983). Furthermore, we have measured pinocytosis of bovine catalase and found that the uptake rate is about 128 ng per 10^6 parasites per hour which, added to an intracellular half-life of about 7.3 h, gives parasites with about 91% of the amino acids required for active multiplication (J.L. Avila & M.A. Casanova, unpublished work).

Nogueira: There is also a paper by Meyer & De Souza (1973) on the interiorization of retinal pigment *in vitro* by *T. cruzi*.

Martinez-Palomo: Yes, but this is through the cytostome, which is a very minor modification of the surface, so the endocytic activity must be practically negligible.

Nogueira: If we accept that the interaction with the monoclonal antibody and the anti-90 K serum is specific for the enzyme then we would say that the enzyme is definitely a parasite product because we know from the biosynthetic label that the 90 K protein is made by the parasite.

Piras: Do you have any experience of treating target cells with sialidase to see what happens to infection with epimastigotes afterwards?

Nogueira: We are testing this on macrophages and using metacyclics as targets, as I mentioned earlier.

Pereira: Infection of myocardial cells *in vitro* is accompanied by release of free sialic acid (M.E.A. Pereira & P. Libby, unpublished observations). The infection is performed in protein-free media; i.e. in the absence of glycoproteins. If we use fetuin at high concentrations (10 mg/ml or more) we do not get an inhibition of infection, but the *release* of sialic acid from the host cells (as detected by metabolically labelling the sialic acid with ^3H) is barely affected by the presence of fetuin. This means that the role of the *T. cruzi* neuraminidase in the host cell infection needs to be determined.

Hernández: Are there any proteolytic enzymes in the preparation?

Pereira: Proteases do not affect the agglutination afforded by peanut agglutinin.

Hernández: How do you remove the neuraminidase from the concanavalin A column?

Pereira: Once the neuraminidase binds to the concanavalin A–Sepharose one cannot remove it with specific sugar haptens. However, if the enzyme-containing supernatant is placed on a concanavalin A–Sepharose column preincubated with bovine serum albumin, then one gets binding and release of the enzyme from the column, especially if the release is done in the presence of 50% ethylene glycol, which is a hydrophobic-breaking reagent.

REFERENCES

Avila JL, Casanova MA, Avila A, Bretaña A 1979a Acid and neutral hydrolases in *Trypanosoma cruzi*. Characterization and assay. J Protozool 26:304-311

Avila JL, Bretaña A, Casanova MA, Avila A, Rodriguez F 1979b *Trypanosoma cruzi*: defined medium for continuous cultivation of virulent parasites. Exp Parasitol 48:27-35

Avila JL, Pérez-Kepp R, Bretaña A 1983 A minimal medium for the cultivation of infective *Trypanosoma cruzi* epimastigotes. J Gen Microbiol 129: in press

Bretaña A, O'Daly JA 1976 Uptake of fetal proteins by *Trypanosoma cruzi*. Immunofluorescence and ultrastructural studies. Int J Parasitol 6:379-386

Brizuela L 1981 Determinación de actividad fosfolipasa en extractos con actividad lítica de *Trypanosoma cruzi*. Degree thesis, Universidad Simón Bolívar, Caracas

Cardoso JE, Brener Z 1980 Hematological changes in mice experimentally infected with *Trypanosoma cruzi*. Mem Inst Oswaldo Cruz Rio de J 75:97-104

Czop JK, Fearon DT, Austen KF 1978 Membrane sialic acid on target particles modulates their phagocytosis by a trypsin-sensitive mechanism on human monocytes. Proc Natl Acad Sci USA 75:3831-3835

De Souza W, Martinez-Palomo A, González-Robles A 1978 Cell surface of *Trypanosoma cruzi*. Cytochemistry and freeze-fracture. J Cell Sci 33:285-299

Galloway CJ, Dean GE, Marsh M, Rudnick G, Mellman I 1983 Acidification of macrophage and fibroblast endocytic vesicles *in vitro*. Proc Natl Acad Sci USA, in press

Hambrey PN, Mellors A, Tizart IR 1981 The phospholipases of pathogenic and non-pathogenic *Trypanosoma* species. Mol Biochem Parasitol 2:177-186

Henricks PAJ, van Erne-van der Tol ME, Verhoef J 1982 Partial removal of sialic acid enhances phagocytosis and the generation of superoxide and chemiluminescence by polymorphonuclear leukocytes. J Immunol 129:745-750

Kipnis TL, David JR, Alper CA, Sher A, da Silva WD 1981 Enzymatic treatment transforms trypomastigotes of *Trypanosoma cruzi* into activators of alternative complement pathway and potentiates their uptake by macrophages. Proc Natl Acad Sci USA 78:602-605

Koide N, Nose M, Muramatsu T 1977 Recognition of IgG by Fc receptor and complement: effects of glycosidase digestion. Biochem Biophys Res Commun 75:838-844

Krettli A, Thomas N, Eisen H 1980 Escape mechanisms of *Trypanosoma cruzi* from the host immune system. In: Israel L et al (eds) Immunologie antitumoral et antiparasitaire. INSERM (Inst Nat Sante Rech Med) Colloq 97:553-558

Matlin KS, Reggio H, Helenius A, Simons K 1981 Infectious entry pathway of influenza virus in a canine kidney cell line. J Cell Biol 91:601-613

Meindl P, Bodo G, Palese P, Schulman J, Tuppy H 1974 Inhibition of neuraminidase activity by derivatives of 2-deoxy-2,3-dehydro-N-acetyl neuraminic acid. Virology 58:457-463

Meyer H, De Souza W 1973 On the fine structure of *Trypanosoma cruzi* in tissue cultures of pigmented epithelium from the chicken embryo. Uptake of melanin granules by the parasite. J Protozool 20:590-593

O'Daly JA, Aso P 1979 *Trypanosoma cruzi*, *Leishmania donovani*, and *Leishmania mexicana*. Extract factor that lyses mammalian cells. Exp Parasitol 47:222-231

Opperdoes FR, Van Roy J 1982 The phospholipases of *Trypanosoma brucei* bloodstream forms and cultured procyclics. Mol Biochem Parasitol 5:309-319

Pereira MEA 1983 A developmentally regulated neuraminidase activity in *Trypanosoma cruzi*. Science (Wash DC) 219:1444-1446

Rangel HA, Araujo PMF, Camargo IJB et al 1981 Detection of a proteinase common to epimastigote, trypomastigote and amastigote of different strains of *Trypanosoma cruzi*. Tropenmed Parasitol 32:87-92

Steiger RF, Opperdoes FR, Bontemps J 1980 Subcellular fractionation of *Trypanosoma brucei* bloodstream forms with special reference to hydrolases. Eur J Biochem 105:163-175

Van Voorhis WC, Kaplan G, Sarno EN et al 1982 The cutaneous infiltrates of leprosy. Cellular characteristics and the predominant T-cell phenotypes. N Engl J Med 307:1593-1597

Toxoplasma gondii: use of mutants to study the host–parasite relationship

E. R. PFEFFERKORN, JOSEPH D. SCHWARTZMAN, and LLOYD H. KASPER

Department of Microbiology, Dartmouth Medical School, Hanover, New Hampshire 03755, USA

Abstract. Toxoplasma gondii, an obligate intracellular parasite, is readily grown in nearly all cultured cells. The host–parasite relationship in these cultures can often be explored by using mutant host cells or mutant parasites. Host cells incapable of incorporating uracil or hypoxanthine, which were excellent precursors for *T. gondii*, allowed the demonstration that the host cell had no access to the purine or pyrimidine nucleotide pools of the parasite. Conversely, a *T. gondii* mutant that was defective in the principal pyrimidine salvage pathway allowed the demonstration that the parasite had no access to pyrimidine nucleotide or deoxynucleotide pools of the host cell. One metabolite that must pass from the host cytoplasm to *T. gondii* is a purine. An absolute defect in purine biosynthesis by the parasite was disclosed by growing *T. gondii* in a mutant host cell that was, itself, incapable of purine synthesis. *T. gondii* grew normally at 40 °C in a mutant host cell that was incapable of protein synthesis at that temperature. Thus, the parasite did not depend on concomitant protein synthesis in the host cell. An antigenic mutant of *T. gondii* was isolated with the aid of parasiticidal monoclonal antibody. This mutant lacked a major parasite surface protein, of relative molecular mass (M_r) 22 000. The antibody used to select this mutant immunoprecipitated a protein of this M_r from the wild-type parasite.

1983 Cytopathology of parasitic disease. Pitman Books, London (Ciba Foundation symposium 99), p 74-91

Cultured cells infected with *Toxoplasma gondii* offer an excellent opportunity to study the host–parasite relationship of an obligate intracellular protozoan parasite. A mammalian cell with *T. gondii* growing inside it is a complex system of one eukaryotic cell within another. Infection with *T. gondii* does not compromise the biosynthetic activity of its host cell; both nucleic acid and protein synthesis continue unabated in human fibroblasts infected with the parasite. A major problem is to distinguish between the biosynthetic activities of the host and the parasite and to determine their importance and interdependence. A further complication is introduced by the parasitophorous vacuole: *T. gondii* does not grow in the cytoplasm of its host cell but in a vacuole that lies in the host cytoplasm. The parasitophorous vacuolar membrane is likely to play an important role in the infection. All biochemical communication between the host cell and the parasite must pass across this membrane. The nature of this metabolic traffic is one aspect of the complex biochemistry of the host–parasite relationship. Our approach to studying this relationship has used mutants in two ways. First, we took advantage of the fact that *T. gondii* grows well in nearly all cultured mammalian cells and we chose mutant host cells from the large repository offered by human genetic studies and by modern cell biology. Alternatively, we have used our own mutants of *T. gondii*, which can readily be isolated because the tachyzoite, the asexual stage grown in cultured cells, is haploid.

Nucleotide exchange

The first clue about the extent of nucleotide exchange between host cell and *T. gondii* was a by-product of our endeavour to devise a simple method for specific radioactive labelling of the nucleic acids of actively growing intracellular parasites. Such a method was required because infection with *T. gondii* does not significantly inhibit the synthesis of host-cell nucleic acids, particularly in the early stages of infection. Thus, in a culture infected with *T. gondii* and labelled with radioactive uridine, hypoxanthine or other precursors, most of the radioactivity will be incorporated into the host cell rather than into the parasite. We found that specific labelling of the nucleic acids of intracellular *T. gondii* could be achieved through the use of mutant human fibroblasts from a patient with Lesch–Nyhan disease. These fibroblasts lack the enzyme hypoxanthine/guanine phosphoribosyltransferase (EC 2.4.2.8) and thus cannot incorporate hypoxanthine supplied in their medium. However, Lesch–Nyhan cultures infected with *T. gondii* show a dramatic exponential increase in the incorporation of radioactive hypoxanthine. We have shown by autoradiography that virtually all the incorporated [^{3}H]hypoxanthine is in the intracellular parasites (Fig. 1a). Since [^{3}H]hypoxanthine must be incorporated into *T. gondii* nucleic acids by way of the parasite purine nucleotide pool, it is clear that this parasite pool is not available to the host cell. If the infected mutant host cells had had access to the purine nucleotides of the parasite, they would have become labelled since their ability to incorporate purine nucleotides was impaired.

Similarly, we were able to examine the flow of pyrimidine nucleotides from the parasite to the host cell without using any mutants, because wild-type human fibroblasts cannot incorporate uracil while *T. gondii* can. Fig. 1b shows the results of incubating infected cultures with [^{3}H]uracil. Although the intracellular parasites were heavily labelled, the host cells that contained

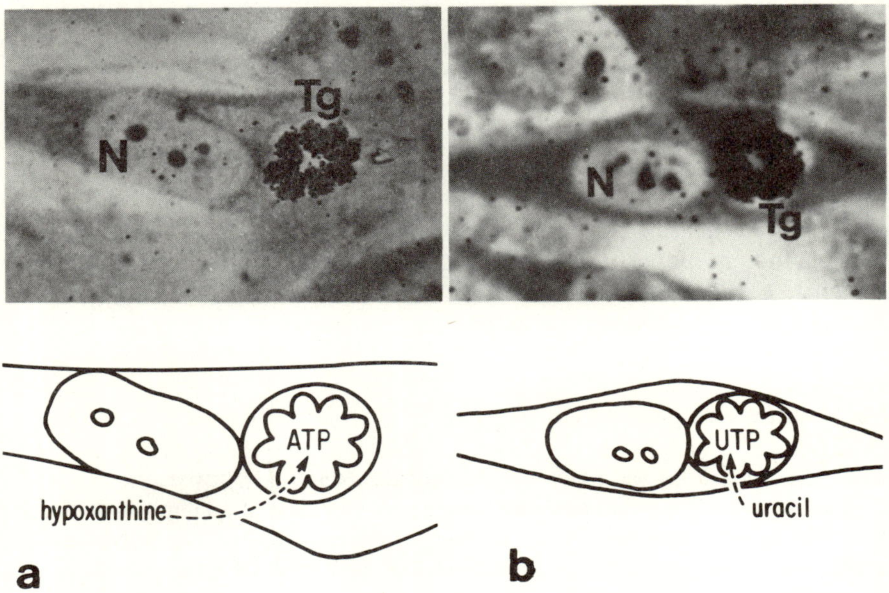

FIG. 1. The unavailability to the host cell of purine and pyrimidine nucleotides within intracellular *T. gondii*, as illustrated by autoradiography (above) and by diagram (below). (a) Lesch–Nyhan fibroblasts infected with wild-type *T. gondii* and incubated with generally labelled [^{3}H]hypoxanthine; (b) human fibroblasts infected with wild-type *T. gondii* and incubated with [5,6-^{3}H]uracil. The cultures were labelled with 10 μCi/ml, during the interval from 16–24 h after infection, and then were prepared for autoradiography. N, host cell nucleus; Tg, a group of eight intracellular *T. gondii*. (Modified from Pfefferkorn & Pfefferkorn 1977a, b.)

them showed no incorporation. We conclude that the host cell has no access to purine or pyrimidine nucleotides of *T. gondii*.

To examine the possibility that pyrimidine nucleotides and deoxynucleotides were supplied to *T. gondii* by the host cell, we turned to the alternative approach of using a mutant parasite. Using chemical mutagenesis, we isolated a mutant that was 100-fold more resistant to 5-fluorodoxyuridine (FUDR) than was the wild-type *T. gondii*. This single step mutant, R-FUDR^R-1, also proved to be resistant to 5-fluorouridine and to 5-fluorouracil (Pfefferkorn & Pfefferkorn 1977a). The biochemical basis for its resistance was shown to be the total lack of the enzyme uracil phosphoribosyltransferase (EC 2.4.2.9) (Pfefferkorn 1978). In wild *T. gondii*, deoxyuridine and uridine (as well as their fluoro analogues) are first converted to uracil, which then enters the pyrimidine nucleotide pool by way of this enzyme. Thus, uracil phosphoribosyltransferase plays a critical role in pyrimidine salvage by *T. gondii*. The observation that mutant R-FUDR^R-1 was incapable of

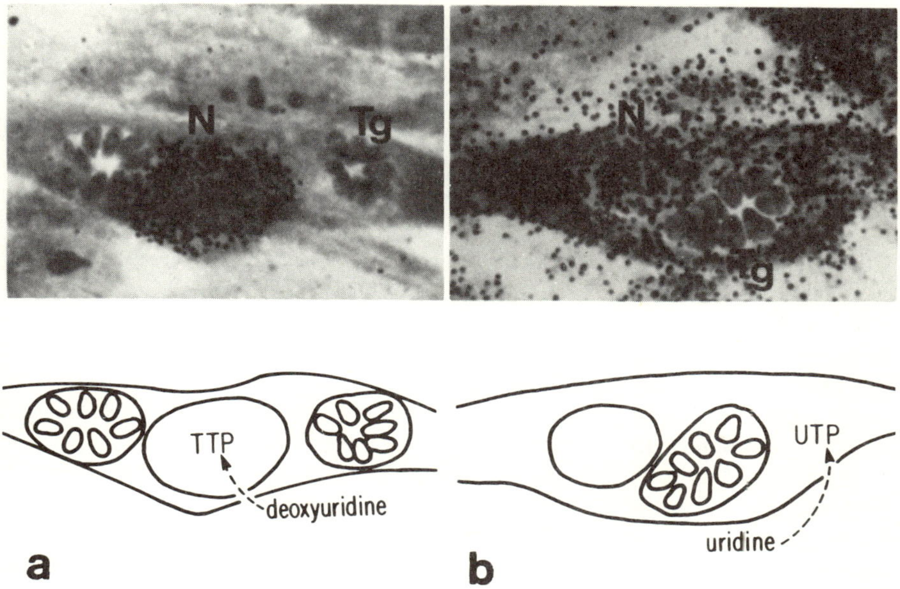

FIG. 2. The unavailability to intracellular *T. gondii* of pyrimidine nucleotides and deoxynucleotides within the host cell, as illustrated by autoradiography (above) and by diagram (below). Human fibroblasts infected with R-FUDR^R-1 *T. gondii* were incubated with (a) [6-^{3}H]deoxyuridine or (b) [5,6-^{3}H]uridine. The cultures were labelled with 10 μCi/ml, during the interval 16–24 h after infection, and then were prepared for autoradiography. N, host cell nucleus; Tg, a group of eight intracellular *T. gondii*. (Modified from Pfefferkorn & Pfefferkorn 1977b.)

incorporating uridine or deoxyuridine allowed us to draw several conclusions about the flow of pyrimidine nucleotides from host cell to *T. gondii*. Fig. 2a shows an autoradiographic analysis of human fibroblasts infected with R-FUDR^R-1. Although intracellular wild-type parasites (data not shown) were heavily labelled with [^{3}H]deoxyuridine, the mutant showed no incorporation. The nucleus of its host cell, however, was heavily labelled because deoxyuridine is a specific precursor for the mammalian pyrimidine deoxynucleotide pool. If these labelled deoxynucleotides had been available to the actively dividing intracellular parasites they, too, would have been labelled. The absence of parasite labelling shows that *T. gondii* has no access to the pyrimidine deoxynucleotide pool of the host cell. Much the same argument can be made concerning the pyrimidine nucleotide pool of the host cell. We examined the availability of this pool by infecting human fibroblasts with R-FUDR^R-1 and then labelling them with [^{3}H]uridine. Again parallel cultures infected with the wild-type parasite showed heavy labelling of the intracellular *T. gondii* (data not shown). However, the cultures infected by the mutant showed little or no incorporation of uridine by the parasite (Fig. 2b). Since the [^{3}H]uridine did label the cytoplasmic and nuclear RNA of the infected cells, their pyrimidine nucleotide pool must also have been labelled. We conclude that pyrimidine nucleotides and deoxynucleotides of the host cell are unavailable to intracellular *T. gondii*.

Purine and pyrimidine synthesis by *T. gondii*

As described above, we have excluded a variety of nucleotide exchanges between *T. gondii* and its host cell. It is reasonable to assume, however, that the host cell must supply *something* to *T. gondii* or else there would be no basis for its obligate intracellular parasitism. Identification of metabolites that must be supplied by the host cell is more complex than simply establishing the nutritional requirement for the growth of an extracellular protozoan. In this case the ability of the free-living organism to carry out a defined series of biosynthetic steps can be determined unequivocally by supplying an appropriate radioactive precursor and detecting its conversion to a particular product. This simple strategy cannot be used to study obligate intracellular parasites because there is no easy way to determine if the observed metabolic conversion is carried out by the intracellular parasite. Since the labelled precursor supplied in the medium must first pass through the cytoplasm of the host cell, the host cell could perform the required biosynthetic steps and export the final radioactive product to its parasite. We have distinguished between the biosynthetic contributions of the host and those of the parasite by using mutant host cells with complete, well defined enzymic defects. Since these host cells have absolute defects in particular biochemical pathways, incorporation into the parasite of a relevant precursor must result from the biosynthetic activity of the parasite. Conversely, the inability of an intracellular parasite to metabolize a precursor while growing in a mutant host with the appropriate enzymic defect is evidence that the parasite must depend on its host cell for the final biosynthetic product.

We have used this approach to study both pyrimidine and purine biosynthesis by *T. gondii*. The experiments on pyrimidine synthesis were done on a mutant isolated from Chinese hamster ovary (CHO) cells with three separate defects in pyrimidine synthesis, the most profound being a total lack of dihydro-orotase (EC 3.5.2.3) (Patterson & Carnright 1977). Uninfected mutant cells showed only a negligible incorporation of [^{14}C]aspartic acid into their pyrimidines. *T. gondii* grew normally in mutant cultures whether or not pyrimidines were supplied in the medium. Moreover, infected cultures showed a marked increase in the incorporation of [^{14}C]aspartate into pyrimidines (Schwartzman & Pfefferkorn 1981). Thus, we concluded that *T. gondii* is capable of pyrimidine synthesis.

Quite the opposite result was obtained when we examined the ability of *T. gondii* to synthesize purines. Here the host was a CHO cell mutant with an absolute defect in the enzyme 5-amino-4 imidazolecarboxamide ribonucleotide formyltransferase (phosphoribosylaminoimidazolecarboxamide formyltransferase, EC 2.1.2.3) (Patterson 1975). This mutant depends on an exogenous source of purines for growth. Nonetheless, *T. gondii* grew normally in this mutant host cell when no purines were supplied in the medium. This observation does not prove that the parasite was capable of purine synthesis; it could have been making its nucleic acids by using preformed purines supplied by the host cell. In order to study purine biosynthesis unequivocally, we added a labelled purine precursor, [^{14}C]formate, to the medium of infected wild-type and mutant host cells. After a long labelling period, the nucleic acids were purified and hydrolysed to free bases. The bases were resolved chromatographically and their radioactivity was measured. Fig. 3 shows that the parasites grown in the wild-type cells contained [^{14}C]formate in their purines and their thymine.

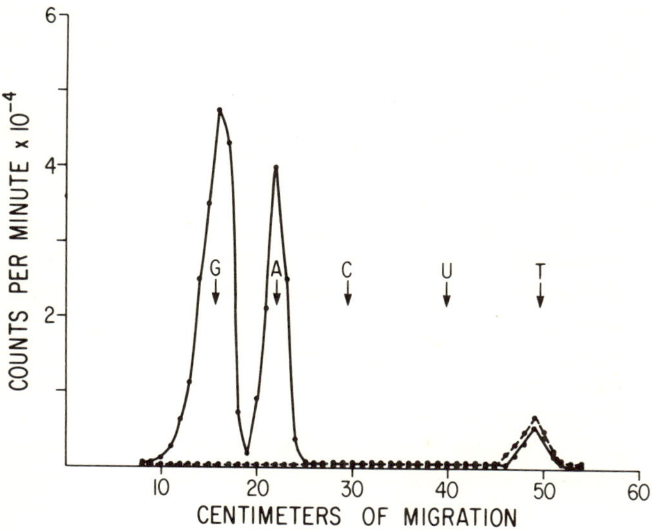

FIG. 3. Incorporation of [^{14}C]formate into nucleic acid bases by wild-type *T. gondii* growing in wild-type Chinese hamster ovary (CHO) cells (————) or in purine-requiring mutant CHO cells (•••••••••••). The cultures were labelled, during the interval from 4–16 h after infection, with 5 μCi/ml [^{14}C]formate. The nucleic acids were hydrolysed to free bases and resolved by paper chromatography. A, adenine; C, cytosine; G, guanine; T, thymine; U, uracil. (From Schwartzman & Pfefferkorn 1982.)

Formate is a good precursor of the methyl group of thymine although it is not used for the pyrimidine ring. The label found in the purines could have been incorporated by either the parasite or by the wild-type host cell. When the same analysis was done on parasites grown in mutant purine-requiring host cells *no* [^{14}C]formate was incorporated into either adenine or guanine, although the methyl group of thymine was labelled to the same extent as seen in infected wild-type cells (Schwartzman & Pfefferkorn 1982). We conclude that *T. gondii* is incapable of purine biosynthesis and must obtain preformed purines from its host cell.

Purines must therefore be part of the biochemical traffic that passes from host cell to *T. gondii*. The mechanism by which the host cell supplies the purines remains unknown. We initially thought that electron microscopic studies of cells infected with *T. gondii* offered a clue. Several investigators, among them Hirsch et al (1974), noted that host-cell mitochondria move to the parasitophorous vacuole and cover nearly all its surface on the host cytoplasmic side. Since the principal product of mitochondria is ATP, we suspected that the perivacuolar mitochondria released their ATP into the parasitophorous vacuole where it served as the purine supply of the growing *T. gondii*. To explore this idea, we examined the ability of extracellular *T. gondii* parasites to incorporate exogenous ATP during the brief interval in which they are capable of limited nucleic acid synthesis. Labelled ATP was incorporated nearly as well as purine bases and nucleosides. However, the ATP was extensively degraded before it entered the parasite. We demonstrated this degradation by following the fate of doubly labelled ATP that contained ^{3}H in the purine ring and ^{32}P in the alpha (innermost) phosphate. The purine ring of ATP was used for parasite nucleic acid synthesis but the phosphate was not (Schwartzman & Pfefferkorn 1982). Nonetheless *T. gondii* was capable of using ATP that we thought might be supplied by the host-cell mitochondria. To determine if these mitochondria played an obligatory role in the growth of the parasite we again used a mutant host cell. This CHO mutant (Ditta et al 1976), which has non-functional mitochondria that are incapable of ATP synthesis by oxidative phosphorylation, supported the growth of *T. gondii* at the same rate that was observed in wild-type host cells. We conclude that the host periparasitophorous vacuolar mitochondria do not play an obligatory role in the supply of purines to *T. gondii*.

The role of host-cell protein synthesis

Purines cannot be the sole contribution of the host cell to *T. gondii* for the parasite fails to grow extracellularly even in the richest of media that include purines among their many nutrients. The additional contributions of the host cell remain undefined. One activity of the host cell that cannot be reproduced in media designed for extracellular growth of *T. gondii* is the synthesis of macromolecules. Can the continued synthesis of nucleic acids and protein in human fibroblasts infected with *T. gondii* play an essential role in supporting the growth of the parasite? The importance of nucleic acid synthesis by the host cell can be excluded because *T. gondii* has been shown to multiply for a short time in enucleated cells (Jones 1973, Sethi et al 1973). Since the nucleus is the site of host-cell DNA and RNA synthesis, these activities are clearly not required by the parasite. However, enucleated host cells continue to synthesize proteins because their preformed mRNA is relatively stable. The dependence of the parasite on host-cell protein synthesis remained to be determined. Most drugs cannot be used to explore this problem because they inhibit all eukaryotic protein synthesis equally well and thus affect the parasite as well as the host. Again, a mutant host cell provided the ideal approach. We used a mutant CHO cell that has a thermolabile leucyl-tRNA synthetase (EC 6.1.1.4) (Thompson et al 1973). As a result of this defect, the mutant cells rapidly lose the ability to synthesize protein at 40 °C. Cultures of wild-type and mutant host cells were infected at 33 °C and then shifted to 40 °C. We measured protein synthesis in the two cultures by the incorporation of [^{3}H]leucine. This amino acid is used equally well by host cell and parasite and thus measures the total (host-cell plus parasite) protein synthesis in the culture. Fig. 4 shows that infection of the wild-type culture caused only a slight increase in the rate of protein synthesis. Most of the [^{3}H]leucine was incorporated by the host cells. In the uninfected mutant cultures, however, there was little or no protein synthesis. Infection of the mutant culture resulted in the same slight increase in [^{3}H]leucine incorporation. Autoradiography of the infected mutant cells showed that protein synthesis in the mutant cells was confined to the intracellular parasites. We measured the growth of *T. gondii* by following the incorporation of [^{14}C]uracil, which is incorporated only by the parasite. As shown in Fig. 4, *T. gondii* grew equally well in the mutant and the wild-type host cells at 40 °C. Thus, *T. gondii* does not depend on protein synthesis by its host cell.

Antigenic mutants

We have recently discovered another class of *T. gondii* mutants that should be useful for studying various aspects of the host–parasite relationship both *in vitro* and *in vivo*. These are antigenic mutants that have altered or absent surface proteins. Although antigenic variation is a prominent feature of some parasitic protozoa such as the African trypanosomes, *T. gondii*

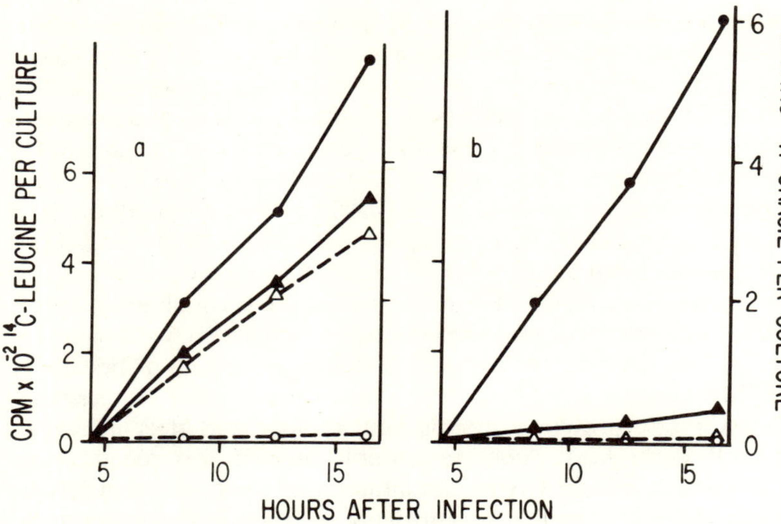

FIG. 4. Incorporation of leucine and uracil by *T. gondii* cultures of (a) wild-type CHO cells and (b) mutant CHO cells with a temperature-sensitive defect in protein synthesis. Both cultures were incubated at 40 °C. Uracil incorporation by uninfected cultures (○); leucine incorporation by uninfected cultures (△); uracil incorporation by infected cultures (●); leucine incorporation by infected cultures (▲); CPM, counts per minute. (From Pfefferkorn & Pfefferkorn 1981.)

appears essentially to be antigenically monomorphic both in various geographical isolates and in the course of individual infections. Polyclonal antisera produced in response to infection with *T. gondii* would be ineffective in selecting an antigenic variant of the parasite. The loss of any one antigenic determinant would offer little selective advantage since such an altered parasite would be attacked by the antibodies that react with its many other surface antigens. Monoclonal antibodies, since they are specific for a single antigenic determinant, offer the opportunity to select antigenic variants of *T. gondii*.

To produce monoclonal antibodies against *T. gondii*, we immunized BALB/c mice with purified tachyzoites that were killed by freezing and thawing. Spleen cells from the immunized mice were fused with an immunoglobulin G(IgG)-secreting myeloma line, and hybridomas were selected in the usual manner. Positive cultures were initially identified by a solid-phase enzyme-linked immunosorbant assay (ELISA) and then recloned. The clones that remained positive were examined for parasiticidal activity in the presence of complement supplied by normal human serum that had no antitoxoplasma activity. Of the several parasiticidal clones identified, two (designated G and B) were studied in detail. Their activity was measured by incubating a mixture

TABLE 1 The effect of monoclonal antibodies and normal human serum on the plaque-forming unit (PFU) titre of wild-type and R-G^R-1 *T. gondii*.

Treatment[a]	*Percent PFU survival*[b] *Wild type*	*R-G^R-1*
Normal human serum only	102	85
Monoclonal antibody G only	91	94
Monoclonal antibody G plus normal human serum	2.2	94
Monoclonal antibody B plus normal human serum	3.0	4.3

From Kasper et al 1982. [a]The monoclonal antibodies were diluted 1/10 and the normal human serum was diluted 1/2. [b]Compared with survival in medium containing only 10% fetal calf serum.

of extracellular *T. gondii*, monoclonal antibody and normal human serum and measuring the reduction in the number of viable parasites by a plaque assay. As shown in Table 1, this activity required the presence of both complement supplied by the normal serum and monoclonal antibody. At a 1/10 dilution, monoclonal antibody G, prepared as ascitic fluid with an ELISA titre of 10^4, produced an exponential fall in plaque-forming unit (PFU) titre for the first 40 min. After this time, the rate of killing progressively decreased, leaving a residual 2–3% *T. gondii* that were notably resistant to further killing (Fig. 5).

The parasiticidal effect of monoclonal antibody G was sufficient to allow the selection of a resistant mutant. We began this selection by treating the exponentially growing intracellular wild-type *T. gondii* with the potent alkylating mutagen, ethylnitrosourea. The surviving parasites were grown for three days and then treated with monoclonal antibody G and normal serum. The survivors, which numbered about 3%, were regrown and again challenged with monoclonal antibody and normal serum. This process was repeated a total of three times without apparent effect, since roughly 3% of the parasites survived each time. However, during each successive cycle of killing and regrowth, mutant parasites must have formed a progressively larger fraction of the population, because the fourth treatment yielded 25% survivors. After a final treatment that resulted in complete survival, a single clone, R-G^R-1, was isolated and studied further. Table 1 shows that R-G^R-1, while resistant to monoclonal antibody G, was sensitive to another monoclonal antibody and thus cannot be generally resistant to complement-mediated lysis.

Our first step in the analysis of the mutation that conferred resistance to monoclonal antibody G was to compare the surface proteins of the wild-type with those of the mutant parasites, since it seemed likely that a change in surface antigenicity was involved. Purified wild-type and mutant parasites were surface-radioiodinated by the lactoperoxidase method, washed free of

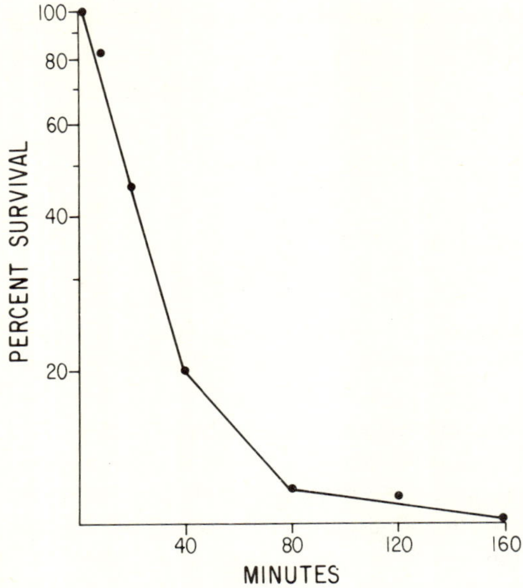

FIG. 5. The kinetics of the parasiticidal effect of monoclonal antibody G (1/10 dilution) plus normal serum (1/2 dilution) as measured by a plaque titration. (From Kasper et al 1982.)

unreacted ^{125}I, and dissolved in sodium dodecylsulphate (SDS), mercapto-ethanol, and buffer. This solution was resolved by SDS acrylamide gel electrophoresis. The gel was dried, and iodinated proteins were located by autoradiography. Fig. 6 shows that the mutant and wild-type parasites were remarkably similar in their patterns of iodinatable surface proteins except for one prominent difference. Mutant R-G^R-1 lacked a major surface protein of relative molecular mass (M_r) 22 000 (P22). This relatively simple picture was shown to be somewhat more complex when the surface-labelled wild-type and mutant parasites were compared by two-dimensional electrophoresis, as described by O'Farrell (1975). With this technique we observed that the mutant parasite actually lacked a family of three proteins that had the same M_r but different isoelectric points (Kasper et al 1982).

We next attempted to immunoprecipitate proteins from wild-type and mutant parasites. The parasites were purified, surface-radioiodinated, and dissolved in a non-ionic detergent. This solution was treated first with monoclonal antibody G and then with a Sepharose–protein-A–goat-anti-mouse-IgG complex designed to precipitate the monoclonal antibody. The precipitate was collected, washed by centrifugation, and dissolved in SDS for analysis by acrylamide gel electrophoresis. Fig. 6 shows that monoclonal

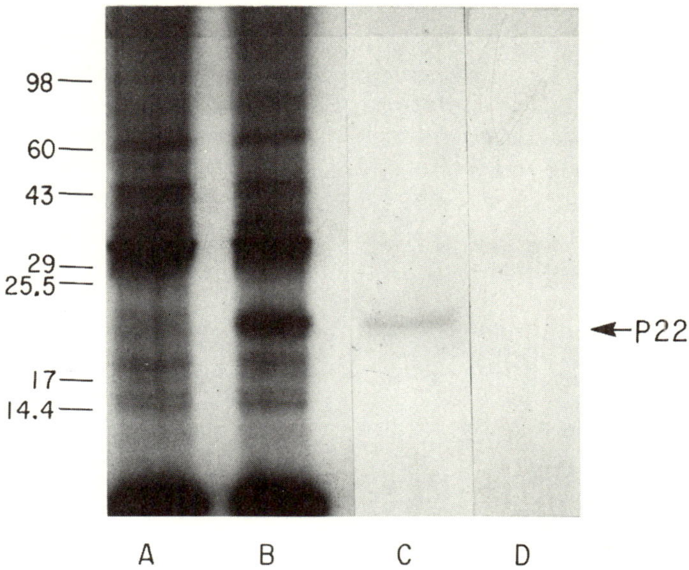

FIG. 6. Autoradiograms of sodium dodecyl sulphate-acrylamide gel electrophoretic analyses of surface-radioiodinated *T. gondii*. A, whole extract of R-G^{R}-1; B, whole extract of wild-type parasites; C, proteins immunoprecipitated from wild-type parasites by monoclonal antibody G; D, proteins immunoprecipitated from R-G^{R}-1 by monoclonal antibody G. The electrophoretic mobilities of proteins of known M_r values (in 1000s) are indicated at the left. (From Kasper et al 1982.)

antibody G immunoprecipitated the protein P22 from the wild-type parasite but failed to show any specific precipitation with R-G^{R}-1 (Kasper et al 1982). We conclude that the protein P22 is not represented at the surface of the mutant R-G^{R}-1, at least in an iodinatable form.

Conclusions

We have illustrated a variety of ways in which mutants can be useful in the study of *T. gondii*. Rather than summarizing our conclusions here, it is more valuable to emphasize the versatility and generality of this genetic approach to the study of host–parasite relationships. Mutant host cells or parasites should prove to be useful in studies of other intracellular parasites. A wide variety of mutant cultured cells remains to be explored. For example, the various mutant macrophage-like cell lines that have recently been characterized deserve to be more widely used in parasitology. Antigenic mutants could be selected from other protozoan parasites by means of monoclonal antibodies. Such mutants may be particularly valuable in the study of *Trypanosoma cruzi* and *Leishmania* species that can be grown *in vitro* in both their extracellular and intracellular stages. It may be possible to select an antigenic mutant that grows normally as the extracellular stage but is incapable of binding to and entering host cells. This mutation would identify a protein that is essential specifically for parasite entry into host cells.

Acknowledgements

These investigations were supported by grant number AI-14151 from the National Institutes of Health and by a grant from the March of Dimes Birth Defects Foundation. We are grateful to Academic Press, the American Association of Immunologists, and the American Society of Parasitologists for permission to reproduce figures.

REFERENCES

Ditta G, Soderberg K, Landy F, Scheffler IE 1976 The selection of Chinese hamster cells deficient in oxidative energy metabolism. Som Cell Gen 2:331-344

Hirsch JG, Jones TC, Len L 1974 Interactions in vitro between *Toxoplasma gondii* and mouse cells. In: Parasites in the immunized host: mechanisms of survival. Associated Scientific Publishers, Amsterdam (Ciba Found Symp 25) p 205-223

Jones TC 1973 Multiplication of toxoplasmas in enucleate fibroblasts. Proc Soc Exp Biol Med 142:1268-1271

Kasper LH, Crabb JH, Pfefferkorn ER 1982 Isolation and characterization of a monoclonal antibody-resistant antigenic mutant of *Toxoplasma gondii*. J Immunol 129:1694-1699

O'Farrell PH 1975 High resolution two-dimensional electrophoresis of proteins. J Biol Chem 250:4007-4021

Patterson D 1975 Biochemical genetics of Chinese hamster cell mutants with deviant purine metabolism: biochemical analysis of eight mutants. Som Cell Gen 1:91-110

Patterson D, Carnright DV 1977 Biochemical genetic analysis of pyrimidine biosynthesis in mammalian cells. I: Isolation of a mutant defective in the early steps of de novo pyrimidine synthesis. Som Cell Gen 5:483-495

Pfefferkorn ER 1978 *Toxoplasma gondii*: the enzymatic defect of a mutant resistant to 5-fluorodeoxyuridine. Exp Parasitol 44:26–35

Pfefferkorn ER, Pfefferkorn LC 1977a *Toxoplasma gondii*: specific labeling of nucleic acids of intracellular parasites in Lesch-Nyhan cells. Exp Parasitol 41:95-104

Pfefferkorn ER, Pfefferkorn LC 1977b *Toxoplasma gondii*: characterization of a mutant resistant to fluorodeoxyuridine. Exp Parasitol 42:44-45

Pfefferkorn ER, Pfefferkorn LC 1981 *Toxoplasma gondii*: growth in the absence of host cell protein synthesis. Exp Parasitol 52:129-136

Schwartzman JD, Pfefferkorn ER 1981 Pyrimidine synthesis by intracellular *Toxoplasma gondii*. J Parasitol 67:150-158

Schwartzman JD, Pfefferkorn ER 1982 *Toxoplasma gondii*: purine synthesis and salvage in mutant host cells and parasites. Exp Parasitol 53:77-86

Sethi KK, Pelster B, Piekarski G, Brandis H 1973 Multiplication of *Toxoplasma gondii* in enucleated L cells. Nature New Biol 243:255-256

Thompson LH, Harkins JL, Stanners CP 1973 A mammalian cell mutant with a temperature-sensitive leucyl-transfer RNA synthetase. Proc Natl Acad Sci USA 70:3094-3098

DISCUSSION

Gutteridge: A number of years ago when we started to work on the intracellular forms of *Trypanosoma cruzi* we considered the very question that you were considering in relation to *Toxoplasma gondii*. The one advantage we had with *T. cruzi* is that we could isolate the intracellular forms of *T. cruzi* from infected muscle cells and maintain them in a viable condition for a number of hours (Gutteridge et al 1978). We did experiments similar to those you have described with *T. gondii*. We are thus comparing the two ends of protozoan classification (the flagellates and the sporozoa), and two intracellular parasites, one of which remains in its parasitophorous vacuole (*T. gondii*) and the other which becomes free in the cytosol (*T. cruzi)*. Yet your conclusions about the intracellular forms of *T. gondii* are exactly the ones that we drew for *T. cruzi* (Gutteridge & Rogerson 1979, Gutteridge 1981): we do not know why this parasite grows intracellularly and what significance this development has. In *T. cruzi* we can find no major biochemical differences between the extracellular and intracellular forms. Do you have any ideas about why *T. gondii* is an obligate intracellular parasite?

Pfefferkorn: We have no answer to this. We have used the richest medium that we could devise and it had absolutely no growth-promoting effect. We used the incorporation of labelled uracil, which is specific for *T. gondii*, to eliminate the possibility of background activity from residual host cells. We could have detected growth by even a fraction of the population, but we saw none at all in this rich medium. One conceivable answer is that the host cell supplies the appropriate ionic environment—that is, that the fluid in the parasitophorous vacuole does not have the ionic composition of the extracellular medium but, rather, reflects the intracellular high-potassium, low-sodium environment. I don't know the composition of the vacuolar fluid but if one concocts a medium that has the ionic composition of cytoplasm it doesn't work, and the parasites do not survive as well as they do in a medium with ordinary sodium and potassium concentrations.

Sharma: What do you think is required inside the cell for *T. gondii* to survive, if you have tried protein synthesis, purine synthesis, the pyrimidine pathway and ATP requirements? How does the intracellular enzyme metabolic pathway differ from that for any other parasite, such as *T. cruzi*, which can adapt to *in vitro* growth?

Pfefferkorn: The TCA cycle is, as far as one can tell, entirely normal in *T. gondii*, so the question is essentially unanswered.

Sharma: Does the 22 K protein react with human IgG or IgM antibody?

Pfefferkorn: Yes; this protein is precipitated by 'convalescent' human serum, and it is present not only in our rather artificial laboratory strain of *T. gondii* (RH) but also in freshly isolated strains from clinical cases, and from naturally infected cats.

Sher: Was the original population that you used cloned?

Pfefferkorn: Yes, and in fact it was re-cloned before these experiments.

Sher: Your antibody-selection experiments are extremely elegant but I have the feeling that you were lucky in that the surface component you selected against was not important for the survival of the organism. Do you know what the monoclonal antibody recognizes? Is it a carbohydrate, or protein determinant?

Pfefferkorn: I doubt that the monoclonal is directed against a carbohydrate component because *T. gondii* is free or virtually free of surface glycoproteins that are accessible to lectins. It is a remarkable organism in this respect. I guess we were indeed lucky because the first monoclonal antibody that we began working with recognizes a parasite protein that is not essential. It may be much more difficult to get antigenic mutants in essential parasite surface proteins. But I should think it is not impossible because antibodies are specific for very short stretches of the amino acid sequence. So we may be able to get a mutation in the antigenic site with which the monoclonal antibody reacts and yet retain the functional activity of the protein. So I think that it is likely that we shall be able to get mutants in other cell-surface proteins. These mutants might be useful to people who work with organisms such as *T. cruzi* or the *Leishmania* species, which can be cultivated both in extracellular and in intracellular stages. It may be possible to isolate an antigenic mutant in the extracellular form which makes the parasite incapable of entering cells because one has eliminated the protein that is essential for invasion and establishment of the intracellular stage.

Wyler: Do you have any information about the behaviour of this isolate in mice with regard to cyst formation?

Pfefferkorn: We could not study cyst formation because the isolate came from a mutant strain that is itself incapable of cyst formation. However, it will be useful to study this mutant with respect to the immunity. First, one can use the purified protein (from immunoabsorbant chromatography) to immunize mice and to see whether they are immune to the wild type but not to the mutant. Alternatively one can use a killed vaccine, derived from the wild-type parasites, which elicits antibody to all the surface components of the parasite and then determine the degree of immunity to mutant parasites that lack an important surface antigen.

Urbina: I would like to discuss why it is necessary to consider the amastigote as intracellular. In *Leishmania* species we have recently completed studies in which we compared the energy metabolism of promastigotes with that of amastigotes. There were few differences, and we found that both of them were more prepared to degrade amino acids than carbohydrates. The intracellular condition may be necessary for evasion of the host immune response but this still doesn't explain why the amastigote, being very similar metabolically, would not survive outside the host cell. The amastigote has an extreme osmotic fragility that is not present in the promastigote or epimastigote forms.

Pfefferkorn: We have looked at the osmotic fragility of parasites that have been outside the host cell for some time and compared it with that of parasites freshly released by lysis of host cells. Although this is not a good comparison with your experiments, both types seem to be equally fragile.

Nogueira: Parasites may not need to invade the host cell in order to survive; they may have the whole machinery for survival outside so that they could adapt to whatever environment they were in. In the host, the only way they could survive outside would be if they evolved mechanisms like the African trypanosomes, i.e. changing surface antigens to evade the host's immune response. So from the immunologist's point of view one need not ask what makes them obligate intracellular parasites. It need not be a biochemical difference but just a way of surviving in the host without killing the host as well.

Pfefferkorn: But in tissue culture we have completely eliminated the influence of the immune response and yet the parasites are unable to grow outside the host cell.

Nogueira: T. gondii can encyst and survive outside until they find a more favourable environment again. *T. cruzi* and *Leishmania* organisms can grow extracellularly according to the host they are in.

Warren: What about physical factors like pH—have you tried mimicking changes in some physical factors with your media?

Pfefferkorn: We have varied pH over the range of 6 to 8 and it seems to have no effect at all. We don't know the pH of the intravacuolar space, however.

Mirelman: Microenvironments for enzymic activity have been found to be extremely important. The work of Goldman et al (1968), using artificial membranes, revealed conditions of intracellular microenvironments that would provide the right milieu for enzyme activity. Perhaps these could be tried, by isolating membranes from the vacuoles, and hooking them onto polymeric carriers. This could provide the environment and would mean that one was not taking them all at once from inside the cell to a free medium, but was providing some artificial conditions that would be similar to those found in the vacuoles.

Pfefferkorn: That is an excellent suggestion. We find the vacuolar membrane to be exceedingly elusive. In our hands it is much more fragile than any other membranous components of the cell. Our efforts to purify something that represents fragments of the vacuolar membrane have not been successful.

Klebanoff: Perhaps you might look at 'professional' phagocytes, where the phagosome has been isolated in a number of instances. You might be able under those circumstances to have a preparation in which the organism is surrounded by the membrane but is essentially cell-free.

Pfefferkorn: That is possible, but the fate of *T. gondii* in professional phagocytes seems to follow two pathways. Those that enter by what one might call facilitated phagocytosis, or parasite-induced endocytosis, end up in a vacuole that does not fuse with lysosomes. On the other hand, those (perhaps already dead) that are phagocytosed by what one thinks of as classical phagocytosis are destroyed after lysosomal fusion.

Hudson: You mentioned looking for mutants that cannot invade host cells. David Snary and I (unpublished results) did some work on *T. cruzi* invasion into muscle cell tumours. We found, in essence, that amastigotes were released from host cells and never got back inside, but host and parasite cells both continued proliferating. I have always interpreted this as being because the amastigote had no active method of penetration, and that the muscle cells were not phagocytic. The interesting point, which is relevant to what Dr Nogueira was saying about sequestration being enough for the immunologist, is that the extracellular parasite under these conditions still had an absolute dependence on host cells. If we took the host cells away the parasite died.

Pfefferkorn: At least that is an easier problem to resolve because one is using an extracellular medium with identifiable components.

Gutteridge: The work of David Snary and Leslie Hudson may reveal a problem that is not necessarily related to the *in vivo* phenomenon of obligate intracellular development. The same problem has been observed in work on the cultivation of trypomastigotes of *Trypanosoma brucei*, an extracellular parasite: one has to have a monolayer of tissue cells to provide adequate growth *in vitro* at 37 °C.

Sher: One does not necessarily have to have cells around in order to grow amastigotes. Juan Carlos Engel, in Jim Dvorak's lab, has derived some lines of pure amastigotes that grow in regular cell-free medium (unpublished results). As long as the cell density is maintained at the right level, the organisms remain as amastigotes.

Hudson: The trouble with *T. cruzi* is that one can never be sure that one really has got amastigotes. We have spent three years trying to show that the extracellular amastigotes are immunochemically and biochemically similar to intracellular amastigotes.

Nogueira: In relation to what Dr Pfefferkorn has said about *T. gondii*, Jones et al (1972) showed initially that about 50% of the organisms ended up in phagolysosomes. The current thinking now, from work on acridine orange to study the viability of the organisms, is that those *T. gondii* were already killed. So in professionally phagocytic cells there is only one fate for viable *T. gondii*—the organisms are within phagosomes that are not fused with lysosomes. So it may be appropriate to study the role of the parasitophorous vacuole in survival.

REFERENCES

Goldman R, Kedem O, Silman HI, Kaplan SR, Katchalski E 1968 Papain collodion membranes. I: Preparation and properties. Biochemistry 7:486-500

Gutteridge WE 1981 *Trypanosoma cruzi*: recent biochemical advances. Trans R Soc Trop Med Hyg 75:484-492

Gutteridge WE, Rogerson GW 1979 Biochemical aspects of the biology of *Trypanosoma cruzi*. In: Lumsden WHR, Evans DA (eds) Biology of the kinetoplastida. Academic Press, London, vol 2:619-652

Gutteridge WE, Cover B, Gaborak M 1978 Isolation of blood and intracellular forms of *Trypanosoma cruzi* from infected rats and other rodents and preliminary studies of their metabolism. Parasitology 76:159-176

Jones TC, Yeh S, Hirsch JG 1972 The interaction between *Toxoplasma gondii* and mammalian cells. J Exp Med 136:1157-1172

Oxidative response of phagocytes to parasite invasion

S.J. KLEBANOFF, R. M. LOCKSLEY, E.C. JONG and H. ROSEN

Department of Medicine, Rm-16, University of Washington School of Medicine, Seattle, Washington 98195, USA

Abstract Phagocytes destroy intracellular pathogens and extracellular targets in part by the production of toxic oxygen metabolites—namely, superoxide, hydrogen peroxide, hydroxyl radicals and possibly singlet molecular oxygen. The toxicity of hydrogen peroxide is increased greatly by peroxidase and a halide. A peroxidase that can be used for this purpose is present in neutrophils and monocytes (myeloperoxidase), but is lost when the monocyte matures into a macrophage; a different peroxidase is present in eosinophils. The latter enzyme, because of its strong positive charge, binds to the surface of parasites; any phagocyte in the region, when appropriately stimulated, may provide the hydrogen peroxide required for completion of the peroxidase system. Further, peroxidase-coated organisms are more readily killed when ingested by macrophages than are uncoated organisms. Oxygen-dependent toxicity requires the production of toxic oxygen products by phagocytes in amounts sufficient to overcome the protective capacity of endogenous scavengers in the parasite. The latter include catalase and glutathione peroxidase, which degrade hydrogen peroxide, and superoxide dismutase which dissipates superoxide. The host defence against parasites appears to depend in part on this balance between toxic oxygen metabolites and scavengers.

1983 Cytopathology of parasitic disease. Pitman Books, London (Ciba Foundation symposium 99), p 92-112

The ability of phagocytes to destroy intracellular pathogens such as protozoa and extracellular targets such as helminths depends in part on the capacity of the phagocytes to generate toxic oxygen products, namely superoxide ($O_2^{\overline{\cdot}}$), hydrogen peroxide (H_2O_2), hydroxyl radicals ($OH^{\cdot}$) and, possibly, singlet molecular oxygen ($^1O_2$) (for review see Klebanoff 1982). All phagocytes (neutrophils, eosinophils, monocytes and macrophages) contain an enzyme or enzymes, which is dormant when the cell is at rest but is activated when the cell is exposed to an appropriate stimulus, with a resulting increase in oxygen consumption. Oxygen is reduced ultimately to water by the acceptance of four electrons. However, partial reduction can occur as follows:

$$O_2 \xrightarrow[e^-]{} O_2^{\overline{\cdot}} \xrightarrow[e^-]{} H_2O_2 \xrightarrow[e^-]{} OH^{\cdot} \xrightarrow[e^-]{} H_2O$$

with the formation of highly reactive intermediates. Excitation of oxygen to its singlet molecular form by phagocytes has also been proposed. The role of the respiratory burst and its oxygen products in the antiparasitic activity of phagocytes will be considered here.

Respiratory burst

The respiratory burst and, as a result, the level of toxic oxygen products correlate with the antiparasitic activity of phagocytes. Thus, resident macrophages have a weak respiratory burst as compared to granulocytes, and certain protozoa survive and replicate in these macrophages, whereas macrophages activated either *in vivo* or *in vitro* by lymphokines have both an increase in antiparasitic activity and in the respiratory burst (Murray et al 1979, Nathan et al 1979, Murray & Cohn 1980, Buchmuller & Mauel 1981, Haidaris & Bonventre 1982). Organisms vary in their ability to induce a respiratory burst and this may be one of the factors influencing their survival in the phagosome. Thus, the respiratory burst resulting from the ingestion of *Toxoplasma gondii* by macrophages is low (Wilson et al 1980, Murray & Cohn 1980) as compared to that produced by ingestion of *Leishmania* species (Murray 1981a). Although both *Leishmania donovani* promastigotes and amastigotes induce a respiratory burst in macrophages, the response to amastigotes is less than to promastigotes (Murray 1982a, Haidaris & Bonventre 1982, Pearson et al 1982), which correlates well with the greater susceptibility of promastigotes to the toxic systems of macrophages. Finally, macrophage cell lines with deficient oxidative activity (Murray 1981b, Tanaka et al 1982), phagocytes from patients with chronic granulomatous disease, which lack a respiratory burst (Wilson et al 1980, Chang 1981, Pearson & Steigbigel 1981, Kazura et al 1981, Locksley et al 1982), and macrophages depleted of the capacity to generate a respiratory burst by pretreatment with a strong stimulus (Murray 1982b) all have decreased antiparasitic activity. If, as these studies suggest, a respiratory burst is required for optimum destruction of parasites, what are the toxic oxygen species involved?

Superoxide anion

Oxygen initially accepts a single electron and is converted to the perhydroxyl radical ($HO_2^{\cdot}$) or its ionized form, the superoxide anion ($O_2^{\cdot-}$). The pK_a of the ionization is 4·8 so that the radical exists almost entirely as $O_2^{\cdot-}$ at neutral pH. $O_2^{\cdot-}$ is both a reductant and an oxidant. When it acts as a reductant, $O_2^{\cdot-}$ gives up an electron and is converted back to oxygen; when it acts as an oxidant, it accepts a second electron and is immediately protonated to form hydrogen peroxide (H_2O_2). When two radicals interact, one is oxidized and the other reduced to form O_2 and H_2O_2. This dismutation can occur spontaneously or be catalysed by the enzyme superoxide dismutase. Spontaneous dismutation occurs best at pH 4.8 where $HO_2^{\cdot}$ and $O_2^{\overline{\cdot}}$ are present in equal concentrations, so the reaction can best be written:

$$O_2^{\overline{\cdot}} + HO_2^{\cdot} + H^+ \rightarrow O_2 + H_2O_2$$

The rate of spontaneous dismutation falls as the pH is raised and $O_2^{\overline{\cdot}}$ predominates. Superoxide dismutase is catalytic over a wide pH range but its effect is most pronounced at neutral or alkaline pH where the rate of spontaneous dismutation is relatively low.

The role of $O_2^{\overline{\cdot}}$ as a primary toxic agent has been the subject of some controversy (Fridovich 1981, Fee 1981). The wide distribution of superoxide dismutase in nature raised the possibility that the primary function of this enzyme is to protect cells from the toxic effect of $O_2^{\overline{\cdot}}$, generated either endogenously or by adjacent cells such as phagocytes. Under some circumstances $O_2^{\overline{\cdot}}$ appears to be directly toxic. However, for many biologically important compounds the reaction with $O_2^{\overline{\cdot}}$ is exceedingly slow, suggesting that $O_2^{\overline{\cdot}}$ itself is not reactive enough to be directly toxic in most instances but, rather, that it exerts its toxicity through more distal oxygen products (Fig. 1).

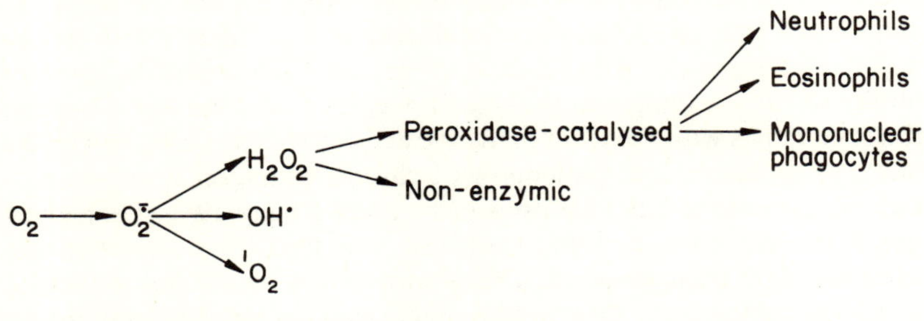

FIG. 1. Oxygen-dependent antimicrobial systems

Parasite superoxide dismutase can, theoretically, protect organisms from the direct toxicity of $O_2^{\overline{\cdot}}$ or from more distal oxygen products that depend on $O_2^{\overline{\cdot}}$ for their formation (see below). The role of endogenous superoxide dismutase in the resistance of parasites to cellular microbicidal systems is unclear. The majority of *Leishmania* promastigotes ingested by mouse peritoneal macrophages are killed, whereas *Toxoplasma* can replicate in these cells, despite the comparable levels of superoxide dismutase in the two organisms (Murray 1981a). *L. donovani* amastigotes have a higher level of superoxide dismutase than do promastigotes and are more resistant to destruction by macrophages. However, amastigotes also have higher levels of catalase and glutathione peroxidase which scavenge H_2O_2 (Murray 1982a). The superoxide dismutase of *Leishmania tropica* promastigotes has been partially characterized; it appears to differ in metal content from the host-cell enzymes (Meshnick & Eaton 1981).

Hydrogen peroxide

The dismutation of $O_2^{\dot{-}}$ results in the formation of H_2O_2. Spontaneous dismutation would be expected to be rapid particularly if, as has been proposed, the pH progressively falls in the phagosome. Superoxide dismutase is present in phagocytes, but there is no evidence that this cellular enzyme is discharged into the phagosome. Superoxide dismutase can, however, be introduced as a component of the ingested microorganism. The protective role of superoxide dismutase in parasites is considered elsewhere in this paper; there is currently no evidence that superoxide dismutase, by catalysing the conversion of $O_2^{\dot{-}}$ to H_2O_2, increases toxicity. The dismutation of $O_2^{\dot{-}}$ to H_2O_2 does not appear to be a limiting factor in the microbicidal activity of phagocytes.

H_2O_2 generated by phagocytes has been implicated in their antiparasitic activity. Thus, when compared to *Toxoplasma gondii*, both *L. tropica* and *L. donovani* promastigotes are more sensitive to H_2O_2, and both contain comparable levels of superoxide dismutase but considerably lower levels of catalase and glutathione peroxidase than do *Toxoplasma*. Possibly as a result, most *Leishmania* promastigotes are killed and digested by resident mouse peritoneal macrophages under conditions in which intracellular *Toxoplasma* replicate. Either added catalase or glucose deprivation (which decreases H_2O_2 production) inhibit the leishmanicidal activity of the macrophages, whereas superoxide dismutase, the $OH^{\cdot}$ scavengers mannitol and benzoate, and the $^1O_2$ scavengers triethylenediamine (DABCO) and histidine do not (Murray 1981a). Similarly, addition of catalase and deprivation of glucose inhibit the leishmanicidal activity of the lymphokine-treated macrophage cell line J774G8 but neither superoxide dismutase nor $OH^{\cdot}$ scavengers do so (Murray 1981b). A variant macrophage cell line defective in the respiratory burst was also unable to kill epimastigotes of *Trypanosoma cruzi* under conditions in which the parental cell line was effective (Tanaka et al 1982). The antiparasitic activity of the variant cells could be reconstituted by phagocytosis of zymosan particles that had glucose oxidase covalently linked to their surface. Glucose oxidase, when provided with its substrate, glucose, generates H_2O_2 without the intermediate formation of superoxide, suggesting that H_2O_2 is the effective oxygen species under these conditions.

When compared to other toxic products formed by phagocytes (e.g. $OH^{\cdot}$ and hypochlorous acid), the reactivity of H_2O_2 is rather low. This relative weakness gives to H_2O_2 an important property; it can pass through complex biological fluids, rebounding intact from collisions, to be toxic at a distance under conditions in which the more reactive oxygen products are readily scavenged. Thus, in one study (Bass & Szejda 1979), the newborn larvae of *Trichinella spiralis*, suspended in a complex medium containing serum, were sensitive to H_2O_2-generating systems. This toxicity was not potentiated by the addition of peroxidase-positive eosinophil or neutrophil granule preparations despite the ability of peroxidases to increase the toxicity of H_2O_2 by many orders of magnitude (see below). The highly reactive products of the peroxidase system are more readily scavenged than is the less reactive H_2O_2. Therefore the addition of peroxidase to H_2O_2 in a complex medium, by utilization of H_2O_2 to form products that are subsequently scavenged, might be expected to inhibit rather than to potentiate the toxicity of H_2O_2, and this has indeed been observed (Bass & Szejda 1979). Similarly toxicity may be decreased by conversion of H_2O_2 to the more reactive $OH^{\cdot}$, if the latter species are immediately scavenged by components of the reaction mixture.

This emphasizes the importance of the microenvironment in the interaction between phagocyte and parasite. Certainly, if toxicity is to occur at a distance through a fluid rich in protein and other scavengers, then H_2O_2 would be expected to be the chief, perhaps only, oxygen product that is toxic. However, when oxygen products are formed where there is close apposition between phagocyte and parasite, as would occur within a phagosome or when phagocytes adhere to the surface of the target, then distances are short and protein and other scavengers may be excluded, thus favouring the involvement of the more reactive oxygen products in the toxicity.

The sensitivity of parasites to H_2O_2 varies widely, and among the factors that influence sensitivity is the concentration of scavengers of H_2O_2 in the parasite. The scavengers are cellular components that react with H_2O_2 to form harmless products. Cells have devised mechanisms for protection against H_2O_2 formed endogenously or by adjacent phagocytes. Chief among these mechanisms are the presence of catalase, which breaks down H_2O_2 to oxygen and water and, in some cells at least, the presence of the more important glutathione cycle (Fig. 2). The latter is a sequence of reactions initiated by the oxidation of glutathione by H_2O_2, catalysed by glutathione peroxidase. The oxidized glutathione formed is then reduced by glutathione reductase in the presence of NADPH, with the latter being oxidized to NADP, which drives the hexose monophosphate shunt. The first two enzymes of the hexose monophosphate shunt, glucose-6-phosphate dehydrogenase and 6-phosphogluconate dehydrogenase reduce NADP to NADPH and the continued activity of the shunt depends on the reoxidation of

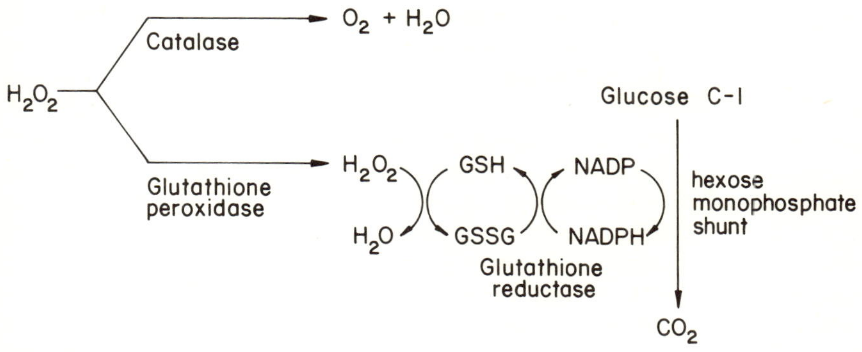

FIG. 2. Cellular protection from H_2O_2

NADPH. The hexose monophosphate shunt is thus an escape valve for the protection of the cell from excess H_2O_2, with the oxidation of the first carbon of glucose to CO_2 as evidence that this escape valve is being used.

Parasites vary in their concentration of these scavenging systems and this has been correlated with sensitivity to H_2O_2. Thus, *T. gondii* are rich in catalase and glutathione peroxidase and are relatively resistant to destruction by H_2O_2 (Murray et al 1980). In contrast, *L. donovani* or *L. tropica* promastigotes contain 100-fold less catalase and glutathione peroxidase than *Toxoplasma* and they are considerably more susceptible to the toxic effect of H_2O_2 (Murray 1981a). Furthermore, *L. donovani* amastigotes have higher levels of catalase and glutathione peroxidase than do promastigotes, and they are correspondingly more resistant to H_2O_2 and to the toxic activity of macrophages (Murray 1982a).

Potentiation of the toxicity of H_2O_2 by peroxidase

The toxicity of H_2O_2 is increased many fold by peroxidase and a halide, a catalysis which is of special interest because peroxidases are present in high concentration in the cytoplasmic granules of some phagocytes. Cells containing a granule peroxidase can release this enzyme into the phagosome, or under some conditions into the extracellular fluid, where it reacts with H_2O_2 generated by the phagocytosis-induced respiratory burst to form an enzyme–substrate complex which oxidizes the halide to a toxic agent or agents. The halide used can be chloride, bromide, iodide or the pseudohalide thiocyanate, with the effectiveness of the halide varying, to some degree, with the peroxidase. The primary product formed, at least for some halides, appears to be the corresponding hypohalous acid with toxicity resulting from halogenation and oxidation of cell-surface components.

Neutrophil. The azurophil (or primary) granules of the neutrophil contain a peroxidase (myeloperoxidase) in high concentration, and this enzyme has been implicated in the microbicidal activity of the cell. Certain parasites are ingested and killed by neutrophils, and in some instances the peroxidase system has been implicated. Thorne et al (1978) found that trypomastigotes and epimastigotes of *Trypanosoma dionisii*, bat-infecting trypanosomes similar to *T. cruzi*, are readily killed by myeloperoxidase and H_2O_2. They also found that *T. dionisii* destruction by intact neutrophils is associated with H_2O_2 production and is prevented by peroxidase inhibitors. They conclude that the neutrophils are toxic to the trypanosomes via the peroxidase system. Similarly, Pearson & Steigbigel (1981) and Chang (1981) have reported that *L. donovani* amastigotes or promastigotes are ingested and killed by human neutrophils and by the isolated peroxidase system. Chang (1981) detected both H_2O_2 and peroxidase in the phagosome by cytochemical techniques and concluded that this system was responsible for the toxicity. The schistosomula of *Schistosoma mansoni* also are killed by the myeloperoxidase–H_2O_2–halide system (Jong et al 1981), and by intact neutrophils in the presence of specific antibody and complement. In one study (Kazura et al 1981), neutrophil-mediated killing of schistosomula was inhibited by catalase and by the haemoprotein inhibitors azide, cyanide and aminotriazole, thus implicating the peroxidase system. The killing of schistosomula by neutrophils is increased when the organisms are pre-coated with eosinophil peroxidase (Jong et al 1982).

Eosinophil. Eosinophils contain a peroxidase in high concentration in cytoplasmic granules, and this enzyme differs from the myeloperoxidase of neutrophils (and monocytes) in its structure and properties. However, like myeloperoxidase, eosinophil peroxidase combines with H_2O_2 and a halide to form an antiparasitic system. Among the parasites susceptible to the cell-free eosinophil peroxidase–H_2O_2–halide system are the schistosomula of *S. mansoni* (Jong et al 1981), the newborn larvae of *T. spiralis* (Buys et al 1981), *T. cruzi* trypomastigotes (Nogueira et al 1982), *T. gondii* (Locksley et al 1982) and the amastigotes and promastigotes of *L. tropica* (R. M. Locksley, C. A. Nacy & S. J. Klebanoff, unpublished data). Eosinophil peroxidase is considerably less effective with chloride (relative to iodide or bromide) than is myeloperoxidase; however chloride can be used as the halide particularly at low pH and relatively high enzyme concentrations (Jong et al 1981, Buys et al 1981).

Eosinophil peroxidase is a highly basic protein which, when preincubated with the target cells, binds firmly to their surface. Targets coated in this way are readily killed after the addition of H_2O_2 and a halide. This has been observed with *Staphylococcus aureus* (Ramsey et al 1982), *T. gondii*

(Locksley et al 1982), *T. cruzi* (Nogueira et al 1982), *L. tropica* (R. M. Locksley, C. A. Nacy & S. J. Klebanoff, unpublished data), schistosomula of *S. mansoni* (Jong et al 1982) and tumour cells (Nathan & Klebanoff 1982). The data from *L. tropica* are shown in Table 1. Protein strongly inhibits the

TABLE 1 Binding of eosinophil peroxidase to *Leishmania* and sensitivity of the complex to added H_2O_2 and iodide[a]

	Percent viable	
Supplements	*Amastigote*	*Promastigote*
LT/EPO	77 ± 5 (8)[b]	93 ± 2 (4)
LT/EPO + H_2O_2	77 ± 4 (6)	90 ± 5 (4)
LT/EPO + iodide	78 ± 3 (6)	92 ± 6 (2)
LT/EPO + H_2O_2 + iodide	2 ± 3 (8)	1 ± 3 (4)
LT/EPO + H_2O_2 + iodide + azide	74 ± 7 (4)	88 ± 3 (4)
LT/EPO + H_2O_2 + iodide + aminotriazole	68 ± 9 (4)	91 ± 4 (4)
LT/EPO + H_2O_2 + iodide + catalase	77 ± 2 (4)	86 ± 7 (4)

[a]*L. tropica* (LT) amastigotes (81% viable) or promastigotes (99% viable) were coated with eosinophil peroxidase (EPO) by preincubation (Locksley et al 1982) and 5×10^6 of the coated organisms (LT/EPO) were incubated for 60 min (amastigotes) or 30 min (promastigotes) in 0.1 M-sodium phosphate buffer at pH 7.0 in a final volume of 0.5 ml with the supplements shown, as follows: H_2O_2, 5×10^{-5} M (amastigotes) or 10^{-5} M (promastigotes); potassium iodide, 10^{-5} M; sodium azide, 10^{-3} M; aminotriazole, 10^{-3} M; catalase, 60 μg/ml. Viability was determined by acridine orange–ethidium bromide staining (Locksley et al 1982). [b]Mean ± 1 SEM of (n) experiments.

toxicity of the free peroxidase–H_2O_2–halide system, presumably by competing with the target cell for the toxic products of the peroxidase system. Protein inhibition, however, is considerably reduced when the peroxidase is bound to the target-cell surface (Nathan & Klebanoff 1982, Jong et al 1982).

Intact eosinophils are toxic to certain parasites, and in some instances the peroxidase system has been implicated. For example, eosinophils are potent effector cells against the schistosomula of *S. mansoni* (Dessein & David 1982), and in one study (Kazura et al 1981) this toxicity was associated with H_2O_2 production, was decreased when chronic granulomatous disease leucocytes were used, and was inhibited by the addition of catalase or the peroxidase inhibitors azide and aminotriazole. Pincus et al (1981), however, could not detect a decrease in the antischistosomal activity of eosinophils on the addition of catalase or by the substitution of anaerobic for aerobic conditions. Eosinophils incubated with antibody-coated schistosomula adhere to their surfaces. Degranulation occurs and peroxidase can be detected on the surface of the organisms by electron microscope cytochemistry (McLaren et al 1977).

Mononuclear phagocytes. Peroxidase-positive granules are present in the blood monocyte of most species; they are, however, fewer in number than in the neutrophil. The monocyte peroxidase appears to be identical to that of the neutrophil, i.e. myeloperoxidase. The antiparasitic activity of monocytes is, in general, intermediate between that of neutrophils and resident macrophages and, in some instances, the peroxidase system has been implicated as a contributor to the toxicity. Thorne et al (1981) found that monocytes are able to kill *T. dionisii* epimastigotes but not trypomastigotes, whereas both forms are killed readily by neutrophils. They concluded that the decreased activity of monocytes is due to the lower level of H_2O_2 and myeloperoxidase in these cells. Human monocytes were found by Wilson et al (1980) to ingest and kill *T. gondii* in contrast to their survival and replication in resident mouse peritoneal macrophages. Monocytes from patients with chronic granulomatous disease have a decreased phagocytosis-induced respiratory burst and an impaired toxoplasmacidal activity, thus implicating oxygen-dependent antimicrobial systems (Wilson et al 1980, Locksley et al 1982). A contribution by the myeloperoxidase-mediated antimicrobial system was suggested by an early defect in toxoplasmacidal activity in leucocytes with a genetic absence of myeloperoxidase; this defect was not seen when organisms coated with eosinophil peroxidase were used (Locksley et al 1982).

Peroxidase-positive granules are retained for a time after monocytes have passed into the interstitial space, and peroxidase can be found in the phagosomes of these tissue monocytes. Since many of the mononuclear phagocytes present in granulomatous lesions have recently emigrated from the bloodstream, peroxidase may contribute to their toxic activity. However, as the monocyte matures into a macrophage, either *in vivo* or *in vitro*, the granule peroxidase is lost as is this mechanism for amplifying the toxicity of H_2O_2.

Mature macrophages can acquire peroxidase by endocytosis; that is, by the pinocytosis of fluid-phase peroxidase or by the phagocytosis of particulate peroxidase. An example of the latter is the ingestion of organisms with peroxidase on their surface. As indicated above, the positively-charged eosinophil peroxidase binds by ionic linkage to negatively-charged surface components of parasites (as well as of other targets), and the organisms coated in this way become exquisitely sensitive to the toxic effect of added H_2O_2 and a halide. The organisms are also more readily killed by macrophages. Thus, *T. gondii* normally survive and replicate in resident mouse peritoneal macrophages. These cells have a weak respiratory burst and lack a granule peroxidase and thus are unable to utilize endogenous peroxidase to amplify the microbicidal activity of the small amount of H_2O_2 formed. However, when the macrophages ingest *Toxoplasma* coated with eosinophil peroxidase, there is significant toxoplasmacidal activity which is inhibited by the haemoprotein inhibitors aminotriazole and azide (Locksley et al 1982). The coated organisms are ingested by the macrophages at a normal rate.

T. cruzi trypomastigotes also survive ingestion by normal mouse peritoneal macrophages. The trypomastigotes, however, are killed by macrophages activated *in vivo* or *in vitro* by lymphokines, and this increased trypanocidal activity correlates well with the amount of H_2O_2 released on stimulation of the cells with phorbol myristate acetate (Nathan et al 1979). The trypanocidal activity of resident mouse peritoneal macrophages or of human monocyte-derived macrophages is also increased by coating the trypomastigotes with eosinophil peroxidase prior to ingestion (Nogueira et al 1982). The killing of coated trypomastigotes by mouse peritoneal macrophages is inhibited by catalase and azide, implicating the peroxidase system. When the phagocytic load is increased either by adding a large multiplicity of coated organisms or by the simultaneous addition of a second particle (e.g. opsonized zymosan), extracellular killing of *T. cruzi* occurs, suggesting reaction of the surface peroxidase with the H_2O_2 released into the medium by the high phagocytic load to form a trypanocidal system. H_2O_2 formed by the trypanosomes may also contribute to the toxicity. As with the other targets, *T. cruzi* trypomastigotes coated with eosinophil peroxidase are readily killed by H_2O_2 and iodide; however, in this instance deletion of H_2O_2 decreases but does not abolish the toxicity. The residual toxicity in the absence of added H_2O_2 is prevented by the addition of catalase, suggesting the formation of H_2O_2 by the parasite and its utilization as a component of a cytotoxic system in the presence of surface-bound peroxidase.

The studies described above indicate that eosinophil peroxidase bound to the surface of certain pathogens can increase the susceptibility of the organisms to the H_2O_2 formed by phagocytes. Can parasites acquire peroxidase on their surface from intact eosinophils? A morphological study by Sanderson & De Souza (1979) of the interaction between *T. cruzi* trypomastigotes and rat neutrophils, eosinophils and macrophages may be relevant to this. The trypomastigotes were transformed into the intracellular amastigote form in the phagosome of macrophages and they replicated. Transformation to amastigotes also occurred in neutrophils, but in these cells degeneration of the organism rapidly followed, and was associated with the accumulation of material of granule origin in the phagosome. The trypomastigotes were also ingested by eosinophils in the presence of specific antibody and, as in the neutrophil, they were transformed to the amastigote form in the phagosome; electron-dense material, which appeared to be of granule origin, accumulated around the ingested organism. However, in the eosinophil preparation, the organisms appeared to be expelled, since amastigotes coated with a layer of granule material similar to that seen accumulating in the phagosomes were found in the extracellular fluid. Should these organisms contain eosinophil peroxidase on their surface, as seems likely, then this enzyme would be available to macrophages (or other phagocytes) for use in the destruction of the ingested organism. Peroxidase also can be released from intact eosinophils by exocytosis or cell lysis, and may bind to the surface of an adjacent parasite. Under these conditions, any phagocyte in the region, neutrophil, eosinophil or macrophage, when appropriately stimulated, may serve as the source of H_2O_2 for the cytotoxic system.

These findings indicate that peroxidase bound to the surface of certain pathogens can increase their susceptibility to the H_2O_2 formed by macrophages. Does this mechanism for potentiation of macrophage toxicity operate *in vivo* against intracellular parasites, particularly in infections where eosinophils are not the major cellular component of the inflammatory response? This question cannot yet be answered.

Hydroxyl radicals

A second mechanism by which the toxicity of H_2O_2 may be increased is by reaction with ferrous (Fe^{2+}) ions (Fenton's reagent) to form OH as follows:

$$H_2O_2 + Fe^{2+} \rightarrow Fe^{3} + OH^- + OH^{\cdot}$$

The conversion of H_2O_2 to $OH^{\cdot}$ can go to completion when the Fe^{2+} concentration is equal to, or greater than, that of H_2O_2. However when the Fe^{2+} concentration is limiting, the reduction of the ferric ion (Fe^{3+}) formed is needed for the complete degradation of H_2O_2. This can be accomplished by $O_2^{\overline{\cdot}}$ as follows:

$$\begin{array}{c} H_2O_2 + Fe^{2+} \rightarrow Fe^{3+} + OH^- + OH^{\cdot} \\ \underline{O_2^{\overline{\cdot}} + Fe^{3+} \rightarrow Fe^{2+} + O_2} \\ H_2O_2 + O_2^{\overline{\cdot}} \rightarrow O_2 + OH^- + OH^{\cdot} \end{array}$$

The latter reaction has been termed the Haber-Weiss reaction and from it has come the working hypothesis that when microbicidal activity is initiated by a $O_2^{\overline{\cdot}}$-generating system, and is inhibited by superoxide dismutase, catalase and $OH^{\cdot}$ scavengers such as mannitol and ethanol, this can be taken as presumptive evidence that $OH^{\cdot}$ generated by the Haber–Weiss reaction is required (Rosen & Klebanoff 1979, 1981). Since both H_2O_2 and $O_2^{\overline{\cdot}}$ are generated by phagocytes, it might be anticipated that their interaction in a metal-catalysed Haber–Weiss reaction would result in the generation of $OH^{\cdot}$ and, indeed, a number of investigators have reported the generation of $OH^{\cdot}$ by stimulated phagocytes (Klebanoff 1982).

Do $OH^{\cdot}$ contribute to the antiparasitic activity of phagocytes? Supporting evidence comes from studies with model systems. *T. gondii*, for example, are killed by the xanthine + xanthine oxidase system, and this toxicity is inhibited by catalase, superoxide dismutase and the $OH^{\cdot}$ scavengers mannitol and benzoate, implicating $OH^{\cdot}$ in the toxicity (Murray & Cohn 1979). Intact macrophages from chronically infected immune mice or these mice immune-boosted by an intraperitoneal injection of heat-killed *Toxoplasma* are also toxic to *T. gondii*. This toxicity is decreased by the same inhibitors that inhibit the toxoplasmacidal activity of the xanthine oxidase system (Murray et al 1979). Although *in vitro*-activated macrophages have increased production of O_2^{-} and H_2O_2, they do not exhibit antitoxoplasma activity unless the macrophages are co-cultivated with lymphokine and brain–heart infusion broth (Murray & Cohn 1980). Scavengers of O_2^{-}, H_2O_2 and $OH^{\cdot}$ inhibit the antitoxoplasma activity. Finally, the presence of scavengers such as superoxide dismutase, glutathione peroxidase and catalase in the *Toxoplasma* and in the phagocyte may help to determine the outcome of the interaction between parasite and host cell (Murray et al 1980). These studies suggest that under some conditions $OH^{\cdot}$ can contribute to the antitoxoplasma activity of intact macrophages.

Singlet oxygen

The formation of $^1O_2$ by phagocytes and its role in the cidal activity of the cell has not yet been definitively established. Singlet oxygen is an excited state of oxygen which is formed when an absorption of energy shifts one of the unpaired valence electrons of oxygen to an orbital of higher energy, with an accompanying inversion of spin (Klebanoff 1982). That $^1O_2$ can be toxic is suggested by the photodynamic action of dyes, a process by which certain dyes in the presence of light and oxygen are toxic to cells, partly through the formation of $^1O_2$. Singlet oxygen can dissipate its excess energy by the emission of light. Interest in the possible formation of $^1O_2$ by phagocytes stemmed from the finding of chemiluminescence by stimulated phagocytes (Allen et al 1972). However, chemiluminescence *per se* is not a measure of $^1O_2$ formation but, rather, of the formation of an excited state. Analyses to date have not revealed the characteristic spectrum of $^1O_2$ decay but a rather broad peak activity. The products of the respiratory burst would be expected to react with cell or particle components to form excited products and it is presumably the decay of these secondary excitations that is responsible for the light emission. Additional evidence for the formation of $^1O_2$ would be the detection of a specific singlet oxygen product after incubation of phagocytes with an appropriate substrate. This has not yet been done.

Both the formation of $^1O_2$ by the Haber–Weiss reaction

$$O_2^{\cdot -} + H_2O_2 \rightarrow {}^1O_2 + OH^- + OH^{\cdot}$$

and its involvement in toxicity have been proposed on the basis of inhibition of toxicity by agents that scavenge $^1O_2$ (Kellogg & Fridovich 1977, Rosen & Klebanoff 1979). The destruction of *T. gondii* by the xanthine oxidase system (Murray & Cohn 1979) and by macrophages (Murray et al 1979, Murray & Cohn 1980) is inhibited by both OH and $^1O_2$ scavengers, suggesting that both these products of the Haber–Weiss reaction may be involved. Some caution however should be exercised, as the $^1O_2$-scavengers lack absolute specificity.

In summary, we have considered the role of oxygen products in the antiparasitic activity of phagocytes. Although accumulating evidence suggests that these agents play an important part in host defence against parasites, we must emphasize that other oxygen-independent antimicrobial systems are also involved. The most extensively studied of these are the basic proteins of eosinophils, which are toxic to the schistosomula of *S. mansoni*, the newborn larvae of *T. spiralis* and the trypomastigotes of *T. cruzi* (Ackerman et al 1982), and which presumably contribute to the toxicity of the intact cell. The release of arginase by activated macrophages has also been implicated in antischistosomal activity (Olds et al 1980). These findings indicate that phagocytes contain a variety of antimicrobial systems effective against parasites but that the parasites in turn have devised a number of mechanisms for evasion of the host response. The outcome may be the eradication of infection, a symbiosis as indicated by infection without evidence of illness, or the overt signs of disease.

Acknowledgements

Grant support from the National Institutes of Health, the Rockefeller Foundation and the Edna McConnell Clark Foundation, and the secretarial assistance of Caroline Wilson, are very gratefully acknowledged.

REFERENCES

Ackerman SJ, Durack DT, Gleich GJ 1982 Eosinophil effector mechanisms in health and disease. In: Gallin JI, Fauci AS (eds) Advances in host defense mechanisms. Raven Press, New York, vol 1:269-293

Allen RC, Stjernholm RL, Steele RH 1972 Evidence for the generation of an electronic excitation state(s) in human polymorphonuclear leukocytes and its participation in bactericidal activity. Biochem Biophys Res Commun 47:679–684

Bass DA, Szejda P 1979 Mechanisms of killing of newborn larvae of *Trichinella spiralis* by neutrophils and eosinophils. Killing by generators of hydrogen peroxide *in vitro*. J Clin Invest 64:1558–1564

Buchmuller Y, Mauel J 1981 Studies on the mechanisms of macrophage activation: possible involvement of oxygen metabolites in killing of *Leishmania enriettii* by activated mouse macrophages. J Reticuloendothel Soc 29:181-192

Buys J, Wever R, van Stigt R, Ruitenberg EJ 1981 The killing of newborn larvae of *Trichinella spiralis* by eosinophil peroxidase *in vitro*. Eur J Immunol 11:843-845

Chang K-P 1981 Leishmanicidal mechanisms of human polymorphonuclear phagocytes. Am J Trop Med Hyg 30:322-333

Dessein AJ, David JR 1982 The eosinophil in parasitic diseases. In: Gallin JI, Fauci AS (eds) Advances in host defense mechanisms. Raven Press, New York, vol 1:243-268

Fee JA 1981 Is superoxide toxic and are superoxide dismutases essential for aerobic life? In: Rogers MAJ, Powers EL (eds) Oxygen and oxy-radicals in chemistry and biology. Academic Press, New York, p 205-221

Fridovich I 1981 The biology of superoxide and of superoxide dismutase—in brief. In: Rogers MAJ, Powers EL (eds) Oxygen and oxy-radicals in chemistry and biology. Academic Press, New York, p 197-204

Haidaris CG, Bonventre PF 1982 A role for oxygen-dependent mechanisms in killing of *Leishmania donovani* tissue forms by activated macrophages. J Immunol 129:850-855

Jong EC, Mahmoud AAF, Klebanoff SJ 1981 Peroxidase-mediated toxicity to schistosomula of *Schistosoma mansoni*. J Immunol 126:468-471

Jong EC, Chi EY, Klebanoff SJ 1982 Human neutrophil-mediated killing of schistosomula of *Schistosoma mansoni*: augmentation by schistosomal binding of eosinophil peroxidase. Clin Res 30:370A

Kazura JW, Fanning MM, Blumer JL, Mahmoud AAF 1981 Role of cell-generated hydrogen peroxide in granulocyte-mediated killing of schistosomula of *Schistosoma mansoni in vitro*. J Clin Invest 67:93-102

Kellogg EW III, Fridovich I 1977 Liposome oxidation and erythrocyte lysis by enzymically generated superoxide and hydrogen peroxide. J Biol Chem 252:6721-6728

Klebanoff SJ 1982 Oxygen dependent cytotoxic mechanisms of phagocytes. In: Gallin JI, Fauci AS (eds) Advances in host defense mechanisms. Raven Press, New York, vol 1: 111-162

Locksley RM, Wilson CB, Klebanoff SJ 1982 Role of endogenous and acquired peroxidase in the toxoplasmacidal activity of murine and human mononuclear phagocytes. J Clin Invest 69:1099-1111

McLaren DJ, Mackenzie CD, Ramalho-Pinto FJ 1977 Ultrastructural observations on the *in vitro* interaction between rat eosinophils and some parasitic helminths (*Schistosoma mansoni, Trichinella spiralis* and *Nippostrongylus brasiliensis*). Clin Exp Immunol 30:105-118

Meshnick SR, Eaton JW 1981 Leishmanial superoxide dismutase: a possible target for chemotherapy. Biochem Biophys Res Commun 102:970-976

Murray HW 1981a Susceptibility of Leishmania to oxygen intermediates and killing by normal macrophages. J Exp Med 153:1302-1315

Murray HW 1981b Interaction of *Leishmania* with a macrophage cell line. Correlation between intracellular killing and the generation of oxygen intermediates. J Exp Med 153:1690-1695

Murray HW 1982a Cell-mediated immune response in experimental visceral leishmaniasis. II: Oxygen-dependent killing of intracellular *Leishmania donovani* amastigotes. J Immunol 129:351-357

Murray HW 1982b Pretreatment with phorbol myristate acetate inhibits macrophage activity against intracellular protozoa. J Reticuloendothel Soc 31:479-487

Murray HW, Cohn ZA 1979 Macrophage oxygen-dependent antimicrobial activity. I: Susceptibility of *Toxoplasma gondii* to oxygen intermediates. J Exp Med 150:938-949

Murray HW, Cohn ZA 1980 Macrophage oxygen-dependent antimicrobial activity. III: Enhanced oxidative metabolism as an expression of macrophage activation. J Exp Med 152:1596-1609

Murray HW, Juangbhanich CW, Nathan CF, Cohn ZA 1979 Macrophage oxygen-dependent antimicrobial activity. II: The role of oxygen intermediates. J Exp Med 150:950–964

Murray HW, Nathan CF, Cohn ZA 1980 Macrophage oxygen-dependent antimicrobial activity. IV: Role of endogenous scavengers of oxygen intermediates. J Exp Med 152:1610-1624

Nathan CF, Klebanoff SJ 1982 Augmentation of spontaneous macrophage-mediated cytolysis by eosinophil peroxidase. J Exp Med 155:1291-1308

Nathan C, Nogueira N, Juangbhanich C, Ellis J, Cohn Z 1979 Activation of macrophages *in vivo* and *in vitro*. Correlation between hydrogen peroxide release and killing of *Trypanosoma cruzi*. J Exp Med 149:1056-1068

Nogueira NM, Klebanoff SJ, Cohn ZA 1982 *T. cruzi*: sensitization to macrophage killing by eosinophil peroxidase. J Immunol 128:1705-1708

Olds GR, Ellner JJ, Kearse LA Jr, Kazura JW, Mahmoud AAF 1980 Role of arginase in killing of schistosomula of *Schistosoma mansoni*. J Exp Med 151:1557-1562

Pearson RD, Steigbigel RT 1981 Phagocytosis and killing of the protozoan *Leishmania donovani* by human polymorponuclear leukocytes. J Immunol 127:1438-1443

Pearson RD, Harcus JL, Symes PH, Romito R, Donowitz GR 1982 Failure of the phagocytic oxidative response to protect human monocyte-derived macrophages from infection by *Leishmania donovani*. J Immunol 129:1282-1286

Pincus SH, Butterworth AE, David JR, Robbins M, Vadas MA 1981 Antibody-dependent eosinophil-mediated damage to schistosomula of *Schistosoma mansoni*: lack of requirement for oxidative metabolism. J Immunol 126:1794-1799

Ramsey PG, Martin T, Chi E, Klebanoff SJ 1982 Arming of mononuclear phagocytes by eosinophil peroxidase bound to *Staphylococcus aureus*. J Immunol 128:415-420

Rosen H, Klebanoff SJ 1979 Bactericidal activity of a superoxide anion generating system. A model for the polymorphonuclear leukocyte. J Exp Med 149:27-39

Rosen H, Klebanoff SJ 1981 Role of iron and ethylenediaminetetraacetic acid in the bactericidal activity of a superoxide anion-generating system. Arch Biochem Biophys 208:512-519

Sanderson CJ, De Souza W 1979 A morphological study of the interaction between *Trypanosoma cruzi* and rat eosinophils, neutrophils and macrophages *in vitro*. J Cell Sci 37:275-286

Tanaka Y, Kiyotaki C, Tanowitz H, Bloom BR 1982 Reconstitution of a variant macrophage cell line defective in oxygen metabolism with a H_2O_2-generating system. Proc Natl Acad Sci USA 79:2584-2588

Thorne KJI, Svvennsen RJ, Franks D 1978 Role of hydrogen peroxide and peroxidase in the cytotoxicity of *Trypanosoma dionisii* by human granulocytes. Infect Immun 21:798-805

Thorne KJI, Glauert AM, Svvennsen RJ, Thomas H, Morris J, Franks D 1981 Evasion of the oxidative microbicidal activity of human monocytes by trypomastigotes of *Trypanosoma dionisii*. Parasitology 83:115-123

Wilson CB, Tsai V, Remington JS 1980 Failure to trigger the oxidative metabolic burst by normal macrophages. Possible mechanism for survival of intracellular pathogens. J Exp Med 151:328-346

DISCUSSION

Warren: You mentioned the relatively small effect of superoxide on parasites and the important role of hydrogen peroxide. Superoxide dismutase is responsible for the production of H_2O_2, which is toxic and an intermediate for even more toxic substances. So the enzyme seems to increase toxicity and yet you raised the question of whether it *decreases* toxicity. Kazura & Meshnick (1982) recently suggested that the more superoxide dismutase and glutathione peroxidase present, the more protected are certain parasitic organisms against the oxygen-derived toxins.

Klebanoff: Superoxide dismutase can theoretically have two effects on toxicity. By catalysing the dismutation reaction and increasing the formation of H_2O_2 it could increase toxicity if H_2O_2 is the crucial toxic product. Spontaneous dismutation is very rapid, particularly at the acid pH reported to be in the phagosome (Jensen & Bainton 1973), and which presumably exists in the pocket of space between an adherent cell and a target too large to be ingested. Under these conditions catalysis by superoxide dismutase may not be biologically important. But it can be important if a substance that can scavenge the superoxide anion is present, such as cytochrome *c*. Using an isolated system, we were able to show that by adding cytochrome *c* one can inhibit the toxicity of the xanthine–xanthine oxidase–myeloperoxidase–chloride system, and that superoxide dismutase increased toxicity under these conditions by preventing this inhibition (Klebanoff 1974). Cytochrome *c* oxidizes superoxide to oxygen and this inhibits its spontaneous dismutation to H_2O_2, a component of the peroxidase system. Superoxide dismutase, by successfully competing with cytochrome *c* for superoxide, increases toxicity by catalysing the formation of H_2O_2.

The second mechanism by which superoxide dismutase can affect the toxicity is by inhibiting the generation of more distal oxygen products such as hydroxyl radicals. The superoxide anion may be toxic under some circumstances but, even more important, it can react with H_2O_2 in a metal-catalysed reaction to form hydroxyl radicals. If one adds superoxide dismutase under conditions in which hydroxyl radicals are the chief toxic agent, then the enzyme will inhibit toxicity by preventing the formation of this toxic agent. Thus, superoxide dismutase can theoretically have either a stimulatory or an inhibitory effect on the toxicity of oxygen metabolites.

Studies in which the levels of scavenging enzymes have been measured have, by and large, not emphasized the importance of the superoxide dismutase level. Promastigotes of *Leishmania* species and *Toxoplasma gondii*, for example, have almost the same levels of superoxide dismutase, whereas the *Leishmania* promastigotes are much more susceptible to destruction by macrophages (Murray 1981). On the other hand, the levels of the H_2O_2 scavengers—catalase and glutathione peroxidase—are considerably higher in *T. gondii* than in *Leishmania* species. Thus, in these studies, the levels of H_2O_2 scavengers correlate more closely with the protection of the organism from the toxic systems of macrophages than does the level of superoxide dismutase.

Wyler: In our hands, phorbol myristate acetate (PMA)-stimulated macrophages do not apparently kill intracellular leishmanial amastigotes and yet they presumably do produce hydrogen peroxide (D.J. Wyler, unpublished observations). Further macrophages, from individuals with chronic granulomatous disease, which are stimulated with lymphokine *in vitro* appear able to kill amastigotes (H.W. Murray, personal communication). Would you comment on these observations in relation to the concept of oxidative killing of *Leishmania* species?

Klebanoff: PMA is a potent stimulus of the respiratory burst, and when the burst of macrophages is exhausted by preincubation with this agent, the antiparasitic activity of the cells is decreased (Murray 1982b). It should be emphasized that PMA has multiple effects on macrophages (Kielian & Cohn 1981) and therefore its effects cannot necessarily be attributed entirely to the stimulation of the respiratory burst. A number of studies indicate that phagocytes from patients with chronic granulomatous disease have decreased antiparasitic activity; however, activity is not lost, which emphasizes (although I have discussed *oxygen-dependent* mechanisms in this paper) that other important mechanisms are certainly involved in the killing of parasites by phagocytes.

Hudson: When we consider that monocytes become macrophages, it seems surprising that nature should have evolved a system in which a cell that can generate a good respiratory burst is converted into one that does not. Presumably, macrophages are important cells in host defence. Is the ability to generate a respiratory burst restored by the action of lymphokines on the macrophages?

Klebanoff: The macrophage acquires a large number of properties as a consequence of this maturation. The neutrophil has one primary function: it is uniquely and beautifully designed to ingest and kill microorganisms. The monocyte also has pronounced microbicidal activity. The macrophage, on the other hand, has many functions: it is, for example, a major secretory cell. It appears that during the acquisition of all these other properties, the macrophage loses some of its toxicity against ingested organisms. When activated by lymphokines, the macrophage does acquire a more pronounced respiratory burst and is a more efficient killer.

Hudson: Is the activation of macrophages by lymphokines a membrane event?

Klebanoff: I don't know.

Sher: There is evidence against a role for oxidative mechanisms in the killing by granulocytes and macrophages of certain parasitic targets. In the case of the eosinophil, an alternative mediator of toxicity is the eosinophil major basic protein. What non-oxidative killing mechanisms could the activated macrophage employ against a parasitic target?

Klebanoff: In addition to oxidative mechanisms, there are reports of basic proteins in macrophages with possible microbicidal activity (Lehrer et al 1981) but they appear to be in lower concentrations than in eosinophils or neutrophils. In addition, there is a fall in pH to 4 or 5 in the phagosomes of macrophages, and this may influence the viability of organisms. Hydrolases can also be released as a consequence of lysosome–phagosome rupture. The hydrolytic enzymes do not appear to be generally involved in the primary destruction of organisms but, rather, in cleaning up the debris. However, we don't yet know if this is always the case.

Nogueira: Very recently Schreiber et al (1982) have described a T-cell hybridoma that secretes lymphokine after activation with concanavalin A. This lymphokine can activate macrophages to kill tumour cells. The macrophage-activating factor co-purifies with γ-interferon, as shown by their very detailed experiments. This lymphokine that induces the tumour-killing activity of macrophages may be the same as that which induces microbe-killing activity.

Sharma: To my knowledge people have not been able to separate γ-interferon from macrophage activating factor. Is this the same as macrophage Ia antigen-inducing factor?

Nogueira: Schreiber et al (1982) have shown a convincing pattern of purification and parallel activity that would be very difficult to attribute to chance. However, the final evidence should come from the use of purified, or cloned, γ-interferon.

Wyler: The lymphokines that we used to activate macrophages to induce killing of *Leishmania* species (Nacy et al 1981) apparently contain no interferon activity. Furthermore, L-cell mouse interferon, added to cultures of murine peritoneal macrophages, failed to induce killing of intracellular *Leishmania tropica* (Wyler et al 1982).

Warren: Another killing mechanism studied is arginase secreted by macrophages activated by BCG or other substances (Olds et al 1980). Your lymphokine may stimulate release of arginase, which has been demonstrated to kill both tumour cells and multicellular organisms like *Schistosoma* species.

Butterworth: In relation to the neutrophil killing of schistosomula, although Anwar et al (1979) and Kazura et al (1981) have reported that human neutrophils can kill schistosomula, we have consistently found under a variety of different experimental conditions that, when the schistosomula are intact in the starting culture, then neutrophils have no detectable *primary* effect (Butterworth et al 1982). If the schistosomula were to be damaged either by poor preparation or by some other effector elements such as antibody and complement, then the neutrophils might be able to accelerate the destruction of these already damaged organisms. You showed some results on killing of schistosomula by neutrophils in the presence of antibody and complement; what was the background level of mortality that you had with antibody and complement alone?

Klebanoff: In the data shown, the incubation period was 18 h; the neutrophil-to-schistosomula ratio was 5000:1; and the background chromium release, with antibody and complement but no cells, was about 10%. If our incubation is for a shorter period, then the background falls. With eosinophil peroxidase-coated schistosomula we detected killing at 2 h and neutrophil-to-schistosomula ratios were down to 500:1. We used either fresh schistosomula, prepared on the same day by skin-penetration, or cells kept in culture fluid overnight, with comparable results.

Butterworth: You suggest that an intracellular parasite may first be taken up by an eosinophil, then coated with peroxidase, then released, taken up by the macrophage and killed. Colin Sanderson has some interesting time-lapse photographs of eosinophils behaving differently from, say, neutrophils, in that they do show a tendency to phagocytose red cells, degranulate, and then release the red cells (Sanderson & Thomas 1978). In some cases, they even re-phagocytose them again. Do you have this sort of observation in your *T. gondii* experiments?

Klebanoff: The experiments I referred to were those of Sanderson & De Souza (1979). They found that the trypomastigotes of *Trypanosoma cruzi*, in the presence of antibody, are ingested by granulocytes *in vitro* and are transformed intracellularly into amastigotes. Degranulation occurs with the release of electron-dense material into the phagosome. In the neutrophil, degeneration of the *T. cruzi* occurs rapidly whereas, in the eosinophil, the phagosome opens to the outside and amastigotes with granular material on their surface can be seen extracellularly. Although the preparations were not stained for peroxidase, this enzyme is probably included in the material on the organism surface. If a macrophage happened to come along at that instant, it could theoretically ingest this complex and kill the organism through the action of the bound peroxidase. These and other studies raise the possibility that resident macrophages, which have a very weak respiratory burst, can be activated in two ways: by classical lymphokine activation and by acquiring peroxidase on the surface of ingested organisms; the latter activation greatly amplifies the toxicity of the small amount of hydrogen peroxide generated within the phagosome. Whether this latter mechanism occurs *in vivo* has yet to be shown.

Sharma: Have you been able to isolate the superoxide-producing enzyme from macrophages?

Klebanoff: There has been a lot of work on the isolation of the oxidase from neutrophils. Isolation is difficult because the enzyme seems to be membrane-associated and is not easy to solubilize and characterize; it loses its activity very quickly. There have not been many studies on the purification and characterization of the macrophage oxidase but it is presumably similar to the enzyme in neutrophils. We have not been directly involved in these studies.

Chang: Does the coating of *T. cruzi* or other parasites with the enzyme influence their uptake rate by macrophages?

Klebanoff: All the measurements to date indicate that the rate of phagocytosis by macrophages is unaffected by the binding of the eosinophil peroxidase to the surface of *T. cruzi.*

Nogueira: We did investigate in detail a possible enhancement of uptake by coating the organisms with eosinophil peroxidase. Actually, an assumption that it might do so was what led us to try it. When I described a few years ago the relationship between the acidic 90 K glycoprotein on the surface and the antiphagocytic effect displayed by the trypomastigotes, Dr Klebanoff asked me if the charge had anything to do with the inhibition of phagocytosis. He suggested that we should coat the organisms with eosinophil peroxidase to see if phagocytosis would be enhanced once the negative charges were neutralized. We could not see any effect on phagocytosis.

Gutteridge: It is curious that many *Leishmania* and *Trypanosoma* species parasitize phagocytic cells but have only low levels of catalase or no catalase at all.

Klebanoff: The catalase level increases approximately 3-fold when *Leishmania donovani* promastigotes transform into amastigotes (Murray 1982a). Superoxide dismutase levels undergo a comparable increase whereas glutathione peroxidase levels increase about 15-fold. The promastigotes are readily killed by macrophages under conditions in which amastigotes are resistant. It is not clear whether the increased concentration of scavengers seen is sufficient to account for this difference. Trypanosomes appear to have little or no catalase (Docampo et al 1976).

Chang: How do you express the enzyme activity? Some workers express activity in terms of mg of protein, while others express it in terms of cell number. This is important because the amastigotes are much smaller, and they probably have much less protein, than the promastigotes. Individual amastigotes and promastigotes may well have the same amount of enzyme activity in terms of their functional need. How do you correlate this with your data? Is the catalase activity higher in the amastigotes regardless of how it is expressed?

Klebanoff: The measurement of increased catalase levels in amastigotes was done by Henry Murray (1982a) who expressed the activity per mg protein.

REFERENCES

Anwar ARE, Smithers SR, Kay AB 1979 Killing of schistosomula of *Schistosoma mansoni* coated with antibody and/or complement by human leukocytes *in vitro*: requirement for complement in preferential killing by eosinophils. J Immunol 122:628-637

Butterworth AE, Taylor DW, Veith MC et al 1982 Studies on the mechanisms of immunity in human schistosomiasis. Immunol Rev 61:5-39

Docampo R, DeBoiso JF, Boveris A, Stoppani AOM 1976 Localization of peroxidase activity in *Trypanosoma cruzi* microbodies. Experientia (Basel) 32:972-975

Jensen MS, Bainton DF 1973 Temporal changes in pH within the phagocytic vacuole of the polymorphonuclear leukocyte. J Cell Biol 56:379-388

Kazura JW, Meshnick SR 1982 Oxidant mediated killing of *Trichinella spiralis*: stage specificity and mechanisms of differential parasite toxicity. Clin Res 30:371A

Kazura JW, Fanning MM, Blumer JL, Mahmoud AAF 1981 Role of cell-generated hydrogen peroxide in granulocyte-mediated killing of schistosomula of *Schistosoma mansoni* in vitro. J Clin Invest 67:93-102

Kielian MC, Cohn ZA 1981 Phorbol myristate acetate stimulates phagosome–lysosome fusion in mouse macrophages. J Exp Med 154:101-111

Klebanoff SJ 1974 Role of the superoxide anion in the myeloperoxidase-mediated antimicrobial system. J Biol Chem 249:3724-3728

Lehrer RI, Szklarek D, Selsted ME, Fleischmann J 1981 Increased content of microbicidal cationic peptides in rabbit alveolar macrophages elicited by complete Freund adjuvant. Infect Immun 33:775-778

Murray HW 1981 Susceptibility of Leishmania to oxygen intermediates and killing by normal macrophages. J Exp Med 153:1302-1315

Murray HW 1982a Cell-mediated immune response in experimental visceral leishmaniasis. II: Oxygen-dependent killing of intracellular *Leishmania donovani* amastigotes. J Immunol 129:351-357

Murray HW 1982b Pretreatment with phorbol myristate acetate inhibits macrophage activity against intracellular protozoa. J Reticuloendothel Soc 31:479-487

Nacy CA, Meltzer MS, Leonard EJ, Wyler DJ 1981 Intracellular replication and lymphokine-induced destruction of *Leishmania tropica* in C3H/HeN mouse macrophages. J Immunol 127:2381-2386

Olds GR, Ellner JJ, Kearse LA Jr, Kazura JW, Mahmoud AAF 1980 Role of arginase in killing of schistosomula of *Schistosoma mansoni*. J Exp Med 151:1557-1562

Sanderson CJ, DeSouza W 1979 A morphological study of the interaction between *Trypanosoma cruzi* and rat eosinophils, neutrophils and macrophages *in vitro*. J Cell Sci 37:275-286

Sanderson CJ, Thomas JA 1978 A comparison of the cytotoxic activity of eosinophils and other cells by ^{51}chromium release and time-lapse microcinematography. Immunology 34:771-780

Schreiber RD, Altman A, Katz DH 1982 Identification of a T cell hybridoma that produces large quantities of macrophage-activating factor. J Exp Med 156:677-689

Wyler DJ, Liang L-F, Downey E, Krim M 1982 Exogenous interferon administration in experimental leishmaniasis: *in vivo* and *in vitro* studies. Am J Trop Med Hyg 31:740-745

Cell biology of host–parasite membrane interactions in leishmaniasis

K.-P. CHANG* and DUNNE FONG

*Parasitology Laboratory, The Rockefeller University, 1230 York Avenue, New York, NY 10021, USA, *Now at: Department of Microbiology, UHS/Chicago Medical School, 3333 Green Bay Road, North Chicago, Illinois 60064, USA*

Abstract Molecular interactions at the host–parasite interface are crucial for the outcome of microbial infection, particularly in infection by intracellular parasites, such as *Leishmania donovani* and *Leishmania mexicana*, whose natural transmission begins with the delivery of the promastigote stage by the sandfly vector into the susceptible host. The ensuing event is intracellular parasitism of macrophages in the host by the amastigote stage. The establishment of this event in leishmaniasis must follow the sequence: (1) *Leishmania*–macrophage attachment; (2) entry of *Leishmania* species into macrophages; (3) intra-macrophage survival and differentiation of *Leishmania* species; and (4) intracellular multiplication of *Leishmania* species. This sequence precedes all clinical symptoms and pathological consequences in different forms of the disease. Study of these cellular events in *Leishmania*–macrophage systems *in vitro* indicates that host–parasite membrane interactions dictate many of the cellular events. Some morphological and functional changes of macrophages in response to leishmanial infection are related to their membrane activities, i.e. endocytosis and exocytosis. *Leishmania* parasites undergo profound plasma membrane-related changes, on entry into macrophages, at the morphological, antigenic and molecular levels. Most of these changes probably reflect necessary steps for the transition of *Leishmania* species from an extracellular to an intracellular life. The remarkable ability of *Leishmania* species subsequently to live in the secondary lysosome of the macrophage may also be due to certain intrinsic structures and dynamic properties of the parasite plasma membrane. Further analysis of leishmanial surface molecules and their interactions with macrophages is essential in any attempt to understand the pathogenic mechanism in leishmaniasis.

1983 Cytopathology of parasitic disease. Pitman Books, London (Ciba Foundation symposium 99), p 113-137

The surface of parasites is vital in their interactions with the host to bring about successful parasitism. This is the very site where parasites extract nutrients to sustain their life and where they stop the parasiticidal actions of the hosts. Even more demanding are the cell surface-related tasks for intracellular parasites, which must deal with not only extracellular but also intracellular microenvironments of the host. The transit of these organisms between intracellular and extracellular locale and their prolonged intracellular residence entail host–parasite membrane interactions which contribute to the cytopathology of the disease.

Trypanosomatid protozoa of the genus *Leishmania* represent an interesting example of intracellular parasitism (Chang 1983). The organisms cause cutaneous, mucocutaneous and visceral leishmaniases, diseases still widespread, mainly in the tropics. *Leishmania* species have two different stages in their life cycle: promastigotes in the sandfly vector and amastigotes in the mammalian host. The insect stage is a slender, motile cell, equipped with a long flagellum at the anterior end. The mammalian stage is a small, non-motile intracellular cell, with its flagellum concealed in a flagellar pocket. In the natural cycle of transmission, promastigotes are delivered by the vector into the susceptible host where they infect macrophages of its reticuloendothelial system. Intracellular parasitism of host macrophages is an unusual aspect of leishmaniasis, as these cells themselves are specialized in defence against invaders. The plasma membrane of the macrophages is highly active and plays a major part in their antimicrobial activities (Edelson 1980). It can bind microorganisms via specific or non-specific receptors and can interiorize them, by phagocytosis, into phagosomes. Membrane fusion of phagosomes with lysosomes exposes the ingested microbes to the microbicidal factors present in the lysosomes and effects their degradation. Membrane fusion of phagolysosomes with the plasma membrane may ensue to expel non-degradable remnants. How the *Leishmania* parasites can manage not only to escape this elaborate mechanism of intracellular degradation but, instead, to nourish themselves must be related to their pathogenic mechanisms in leishmaniasis.

Previously, we have discussed these questions in terms of the sequential events leading to the establishment of intracellular parasitism, i.e. recognition, intracellular entry, survival and multiplication of *Leishmania* species (Chang 1983). Here, we shall focus on the functions of the plasma membrane, particularly the *Leishmania* membrane and its associated components, in the mechanism of intracellular parasitism in leishmaniasis.

Leishmania plasma membrane complex and related structures

Aside from morphological descriptions, our knowledge of the plasma membrane of *Leishmania* parasites is limited and fragmentary. Most of the biochemical data are available for the promastigote stage only. Dwyer (1981) and Hernández et al (1981) have recently summarized their respective work on the plasma membranes of *L. donovani* and *L. braziliensis*. The following account of the cell-biological aspects of the leishmanial plasma membrane is based mainly on their work and on our own observations.

In general, *Leishmania* species resemble other trypanosomatids in the structural organization of the plasma membrane and its associated components. It is a tripartite unit membrane in both the flagellar and the cell-body sections. The limiting membrane of the flagellar pocket gives rise to both sections, providing continuity between them. Underneath the cell-body section of the plasma membrane are subpellicular microtubules, which run in parallel, along the longitudinal axis of the cell body. These microtubules are connected to each other and to the plasma membrane. The spatial organization of these structures is maintained even in isolated plasma membrane (Dwyer 1980) and after the solubilization of other cellular components with non-ionic detergents. Thus, the subpellicular microtubules form the cytoskeleton of *Leishmania* species which is responsible for its rigidity and cell shape, as for other trypanosomatids. Another major part of the leishmanial microtubules is in the flagella, whose structural organization is identical to that in other organisms. Flagella are organelles of cell motility for *Leishmania* species.

The surface properties and activities of *Leishmania* species generally conform with those of a typical eukaryotic cell. However, the leishmanial cell surface lacks membrane ridges and folds, and is incapable of endocytosis, with the exception of the lining membrane of the flagellar pocket and, possibly, the very posterior end of the cell. A thin layer of coat materials covers the entire surface of promastigotes and is demonstrable by special staining for polysaccharides. Lectins specific to different monosaccharides bind to the surface of promastigotes, and lectin binding reveals the following terminal sugar residues: mannose, fucose, N-acetylglucosamine, N-acetylgalactosamine and N-acetylneuraminic acid (Dwyer 1981). The lectin-binding ligands are randomly distributed on the cell surface and vary with different species. The lateral mobility of lectin-binding and antibody-binding ligands produces patches and bipolar caps of these ligands on the leishmanial surface, indicating a fluidity of the plasma membrane and the presence of discrete protein molecules in the membrane. The lectin-mediated cap formation is energy- and temperature-dependent and is sensitive to cytochalasin B (Hernández et al 1981). Under normal growth conditions, promastigotes of *L. donovani* can shed their surface antigens into the culture medium (Kaneshiro et al 1982). It is also of interest that Fc receptors can be found on the surface of pathogenic trypanosomatids, including *Leishmania* species, but not on that of the non-pathogenic species (Ferreira de Miranda-Santos & Campos-Neto 1981). These results suggest a leishmanial challenge to the host's immune response by modification of the protozoan cell surface.

Biochemical assays for the plasma membrane-associated enzymes have just begun to receive attention. Gottlieb & Dwyer (1981) demonstrated acid phosphatase activity on the surface of *L. donovani* promastigotes, as found in certain members of saprophytic yeasts. Konigk & Putfarken (1980) detected membrane nucleotidases and found them to differ between the two leishmanial stages. These leishmanial enzymes may be parasite-specific and different from the corresponding enzymes in mammalian cells.

Biochemical and antigenic complexity of the leishmanial surface appears to vary with the species studied. Sodium dodecyl sulphate (SDS) gel electrophoresis and autoradiography, in conjunction with radiolabelling of the cell surface, immunoprecipitation and lectin-affinity binding, are the usual approaches for characterization of externally exposed surface molecules of the leishmanial plasma membrane. By surface iodination of living cells, Dwyer (1980) found about 27 peptides or glycopeptides on the surface of *L. donovani* promastigotes, while Hernández et al (1981) found only two major bands on that of *L. braziliensis*. We have studied promastigotes of *L. mexicana amazonensis* and found a heavy band with a relative molecular mass (M_r) of 68 000 and a minor band of M_r 43 000; both bands proved to be cell-surface antigenic glycoproteins (Fig. 1). We have also identified these molecules by using *Leishmania* species that were biosynthetically labelled with [^{35}S]methionine (Fig. 2), which indicates that the molecules are intrinsic to the leishmanial membrane and not medium components adhering to it. Biosynthetically labelled *L. mexicana* gave a triple set of bands instead of a single heavy band, as seen in the iodinated sample at the 68 000 M_r region (Fig. 2). These results suggest that the leishmanial cell surface may consist of a number of protein molecules amenable to detailed analysis.

Recently, the hybridoma technique has been used to prepare monoclonal antibodies against *Leishmania* species for identification and characterization of their surface antigens. McMahon Pratt & David (1981) were the first to produce monoclonal antibodies against *L. braziliensis braziliensis* and *L. mexicana amazonensis* for species differentiation. We made a number of hybridomas for *L. mexicana amazonensis;* the monoclonal antibodies released from most clones recognize the triplet antigenic glycoproteins (Fig. 3) (Fong & Chang 1982). These molecules apparently cover the entire surface of the cells (Fig. 4 A, B) and form bipolar caps after binding with the monoclonal antibody under living conditions (Fig. 4 C, D). Handman & Hocking (1982) also produced a number of monoclonal antibodies against *L. tropica*, most of which were found to be surface-reactive, but the antigens were not characterized. These monoclonal antibodies are potentially very useful for further characterization and purification of leishmanial surface antigens.

To our knowledge, there has been no report on the lipid fraction of the leishmanial plasma membrane. Analysis of total lipid composition and lipid

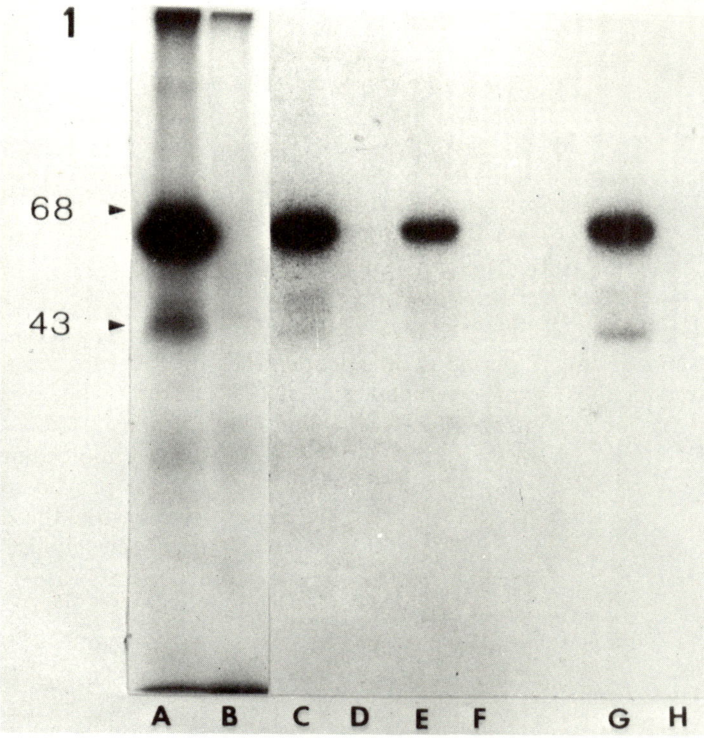

FIG. 1. Autoradiogram after SDS-polyacrylamide gel electrophoresis of radio-iodinated *L. mexicana amazonensis*. *A*, Living promastigotes were surface-iodinated at 4 °C for 10–15 min at 50–100 μCi $Na^{125}I$ per 10^8 cells per ml Hanks' balanced salt solution, in glass tubes coated with IODO-GEN according to the manufacturer's procedures (Pierce Co.); *B*, iodination of living cells in the absence of IODO-GEN; *C*, affinity binding of detergent (Nonidet P-40)-solubilized sample to concanavalin A–Sepharose (Nogueira et al 1981); *D*, same as C, but in the present of 0.1 M-α-methyl-D-mannoside and 0.1 M-α-methyl-D-glucoside; *E*, elution pattern of concanavalin A–Sepharose-bound sample from C with sugar solution in D; *F*, control for *E* without sugars; *G*, immunoprecipitation of Nonidet P-40-solubilized sample followed by affinity binding to protein A–Sepharose (Chang 1983); *H*, control for G using normal mouse serum. M_r 68 K and 43 K are marked.

metabolism of these organisms revealed several interesting aspects, e.g. incorporation of O-alkylglycerols into lipids, leading to changes in the promastigote shape (Hermann & Gercken 1982), and the presence of cyclopropane fatty acids (commonly found in bacteria but not in eukaryotic cells) in the phosphatidylethanolamines (Fish et al 1981). Whether these

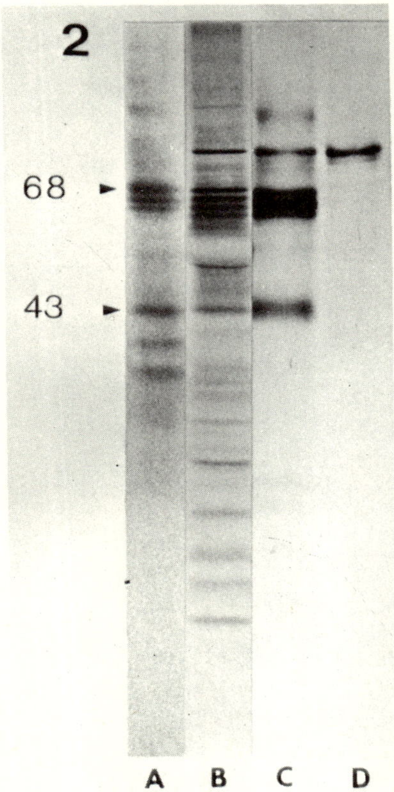

FIG. 2. Autoradiogram after SDS–polyacrylamide gel electrophoresis of [^{35}S]methionine-labelled *L. mexicana amazonensis*. See Fong & Chang (1981) for labelling procedures. *A*, Detergent-solubilized sample bound to concanavalin A–Sepharose as in Fig. 1; *B*, immunoprecipitation of Nonidet P-40-solubilized sample followed by affinity binding to protein A–Sepharose; *C*, immunoprecipitation of cell-surface antigens by the following method: living cells after [^{35}S]methionine labelling were opsonized at 4 °C for 1 h with a 1/10 dilution of anti-*Leishmania* hyperimmune mouse serum and then extensively washed; surface antigen–antibody immune complexes of these cells were released by solubilization in 1% Nonidet P-40 in phosphate buffered saline, cleared by centrifugation and collected by binding to protein A–Sepharose 4B (Nogueira et al 1981); *D*, control for C using normal mouse serum.

findings have some relevance to the leishmanial surface-membrane activity must await detailed analysis of the plasma-membrane lipids.

This brief account of the leishmanial plasma membrane is far from exhaustive. We have simply provided a general coverage of the current work to facilitate our discussion as it relates to the pathogenic mechanisms in leishmaniasis.

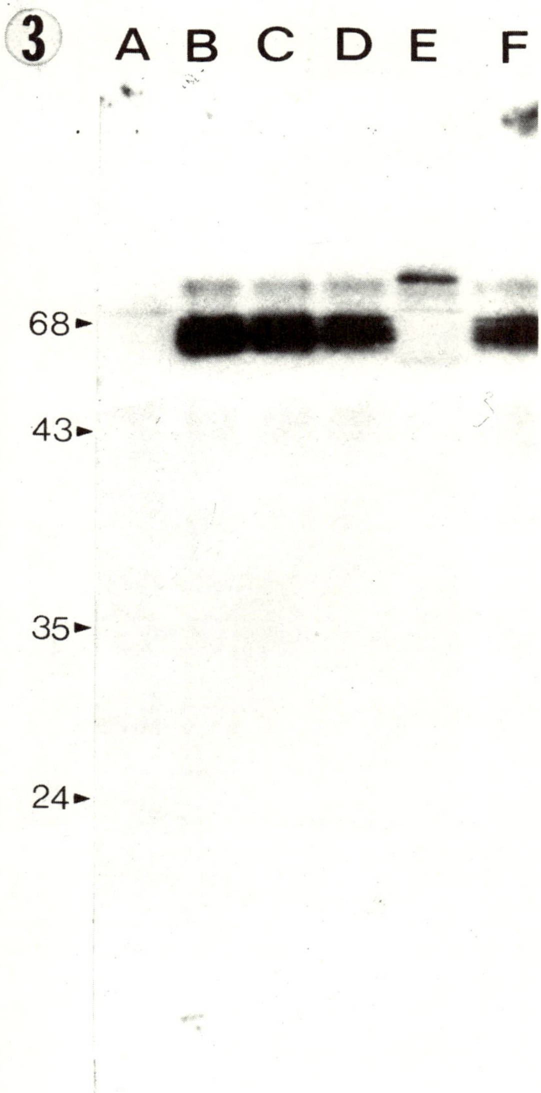

FIG. 3. Immunoprecipitation of [^{35}S]methionine-metabolically-labelled promastigote lysate of *L. mexicana amazonensis* by different hybridoma culture supernatants. *A*, 4G11; *B*, 4D11; *C*, 4H9; *D*, 6A11; *E*, 6G5; *F*, 6H12. Note the similarity of the triplet polypeptides in A–D and F to those in C of Fig. 2 which were identified by polyvalent hyperimmune serum as surface antigens.

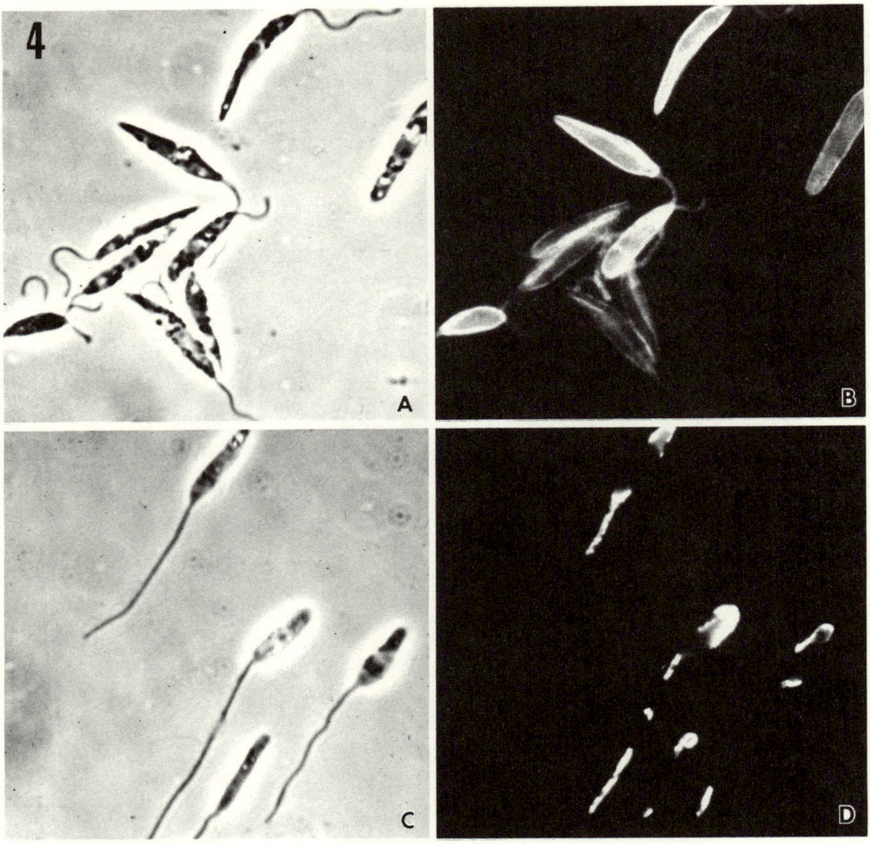

FIG. 4. Indirect immunofluorescent antibody assay of *L. mexicana amazonensis* using hybridoma 6H12 ascites fluid at 1 : 200 dilution. See Fong & Chang (1982) for experimental details. *A*, Glutaraldehyde-treated promastigotes, phase contrast; *B*, immunofluorescent microscopy of A; *C*, living promastigotes, phase contrast; *D*, immunofluorescent microscopy of C, showing the capping phenomenon by living promastigotes.

Plasma-membrane changes and *Leishmania*–macrophage interactions *in vitro*

The establishment of intracellular parasitism in any host–parasite system involves a series of cellular events. In leishmaniasis, promastigotes must first attach themselves to the surface and then enter the macrophages. The subsequent intracellular survival, differentiation and multiplication of *Leishmania* species culminate in all the pathological consequences of the infection. *Leishmania*–macrophage membrane interactions govern most of the cellular events leading to intracellular parasitism. In other instances, the host–parasite interactions result in changes in the plasma membrane of interacting cells. In this section, we shall examine some of these changes during leishmanial infection of macrophages.

Leishmania–*macrophage attachment*

Leishmania species must attach themselves to macrophages before their intracellular entry. The *Leishmania*–macrophage binding is a membrane phenomenon akin to ligand–receptor interactions in a broader sense. Several lines of evidence from *in vitro* studies support this assumption (Chang 1983). Promastigotes bind avidly to macrophages, less well or poorly to lymphocytes and not at all to erythrocytes. Thus, *Leishmania* species preferentially bind to their normal host cells. For studying the binding mechanism, we have used the system of *L. donovani* promastigotes and hamster peritoneal macrophages *in vitro* (Chang 1981). Other workers have studied different aspects of *Leishmania*–macrophage binding in other *in vitro* systems (see Chang 1983). Their results are generally in agreement with our interpretations presented below. In our system, vigorous rinsing with buffer or medium failed to dislodge promastigotes bound to macrophages, suggesting a strong cell–cell adhesion. By using a radioisotopic assay, we found that the binding followed saturation kinetics, required Ca^{2+}, and was temperature-dependent. We also used the same assay to probe the molecular properties of *Leishmania*–macrophage adhesion in binding-competition experiments and in experiments with cells pretreated to modify their surface properties. Sialic acid, glucose, mannose, mannosamine, glucosamine and N-acetylglucosamine compete with *Leishmania* species for binding to the macrophages. Consistent with this interpretation is the effect of pretreating promastigotes with different glycosidases, which specifically cleave these sugars off their surfaces. Most of the monosaccharides that compete with *L. donovani* promastigotes for binding to macrophages have been found, in lectin-binding experiments, to be on the surface as terminal sugar residues (Dwyer 1981). Also, pretreatment of macrophages with anti-macrophage antisera or trypsin significantly reduces their capacity to bind promastigotes. Results from these and other experiments lead to the following interpretations (Chang 1983): (1) the host–parasite binding in our system involves surface ligands of *L. donovani* and membrane receptor(s) of hamster macrophages; (2) the putative 'receptor(s)' of macrophages for *Leishmania* species are antigenic surface proteins; and (3) the binding ligands of *Leishmania* species are their surface antigenic glycoproteins, with a variety of terminal saccharides as possible binding determinants.

Two additional points concerning *Leishmania*-binding ligands in relation to the cell-surface property deserve further discussion. The binding ligands must be present on both the flagellar and the cell-body sections of promastigotes because they can attach to macrophages via either end (Chang 1983, Aikawa et al 1982). This interpretation also conforms with the distribution of other leishmanial surface-binding sites, e.g. the lectin-binding ligands (Dwyer 1981). Pretreatment of *Leishmania* species with cytochalasins, which depolymerize actin, was found to inhibit leishmanial binding to the macrophage (Aikawa et al 1982, Wyler 1982), suggesting that the binding might somehow involve the leishmanial actin filaments. Perhaps actin filament-mediated patch formation or clustering of leishmanial surface ligands facilitates its binding to the macrophage.

From our results, we found similarities between promastigote–macrophage binding and binding in receptor-mediated endocytosis of zymosan granules or lysosomal glycosidases by phagocytes (see Chang 1981, 1983). Presumably, the latter binding is mediated by a mannose/N-acetylglucosamine-specific recognition system which plays an important part in the retrieval of secreted lysosomal enzymes and/or in non-specific cellular defence against invading microbes. Whether the same receptor mechanism mediates all these binding phenomena must await further study. As a working hypothesis, we have proposed the possibility of molecular mimicry whereby leishmanial surface components may fit pre-existing receptor(s) of macrophages for other important biological function(s), e.g. for sequestration of released lysosomal enzymes (Chang 1982). This concept is compatible with the finding of acid phosphatase on the surface of *L. donovani* promastigotes (Gottlieb & Dwyer 1981).

Entry of Leishmania *species into macrophages*

The entry of *Leishmania* species into macrophages appears to depend in large part on the membrane activity of the macrophages. In all aspects, the process of entry resembles phagocytosis of other particles by macrophages (Chang 1983). Electron microscopy shows an exaggerated response of the macrophage surface membrane around the promastigotes, manifested as the formation of extensive ruffles and whorled pseudopodia. In the presence of cytochalasin B, an inhibitor of phagocytosis, macrophages no longer show such membrane activity and ingest very few promastigotes. The entry of promastigotes into macrophages is accompanied by chemiluminescence (Meshnick & Eaton 1981) and the release of hydrogen peroxide (Murray 1981), which are metabolic activities of macrophages triggered by their phagocytic activity.

The role of leishmanial flagella in the infection of macrophages by promastigotes has been a matter of some controversy (Chang 1983). We have suggested that these organelles help the infection indirectly by conferring motility on the promastigotes to increase their chances of encounter with the macrophages (Chang 1983). Moreover, the flagella of certain leishmanial species do function in their entry into non-phagocytic cells or cells with low phagocytic activity (see Chang 1983). How these *Leishmania* species can induce phagocytic activity of otherwise non-phagocytic cells is unknown.

Intracellular survival of Leishmania *species*

Once inside the macrophages, *Leishmania* species must overcome a formidable array of hostile activities with which the macrophages are equipped to kill ingested microbes. The most intriguing of these events is the finding that lysosome–phagosome fusion occurs after leishmanial entry into macrophages, and that *Leishmania* species not only survive but continue to multiply in the phagolysosomes (Alexander & Vickerman 1975; see Chang 1983). *Leishmania* species are thus processed by macrophages as other digestible particles are, but do not suffer the consequences of lysosomal degradation. How *Leishmania* species are able to resist the microbicidal factors present in the lysosomal compartment of macrophages has yet to be elucidated. One possibility is that the leishmanial cell surface may be naturally resistant to enzyme degradation (Alexander & Vickerman 1975; see Chang 1983). To test this possibility, we have subjected antigenic glycoproteins from the surface of *L. mexicana* promastigotes to treatment with solubilized rat liver lysosomes (Fig. 5). At least one of the triplet surface glycoproteins at 68 000 M_r, as well as the other at 43 000 M_r (see Figs 1–2), persisted throughout the entire period of treatment, while other internal proteins became degraded (Fig. 5). When radio-iodinated living promastigotes were fed to macrophages, the labelled surface molecules also persisted for up to 36 h without being digested. These results offer direct evidence for the refractory property of leishmanial surface molecules to lysosomal degradation. These surface molecules may provide a protective 'shield', allowing *Leishmania* species to live normally in the lysosomal compartment of macrophages. The functional and structural integrity of lysosomes is known to depend partly on prevention or the mutual degradation of the constituent enzymes, and the carbohydrate moieties of the lysosomal enzymes may be the stabilizing factors. Whether the acid phosphatase and other glycoproteins on the leishmanial surface may, via a similar mechanism, prevent the activation of lysosomal enzymes deserves consideration. An alternative proposal for the intralysosomal survival of *Leishmania* species is their release of excretory factors as lysosomal enzyme inhibitors (El-On et al 1980). Obviously these possibilities are not mutually exclusive.

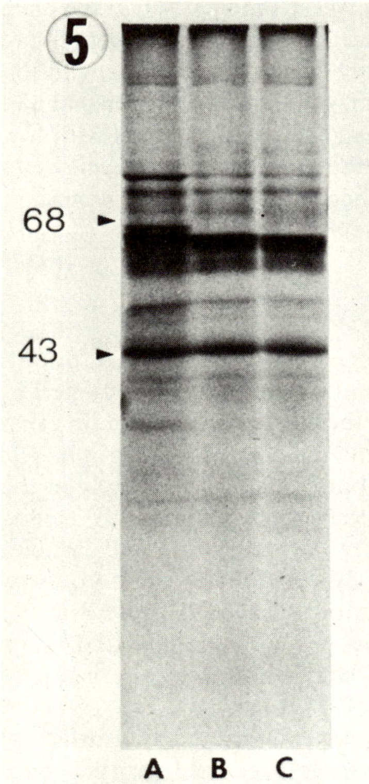

FIG. 5. Autoradiogram after SDS-polyacrylamide gel electrophoresis of [^{35}S]methionine-labelled and detergent-lysed *Leishmania* antigens treated with lysosomal enzymes from rat liver. These lysosomes were obtained as frozen pellets through the courtesy of Dr L. Wang, Laboratory of Biochemical Cytology, the Rockefeller University. Lysosomal fractions (density = 1.1 g/ml) were purified from livers of Triton WR1339-treated rats by zonal ultracentrifugation in a sucrose gradient. Parasite antigens collected in protein A–Sepharose beads were treated at 37 °C with the lysosomal preparations (10^8 promastigotes per mg protein) in 1 ml MES (2-[N-morpholino] ethane-sulphonic acid, sodium salt) buffer, pH 5, containing 0.02% NaN_3 and 1% Triton X-100. *A*, at time zero; *B*, 8 h; *C*, 24 h. Controls at 37 °C in the absence of lysosomal enzymes were identical to A.

Another way to investigate the importance of surface antigens of promastigotes for intracellular survival is through the use of monoclonal-antibody probes. Handman & Hocking (1982) treated *L. tropica* promastigotes with monoclonal antibodies reactive to their surface and fed the promastigotes to peritoneal macrophages cultured *in vitro*. They found that within the 24 h period of study two out of the battery of nine monoclonal antibodies tested

TABLE 1 Monoclonal antibody-mediated inhibition of parasitophorous vacuole formation in murine resident peritoneal macrophages by *L. mexicana amazonensis*

Monoclonal antibody	*Treatment*	*Percent of macrophages with parasitophorous vacuoles*[a] 3 Days	7 Days
none	none	73 ± 6.9	83 ± 5.4
6G5	Inclusion[b] in medium	70 ± 4.2	75 ± 7.4
6H12	Inclusion[b] in medium	31 ± 4.3	40 ± 7.4
4G11	Inclusion[b] in medium	26 ± 3.3	27 ± 4.1
none	none	56 ± 6.4	68 ± 8.2
6G5	Opsonization[c] of promastigotes	66 ± 9.2	78 ± 5.7
6H12	Opsonization[c] of promastigotes	50 ± 10	54 ± 8.3
4G11	Opsonization[c] of promastigotes	27 ± 4.3	22 ± 3.0

Peritoneal exudate cells of BALB/c mice were collected and cultured at 3×10^6 cells per 25 cm^2 tissue-culture flask in RPMI-1640 medium plus 20% heat-inactivated fetal bovine serum at 35 °C for 2–3 days. Each culture was subsequently inoculated with 15×10^6 promastigotes under appropriate conditions of ascites-fluid treatment and incubated at 35 °C for 7 days.

[a]Determined by examining at least 10 microscopic fields or over 1000 cells at × 250 magnification under an inverted microscope. [b]Simultaneous addition of hybridoma-derived ascites fluid to the macrophage culture, with the promastigote inoculum, at a final concentration of 0.5%. [c]10^7 promastigotes were treated with 10% ascites fluid in 1 ml Hanks' balanced salt solution for one hour at 4 °C and washed twice with phosphate buffered saline before use.

resulted in a decrease in the number of intracellular *Leishmania* species. However, whether the effective monoclonals recognize the same or different surface antigens is unknown. We have done similar experiments using three monoclonals, i.e. 6H12, 6G5 and 4G11, which recognize *L. mexicana* surface antigens as a triplet glycopeptide (68 000 M_r), a single heavy band (90 000 M_r) and an unknown, respectively (see Fig. 3). We observed different effects among the three monoclonal antibodies in the inhibition of parasitophorous vacuole formation (Table 1) and in the reduction of the total number of intracellular amastigotes in macrophages (Table 2), the order of effectiveness of the three antibodies being: 4G11 > 6H12 > 6G5 = control. For comparison, we present the data on monoclonal antibody-dependent complement-mediated lysis of *L. mexicana* in Table 3. The order of effectiveness in this lysis experiment among different monoclonals was: 6G5 > 6H12 > 4G11 = control. Thus, our results provide evidence that *L. mexicana* surface antigens have different immunological properties and biological functions which are recognized by these monoclonal antibodies. Handman & Hocking (1982) proposed that the binding of monoclonal antibodies to critical surface antigens of promastigotes may inhibit their differentiation into amastigotes and, hence, that fewer of them can survive in macrophages. This appears to

TABLE 2 Monoclonal antibody-mediated reduction of *L. mexicana amazonensis* in murine macrophage line J774G8 cells

Monoclonal antibody	Treatment	Total intracellular amastigotes ($\times 10^{-6}$)[a] 2 Days	3–4 Days	7–8 Days
none		10 ± 1.5	12 ± 0.7	15 ± 0.8
6G5	Inclusion in medium	8 ± 1.1	11 ± 2.6	14 ± 1.2
6H12	Inclusion in medium	4 ± 0.4	6 ± 0.9	8 ± 1.1
4G11	Inclusion in medium	4 ± 1.0	5 ± 0.1	7 ± 1.3
none		—	12 ± 0.4	21 ± 1.0
6G5	Opsonization of promastigotes	—	17 ± 2.1	21 ± 1.9
6H12	Opsonization of promastigotes	—	9 ± 1.0	11 ± 2.5
4G11	Opsonization of promastigotes	—	7 ± 0.7	10 ± 0.8

[a]Determined by counting the number of J774G8 cells, % of infected cells and the average number of amastigotes per cell (Chang 1980). See footnotes of Table 1 for other details.

TABLE 3 Monoclonal antibody-dependent complement-mediated killing of *Leishmania mexicana amazonensis* promastigotes

Organism[a]	0.5% *Guinea-pig*[b] *serum*	0.5% *Monoclonal antibody*[c]	*% Lysis*	[^{3}*H*]*Leucine incorporation* ($\times 10^{-3}$ *c.p.m*)
L. mexicana	+	–	0.5 ± 0.07	83 ± 2.1
L. mexicana	–	6G5	0.3 ± 0.01	81 ± 3.2
L. mexicana	+	4G11	1.2 ± 0.1	81 ± 1.6
L. mexicana	+	6H12	74.0 ± 2.2	60 ± 7.5
L. mexicana	+	6G5	81.0 ± 6.1	33 ± 3.7
L. mexicana	+	6G5 + 6H12	—	31 ± 4.6
L. donovani	+	6G5 + 6H12	—	83 ± 2.0

Incubation was done with agitation for 20 min at 37 °C in glass tubes containing 10^7 cells/ml in Hanks' balanced salt solution and appropriate amounts of serum and/or ascites fluid. At the end of incubation, viability of promastigotes was determined by incorporation of radioactive precursors and by counting the percentage of lysed promastigotes. In the radioisotopic assay, each tube received 10 μCi [^{3}H]leucine and was incubated for an additional hour at 27 °C; samples were then processed for scintillation counting as before (Chang 1981). For direct examination, each tube received five volumes of a 2% buffered glutaraldehyde solution and the percentage of lysis was determined by counting the numbers of ghosts and intact cells in a haemocytometer, under phase contrast, using a × 40 objective lens. [a]Cultured in a defined medium (see Chang 1981); [b]collected by cardiac puncture and stored at − 100 °C until use; [c]Ascites fluid prepared from hybridoma in BALB/c mice as described by Fong & Chang (1982).

be one of several possible mechanisms, all of which must await further investigations. The monoclonal antibody-dependent killing of *Leishmania* species in macrophages and the killing mediated by complement in all experiments done so far have been incomplete. In our observations, for up to seven days, effective monoclonal antibodies reduce the initial number of intracellular amastigotes but not the growth rate of the survivors (Tables 1–2). The implications of this will be discussed in the last section of this paper.

Leishmanial differentiation

Leishmania species undergo cytodifferentiation in their transmission cycle of vector–mammalian host–vector. This is presumably a necessary feature of adaptation, enabling *Leishmania* species to live alternately in the sandfly gut and in the intralysosomal compartment of mammalian macrophages. Certain changes in the leishmanial limiting membrane may be expected, as this membrane bears the brunt of immediate exposure to the drastic environmental changes incurred during transition between extracellular and intracellular living. During leishmanial differentiation we have, indeed, found changes in the surface antigens of the organisms and their tubulins, which are molecular subunits of flagellar and subpellicular microtubules (Fong & Chang 1981; see Chang 1983). For this study, we have used the system of *L. mexicana amazonensis*–J774G8 macrophages *in vitro* (Chang 1980). As mentioned already, the triplet band of *L. mexicana* at 68 000 M_r represents a cell-surface antigenic glycoprotein (Fig. 2, lane C), which is recognized by the monoclonal antibody 6H12 (Fig. 3, lane F). This antigen is apparently specific to promastigotes, as amastigotes do not bind 6H12 (Fong & Chang 1982). When the amastigotes are induced to differentiate into promastigotes under appropriate conditions, the leishmanial binding to 6H12 increases by 4–8 fold (Fig. 6), concomitantly with the morphological changes (Fong & Chang 1982). The emergence of new antigens on the leishmanial surface during differentiation may signify a molecular reorganization of the plasma membrane, which may be important for the *Leishmania* species to live in the different environments of their life cycle. Differentiation-related changes in the exterior of the plasma membrane may indicate corresponding changes in its interior section. Morphological changes have long been observed during leishmanial differentiation; i.e. lengthening and shortening of the flagella and the subpellicular microtubules take place. Recently, we have been able to put this type of cellular change into a biochemical perspective by demonstrating its correlation with the altered rate of tubulin biosynthesis (Fong & Chang 1981). Obviously, a decrease in demand for the microtubular structures calls for a reduction in tubulin biosynthesis. Of particular interest is our subsequent finding that this process is under post-transcriptional regulation, in contrast to the transcriptional control of tubulin biosynthesis in other systems of eukaryote differentiation (Wallach et al 1982). Molecular and

6

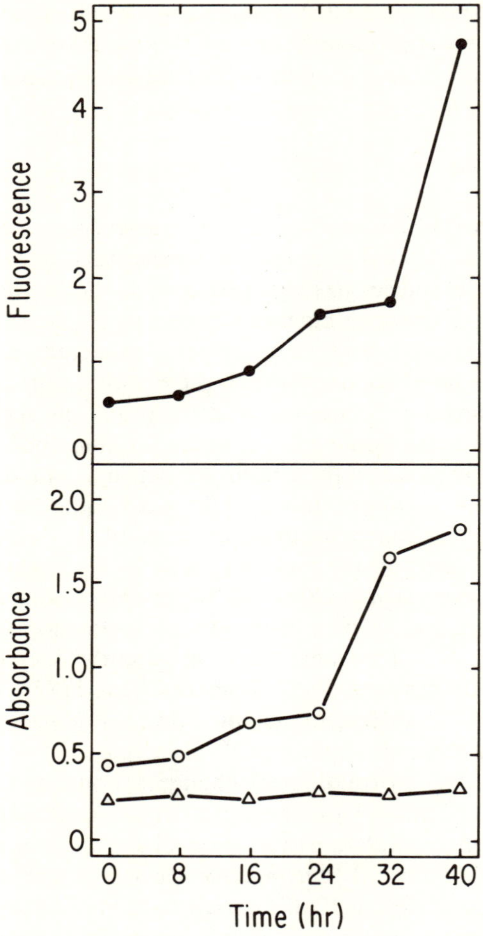

FIG. 6. Antigenic changes during amastigote-to-promastigote differentiation of *L. mexicana amazonensis*. See Fong & Chang (1982) for details. Top panel, binding of hybridoma 6H12-derived ascites fluid (at 1/200 dilution) to differentiating *Leishmania*, as quantitated by fluorometric assay for fluorescein isothiocyanate conjugated antibody; Bottom panel, binding of hybridomas 6H12 (open circles) and 4G11 (open triangles) ascites fluids at 1/200 dilution to differentiating *Leishmania*, as quantitated by sandwich enzyme-linked immunosorbant assay.

antigenic changes in the plasma membrane complex during leishmanial differentiation deserve further detailed study in view of their obvious significance for the survival of *Leishmania* species in their hosts.

Changes induced by leishmanial infection in the plasma membrane of macrophages

We have already discussed the response of the macrophage surface membrane to leishmanial infection during the early host–parasite interactions. The contact between macrophages and promastigotes triggers promastigote uptake or their interiorization into parasitophorous vacuoles and lysosome–phagosome fusion. We understand these events by virtue of their analogy to the well characterized phenomenon of phagocytosis. Beyond this point, *Leishmania*–macrophage membrane interactions have not been studied, with the exception of a few isolated observations. There is an intimate association between amastigotes and the inner lining of the parasitophorous vacuoles (Chang 1983), which is manifested by the formation of gap junction-like structures (Benchimol & de Souza 1981). Leishmanial infection of the macrophages increases their pinocytic rate (see Chang 1983) and results in the expression of leishmanial antigens on their surfaces (Berman & Dwyer 1981). This may happen because the leishmania antigens released may adhere to the parasitophorous vacuolar membrane and may be carried to the surface of the macrophages via exocytosis of vesicles pinched off from the parasitophorous vacuoles. Changes in endocytic and exocytic activities of infected macrophages may be expected, because *Leishmania* species are parasites of the lysosome–phagosome vacuolar system.

Discussion

We have summarized the available information on the properties of the leishmanial plasma membrane, and described membrane changes and their possible roles during *Leishmania*–macrophage cellular interactions that lead to the establishment of intracellular parasitism. While the significance of the leishmanial plasma membrane and its changes in leishmanial infection of macrophages is often self-evident, we need additional information on the membrane's chemical composition and physical properties for a fuller understanding of its contributions to the cytopathology of leishmaniasis. It is particularly urgent to characterize the plasma membrane of intracellular amastigotes, the mammalian stage of *Leishmania* species, and we now have simple methods to purify this stage of the parasites in adequate quantities for such investigations. It is also essential to study the externally exposed surface glycoproteins and glycolipids because their interactions with host cells may result directly or indirectly in the pathological effects observed in leishmaniasis. These molecules participate in both the attachment and the engulfment phases of leishmanial phagocytosis by macrophages. Evidence presented here suggests that some of the surface antigenic glycoproteins may contribute to the protection of *Leishmania* species against their degradation by the lysosomal enzymes in the host. Membrane molecules may also transmit environmental signals that trigger intracellular differentiation of *Leishmania* species and the molecules may serve to transport essential nutrients to sustain the intracellular leishmanial replication. These functions of the leishmanial plasma membrane have yet to be correlated with surface antigens or glycoproteins so far identified there. In the pathogenic mechanisms of leishmaniasis, even more important than such a correlation between molecular structure and function is, perhaps, the dynamic properties of the leishmanial cell surface. For example, the cell-surface ligands in *Leishmania* species can be induced to show a high degree of lateral mobility. This mobility may prove essential for producing immune complexes, so accounting for the immunopathology of cells and tissues. We have observed incomplete effects on cloned *Leishmania* species in their antibody-dependent complement-mediated cytolysis, in their antibody-mediated killing by macrophages and even in their binding to fluorescent antibodies. We propose that these phenomena indicate versatility or variability of leishmanial surface antigens. Whether the individual differences in the expression of cell-surface antigens is cell-cycle-dependent is uncertain. Whatever the mechanism, it may ensure that a small population of *Leishmania* species escape from the host immune surveillance or attack, thereby establishing successful intracellular parasitism in the susceptible hosts.

Acknowledgements

We thank Drs S. J. Karakashian, N. Lanners and W. Trager for suggestions in reviewing this manuscript, and Mr J. Stanorski for skilful stenographic work. The authors' work was supported by NIH, NIAID Grant No. AI-15183.

REFERENCES

Aikawa M, Hendricks LD, Ito Y, Jagusiak M 1982 Interactions between macrophage-like cells and *Leishmania braziliensis in vitro*. Am J Pathol 198:50-59

Alexander J, Vickerman K 1975 Fusion of host cell secondary lysosomes with the parasitophorous vacuoles of *Leishmania mexicana* infected macrophages. J Protozool 22:502-508

Benchimol M, de Souza W 1981 *Leishmania mexicana amazonensis*: attachment to the membrane of the phagocytic vacuole of macrophages *in vivo*. Z Parasitenkd 66:25-29

Berman JD, Dwyer DM 1981 Expression of *Leishmania* antigen on the surface membrane of infected human macrophages *in vitro*. Clin Exp Immunol 44:342-348

Chang KP 1980 Human cutaneous leishmania in a mouse macrophage line: propagation and isolation of intracellular parasites. Science (Wash DC) 209:1240-1242

Chang KP 1981 *Leishmania donovani*–macrophage binding mediated by surface glycoproteins/antigens: characterization *in vitro* by a radioisotopic assay. Mol Biochem Parasitol 4:67-76

Chang KP 1983 Cellular and molecular mechanisms of intracellular symbiosis in leishmaniasis. Int Rev Cytol (Suppl 14):267-302

Dwyer DM 1980 Isolation and partial characterization of surface membranes from *Leishmania donovani* promastigotes. J Protozool 27:176-181

Dwyer DM 1981 Structural, chemical and antigenic properties of surface membranes isolated from *Leishmania donovani*. In: Slutzky GM (ed) The biochemistry of parasites. Pergamon Press, Oxford, p 9-28

Edelson PJ 1980 Monocytes and macrophages: aspects of their cell biology. In: Weissman G (ed) The cell biology of inflammation. Elsevier/North-Holland, Amsterdam, p 469-495

El-On J, Bradley DJ, Freeman JC 1980 *Leishmania donovani*: action of excreted factor on hydrolytic enzyme activity of macrophages from mice with genetically different resistance to infection. Exp Parasitol 49:167-174

Ferreira de Miranda-Santos IK, Campos-Neto A 1981 Receptor for immunoglobulin Fc on pathogenic but not on nonpathogenic protozoa of the trypanosomatidae. J Exp Med 154:1732-1742

Fish WR, Holz GG Jr, Beach DH, Owen E, Anekwe GE 1981 The cyclopropane fatty acid of trypanosomatids. Mol Biochem Parasitol 3:103-115

Fong D, Chang KP 1981 Tubulin biosynthesis in the developmental cycle of a parasitic protozoan, *Leishmania mexicana*: changes during differentiation of motile and non-motile stages. Proc Natl Acad Sci USA 78:7624-7628

Fong D, Chang KP 1982 Surface antigenic change during differentiation of a parasitic protozoan, *Leishmania mexicana*: identification by monoclonal antibodies. Proc Natl Acad Sci USA 79:7366-7370

Gottlieb M, Dwyer DM 1981 Protozoan parasite of humans: surface membrane with externally disposed acid phosphatase. Science (Wash DC) 212:939-941

Handman E, Hocking RE 1982 Stage-specific, strain-specific and cross-reactive antigens of *Leishmania* species identified by monoclonal antibodies. Infect Immun 37:28-33

Hermann HO, Gercken G 1982 Metabolism of 1-*O*-[1′-^{14}C]octadecyl-SN-glycerol in *Leishmania donovani* promastigotes: ether lipid synthesis and degradation of the ether bond. Mol Biochem Parasitol 5:65-76

Hernández AG, Arguello C, Ayesta C et al 1981 The surface membrane of *Leishmania*. In: Slutzky GM (ed) The biochemistry of parasites. Pergamon Press, Oxford, p 47-65

Kaneshiro ES, Gottlieb M, Dwyer DM 1982 Cell surface origin of antigens shed by *Leishmania donovani* during growth in axenic culture. Infect Immun 37:558-567

Königk E, Putfarken B 1980 Stage-specific differences of a perhaps signal-transferring system in *Leishmania donovani*. Tropenmed Parasitol 31:421-424

McMahon Pratt D, David JR 1981 Monoclonal antibodies that distinguish between New World species of *Leishmania*. Nature (Lond) 291:581-583

Meshnick SR, Eaton JW 1981 Leishmanial superoxide dismutase: a possible target for chemotherapy. Biochem Biophys Res Commun 102:970-976

Murray HW 1981 Interaction of *Leishmania* with a macrophage cell line: correlation between intracellular killing and the generation of oxygen intermediates. J Exp Med 153:1690-1695

Nogueira N, Chaplan S, Tydings JD, Unkeless J, Cohn Z 1981 *Trypanosoma cruzi*: surface antigens of blood and culture forms. J Exp Med 153:629-639

Wallach M, Fong D, Chang KP 1982 Post-transcriptional control of tubulin biosynthesis during leishmanial differentiation. Nature (Lond) 299:650-652

Wyler DJ 1982 *In vitro* parasite–monocyte interactions in human leishmaniasis: evidence for an active role of the parasite in attachment. J Clin Invest 70:82-88

DISCUSSION

Wyler: Do the Fab fragments of the monoclonal antibodies have the same effect on *Leishmania* species? Does preincubating parasites with antibody in any way affect lysosomal fusion with the parasitophorous vacuole?

Chang: We know that when *Leishmania* species are inside the macrophage there is a lysosome–phagosome fusion, so I assume that when one coats them with antibody this effect will be indirectly enhanced, and I know of no evidence that it will be inhibited, although we have not tried this in the manner you mentioned.

In the case of *Toxoplasma gondii* there is no phagolysosomal fusion after entry of the parasites into macrophages, and after antibody coating fusion will be induced (Jones et al 1975).

Nogueira: Did you test your monoclonal antibodies with other species of *Leishmania* apart from *L. mexicana amazonensis?*

Chang: The monoclonal antibody 6H12 which, as I mentioned recognizes the triplet surface protein species, is specific to *L. mexicana amazonensis* and unreactive with the strains of *Leishmania donovani*, *Leishmania tropica* and *Leishmania braziliensis* that we have used.

Nogueira: David Lepay, in my laboratory, has been studying the surface antigens of *L. donovani* promastigotes. He identified a major component as being a glycopeptide of 65 000 M_r. This major surface antigen is present in African and Brazilian isolates of *L. donovani*, and is also the major component recognized by immune sera from patients with visceral leishmaniasis. This component was also strongly recognized by immune sera from patients with cutaneous leishmaniasis (*L. braziliensis*).

We found it interesting that the surface profile you have shown for *L. mexicana amazonensis* is so similar to what we found.

Another student in my laboratory, Veronica Colomer, has been continuing these studies and has found that the surface iodination profile of all other *Leishmania* species (*L. tropica*, *L. mexicana*, *L. braziliensis*) is remarkably similar to that of *L. donovani*. Peptide mapping is being done to assess the homologous nature of such peptides. Perhaps the major surface antigen is a primordial *Leishmania* antigen. It is interesting that Howard et al (1982) have shown that immunization with irradiated promastigotes resulted in dramatic cross-protection with *L. tropica*, *L. braziliensis* and *L. mexicana*.

Chang: It is certainly known that different strains or species of *Leishmania* share common antigens. But each strain or species also has unique surface antigens. This property has been used by McMahon Pratt & David (1981) to differentiate *L. braziliensis* from *L. mexicana*. We have studied the surface antigens of *L. donovani* and seen three surface antigens, with M_rs of 65 K, 35 K and 43 K (K.-P. Chang, unpublished work). The 43 K protein is similar in size to one we found in *L. mexicana*. As you know, the sources of molecular markers used by various workers are different, and this may cause a lot of confusion.

Nogueira: Have you looked at the immunological cross-reactivity between the two peptides to see if they are similar? The published work reveals much more similarity than divergence, yet most people are still assuming that the major antigens are different.

Chang: You are right. We are interested in looking at immune cross-precipitation, using our monoclonal antibodies against *L. donovani*.

Warren: One cannot denigrate the idea of looking for different antigens, which is of great importance in immunodiagnosis.

Nogueira: I know, but in terms of *protection* a major antigen seems to be cross-reactive. This antigen may also be common to promastigotes and amastigote stages.

Butterworth: You suggest that the delay of leishmanial division in macrophages, after preincubation of amastigotes with the monoclonal antibodies, may be associated with patching or capping. Earlier you demonstrated that capping could occur. The biological relevance of this effect would depend on whether capping could be achieved in the presence of a *single* layer of antibody; that is, without using an antiglobulin as a second antibody. Also, do you obtain resynthesis after capping?

Chang: We have not tested the first point, but this is suggested by the work of Dwyer (1976) with regard to either antibody-induced or concanavalin A-induced capping of *Leishmania*. Dr Hernández has investigated the second point. *Leishmania* do regenerate their surface ligands after capping and shedding, as other cells do.

Hernández: I was originally worried about our results (Hernández et al 1977, 1981) but I am glad to hear that you have found capping with the antibody because when we did the experiment with concanavalin A we inhibited agglutination by metabolic inhibitors and also by cytochalasin B. On the other hand, Dwyer (1977) reported that these inhibitors did not prevent agglutination in *L. donovani*. He observed agglutination by fixing the parasite with glutaraldehyde, yet we saw none. We have found that the promastigote of this parasite is covered by a cell coat of about 20 nm thickness. Tunicamycin treatment eliminated the coat, as I will describe in my paper (this volume). The conclusion is that this cell coat in the promastigote should be linked to the interior of the cell somehow, and the capping may be selective. We must clarify this because we know that the promastigotes of *L. braziliensis* have two different types of concanavalin A receptor, as defined by their low or high affinity. I believe that we may have minor differences in the glycosidic branch of these glycoproteins, and that this may determine the differences not between *species*, as people have said, but even the differences between *isolates*. My paper emphasizes this. In *L.*

braziliensis the main surface antigen is a complex that ranges in relative molecular mass between 54 and 45 K. We have found four glycoproteins, of 54 K, 50 K, 47 K and 45 K, and these and another component of 63 K are also present in the cell surface. The pattern that Dr Chang obtained with *L. mexicana*, using the same technique and also using reduced gels, as we did, is different from the pattern that we have, even though we have also tested the same strain, and found a different label on the cell surface. The migration of the glycoproteins is definitely altered by the glycosidic composition, so we shall have other problems in comparing different strains. Do you have any idea about the mechanism of transformation from promastigote to amastigote in morphological terms? I am concerned about this because there is a 5-fold reduction in protein content between the promastigote and the amastigote.

Chang: I know that you have proposed a hypothesis concerning the invagination of the surface membrane during promastigote to amastigote differentiation, but I do not know the precise mechanism. If you are talking about the signals received by the cell membrane, I have no information about that. I have results only on antigenic and molecular changes during leishmanial differentiation. There are differences in antigenic composition, but I do not know what they mean in terms of the signals for differentiation until further study.

Pérez: I think that the problem of cross immunity between American *Leishmania* species is more complex than we originally thought. There is no cross immunity between *L. mexicana* and *L. braziliensis*. In your work on promastigotes and amastigotes have you used antibodies obtained from infected animals to check if they interfere with the *in vitro* transformation of amastigotes to promastigotes? In addition, will coating of amastigotes with antibodies interfere with the uptake and intracellular multiplication of amastigotes?

Chang: We have tried this in relation to my previous work with *L. donovani* (K.-P. Chang, unpublished results). If we use hyperimmune serum produced in rabbits to treat amastigotes of *L. donovani* and feed them into macrophages, we see no effect on the uptake or survival of the parasites. I have not done this with *L. mexicana amazonensis,* except for the results with monoclonal antibodies that I already mentioned.

Pérez: I wonder about the possible differences between the antibodies obtained by immunization of animals with killed parasites and the antibodies that are induced by a living infection. Have you ever tried to see the effect of antibodies obtained from immune animals and to look for the effect on the parasites?

Chang: That is difficult for *L. donovani* infections. We have been trying, but unsuccessfully, to cure hamsters infected with *L. donovani*.

Pérez: But surely hamsters are very susceptible to the leishmanial parasites and so they are not a suitable model for studying the effect of antibodies?

Chang: Dr Wallace Peters (personal communication) mentioned to me that if one treats hamsters infected with *L. donovani* five times with amphotericin B, the hamster can be cured.

Pérez: It would be interesting to do the same experiment using antibodies from patients.

Chang: I have not done that because I do not have access to patients' serum, and there would be different kinds of problems.

O'Daly: We are all talking about antigens but not considering how the parasites were cultured. For the last three years we have been culturing these parasites and we have found, for *L. mexicana*, *L. donovani* and *Trypanosoma cruzi*, culture media containing specific peptides. The parasites are tremendously versatile. For example, if we culture *L. mexicana* by several passages in serum and then switch to a culture medium with peptides and make more passages, the parasites acquire the potential to grow without any protein supplement at all. We have successfully grown *L. mexicana* by more than 50 passages through this non-protein medium. *L. donovani* requires different peptides for growth than *L. mexicana* and *T. cruzi*, and the *L. donovani* cannot grow successfully in a medium without peptides (O'Daly et al 1982). We have also been able to grow *T. cruzi* at different temperatures: 26, 30, 34 and 37 °C, but we have not succeeded in switching them to a medium without protein supplements. I wonder whether these different culture conditions in different laboratories can themselves change the antigenic properties of the surface. We know that the requirements at different temperatures are totally different, so the enzymes that they produce are different.

Chang: We have been using a defined medium designed by Steiger & Steiger (1976) to culture our strains of *L. donovani*, *L. mexicana* and *L. tropica*. Protein components in the undefined culture medium may adhere to the surfaces of the parasites and can subsequently be identified as surface antigens. To avoid this problem, we have also used promastigotes grown in this defined medium for our immunofluorescence and immunoprecipitation work. I also have encountered certain strains of *L. donovani* and *L. braziliensis* that do not grow in the defined medium, which tends to support your results. This does pose problems in comparisons of data from different laboratories.

Piras: Dr Hernández has just raised the question of what the signal might be for the differentiation of *Leishmania* species. We could ask, in more general terms, what we really know about the signals for differentiation of other parasites as well.

Sharma: We have been looking at kinetoplast DNA in amastigotes, promastigotes and epimastigotes of *T. cruzi* and found no differences in their restriction enzyme patterns. We have some monoclonal antibodies specific for each strain and are now trying to test for any differences in mRNA between these three forms. We have not been able to get adequate numbers of amastigotes to do the experiments. I would be interested to know what signals trigger the differentiation (see also p 172 and p 254).

Hudson: We have been looking at the control of differentiation and proliferation in a range of human and protozoan cells. Specifically, we have been looking at the activity of the enzyme ADP ribosyl transferase, by using two inhibitors—5-methylnicotinamide and 3-methoxybenzamide. When quiescent lymphocytes are activated and start differentiating, they can rejoin any breaks that are already present in their DNA (Johnstone & Williams 1982). This process can be inhibited by these two chemicals. Exactly the same findings have been shown for *T. cruzi*.

Sher: There seems to be something unique about the amastigote surface. Dr Chang had difficulty raising monoclonal antibodies against amastigotes. Amastigotes, like trypomastigotes, are resistant to killing by the alternative pathway of complement but, even more interestingly, they appear to be resistant to killing by the *classical* pathway of complement. Antibody and complement will not kill amastigotes, an observation which may partly explain the survival of the organisms in the extracellular host environment. Do you have any idea of the changes in the amastigote surface that are responsible for its evasion of immune responses, particularly antibody-mediated immune responses?

Chang: I don't know. This would require purification of the amastigote membranes for comparison with those of the promastigotes. Dr Hernández works more on the chemical aspects of the purified leishmanial membrane. Perhaps he has found chemical differences between promastigotes and amastigotes.

Hernández: Well, when the promastigote is transformed to the amastigote form, the binding of cationic compounds diminishes. Under electrophoretic conditions, however, the two forms migrate similarly. This implies bigger changes in the compounds that confer the negative charge in the transformation from promastigote to amastigote. We found few differences in the cell surface molecular compounds (Hernández et al 1981). Perhaps minor changes in the distribution of the compounds are more important than the new synthesis of compounds.

REFERENCES

Dwyer DM 1976 Antibody-induced modulation of *Leishmania donovani* surface membrane antigens. J Immunol 117:2081-2091

Dwyer DM 1977 *Leishmania donovani*: surface membrane carbohydrates of promastigotes. Exp Parasitol 41:341-358

Hernández AG, Infante RB, La Riva G, De Vera O, Dawidowicz K, Convit J 1977 The surface membrane of *Leishmania*. II: Energy-dependent agglutination of *L. braziliensis* by concanavalin A. Acta Cient Venez 28:380-384

Hernández AG, Arguello C, Ayesta C et al 1981 The surface membrane of *Leishmania*. In: Slutzky GM (ed) The biochemistry of parasites. Pergamon Press, Oxford, p 47-65

Howard JG, Nicklin S, Hale C, Liew FY 1982 Prophylactic immunization against experimental leishmaniasis. I: Protection induced in mice genetically vulnerable to fatal *Leishmania tropica* infection. J Immunol 129:2206

Johnstone AP, Williams GT 1982 Role of DNA breaks and ADP-ribosyl transferase activity in eukaryotic differentiation demonstrated in human lymphocytes. Nature (Lond) 300:368-370

Jones TC, Len L, Hirsch JG 1975 Assessment *in vitro* of immunity against *Toxoplasma gondii*. J Exp Med 141:466-482

McMahon Pratt D, David JR 1981 Monoclonal antibodies that distinguish New World species of *Leishmania*. Nature (Lond) 291:581

O'Daly JA, Rodríguez MB, Caballero H, Garlin G, Serrano LE, Cabrera Z 1982 Biología molecular de *Leishmania mexicana* y *Leishmania donovani*. Bol Of Sanit Panam, in press

Steiger RF, Steiger E 1976 A defined medium for culturing *Leishmania donovani* and *L. braziliensis*. J Parasitol 62:1010

Leishmanial excreted factors and their possible biological role

A. G. HERNÁNDEZ

Facultad de Ciencias, Universidad Central de Venezuela, Apartado 47069, Los Chaguaramos, Caracas 1041, Venezuela

Abstract In the study of interactions between parasites of *Leishmania* species and their environment the release of a variety of materials has been detected. Some of these exo-metabolites are species-specific and may be exploited to characterize different leishmanial isolates. As the plasma membrane is the site of interaction between parasite and host it appears that the presence of metabolic products on, and their subsequent release from, the leishmanial cell surface bears a strong relationship to the biological performance of the parasite. The presence of a shedding mechanism in addition to other means of secretion has been shown in *Leishmania braziliensis* (NR strain). The products shed from the cell surface include glycoproteins and polysaccharide-like complexes. One of these glycoproteins has been purified, and it appears to affect macrophage activity. Because the recognition of these leishmanial metabolic products by antibody is mediated by the glycosylated portion of the secreted macromolecules, a limited repertoire of sugar residues may be common to these types of surface and extra-surface immunogens. Minor changes in the branching or sequence of sugars might constitute a code related to both serotype and biological activity of a given *Leishmania* strain.

1983 Cytopathology of parasitic disease. Pitman Books, London (Ciba Foundation symposium 99), p 138-156

Leishmania species cause leishmaniasis. In unusual hosts, including humans, the disease results in skin lesions—cutaneous and mucocutaneous leishmaniasis—or severe pathological changes in the internal organs—kala-azar—and other forms of visceral leishmaniasis.

During their life cycle these parasites display two different morphological and physiological forms: the amastigote, living intracellularly, with a predilection for cells of the mononuclear phagocyte system of the vertebrate host, and the promastigote in the digestive system of the invertebrate vector as well as in culture medium. One of the most interesting properties of leishmanial parasites is their ability to resist the microbicidal process of even activated macrophages. Moreover, the final outcome seems to depend on the particular host–parasite combination (Mauel 1980).

Leishmanial cell-surface components have been implicated in the protection of the parasite itself against hydrolytic degradation by lysosomal enzymes released into the phagocytic vacuole. The participation of leishmanial released (excreted) products in parasite biology and survival has been proposed by many workers. These propositions fall in two main categories: (a) effects of parasite-excreted factors on the parasite itself (El-On et al 1979, Slutzky & Greenblatt 1979), and (b) effects of the excreted factors on the host cell, such as a conditioning of host susceptibility (Handman & Greenblatt 1977), lysosomal enzyme inhibition (El-On et al 1980) and changes in macrophage metabolism and/or activity (Slutzky & Greenblatt 1977, 1979, Kutish & Janovy 1981, N. Rodríguez et al 1983). Hernández et al (1981), after considering the observed close relationship between parasite-excreted products and parasite membrane components, proposed that specific components in the cell surface of both the promastigote and the amastigote stages may decide the success of the invading organism. This is because some of these components are probably involved in the cellular and biochemical changes that accompany transformation whereas others, once excreted and/or on contact with the host cell, may alter their biological activity. In this paper, I shall outline the specificity, chemistry and production of the excreted factors, their relationship with the parasite cell surface, and the possible biological significance of this relationship. This last point will be speculative because little is known about the molecular mechanisms that regulate invasion, transformation and survival of *Leishmania* species in their host.

Leishmanial excreted factors and strain specificity

Until 1972, one of the accepted means of identifying leishmanial species was based on the known Noguchi–Adler phenomenon (Adler 1964), which consisted in the formation of aggregates of leishmanial promastigotes when cultured in the presence of different concentrations of anti-*Leishmania* serum. The identity of and relationship between different *Leishmania* isolates could be established from the aggregation titre observed in the presence of homologous and heterologous rabbit anti-*Leishmania* sera. In 1972, Schnur et al used gel diffusion on excreted factors (obtained from culture medium freed from parasites) against specific antisera, and monitored the reaction with standard patterns of excreted factor-antisera. From this they were able to assign *Leishmania* strains to different serotypes and sub-serotypes (Schnur & Zuckerman 1977). After the technique was shown to be species-specific, excreted factors became the basis for serotyping *Leishmania* strains and a

TABLE 1 Standard sub-serotypes and the excreted factors of NR and LBY strains of *L. braziliensis*

Antiserum[a]	*Excreted factor*	*Sub-serotype*
LRC-L32	LRC-L36	A_1
LRC-L32	LRC-L32	A_2
LRC-L32	NR[b]	A_3
LRC-L32	LBY[c]	Non-reacting
LRC-L47	LRC-147	B_1
LRC-L47	LRC-L52	B_2
LRC-L47	LBY	Non-reacting

[a]These strains were obtained from the collection of the World Health Organization's Reference Centre for Leishmaniasis (WHO-LRC), maintained in the Department of Medical Protozoology at the Hebrew University, Hadassah Medical School, Jerusalem. Antisera and excreted factors from these strains were kindly supplied by Dr L. F. Schnur. [b]NR strain was isolated from a human case of diffuse cutaneous leishmaniasis. [c]LBY strains were isolated from a human case of cutaneous leishmaniasis and had lost their infectivity.

valuable tool in diagnostic, demographic and ecological studies of the disease. Working in collaboration with Dr L. F. Schnur at The Hebrew University we have established (unpublished results) the the *pathogenic L. braziliensis* (NR strain) belongs to the mixed sub-serotype A_3,B_2 (Table 1). On the other hand, the *non-pathogenic* strain, LBY, does not produce excreted factors capable of being precipitated by any of the so-far tested *Leishmania* antisera of pathogenic strains. The immune precipitate between excreted factors and anti-*Leishmania* serum is inhibited if sugars in the excreted factors are destroyed by treatment with sodium metaperiodate.

The lack of reactivity observed between excreted factors of LBY strain and antisera from the pathogenic strains may therefore be related to the lack of lectin-binding sugars on the cell surface of LBY (Dawidowicz et al 1975) and, thus, to pathogenicity (Dawidowicz et al 1975, Jacobson et al 1982). It is of interest that excreted factors from different Venezuelan strains, which are able to infect mice and hamsters as well as macrophages in culture, belong to serotype A, and that they sub-serotype differently (A_4, A_5, and A_6) from those sub-serotypes so far established (A. G. Hernández et al, unpublished).

Chemistry of excreted factors

At present the number and nature of the products released by the *Leishmania* parasites remains to be determined, and many discrepancies exist among recent reports. The purified product from *L. tropica* (LRC-137) and *L. donovani* (LRC-52) is a polysaccharide-like material of relative molecular mass (M_r) 18 000, containing little or no protein and, despite its content of galactose, glucose and mannose, reacting poorly with concanavalin A. A compound of lower M_r is also secreted by both strains. but in higher proportion by *L. donovani* (El-On et al 1979, Slutzky et al 1979). Decker-Jackson & Honigberg (1978) isolated from the incubation medium of *L. donovani* excreted products called antigenic-active glycoproteins. These macromolecules were found to form precipitin lines with concanavalin A, but not with other lectins tested, in gel diffusion. More recently, Semprevivo & Macleod (1981) argued that the products detected by Decker-Jackson & Honigberg (1978) in *L. donovani* and *L. tropica* could arise either from aggregation and/or degradation processes in media conditioned by growth of promastigotes or during isolation procedures. The results we have obtained with the NR strain do not appear to support the latter hypothesis because we found, as soluble excreted products, at least six glycoproteins of 63 000, 54 000, 50 000, 47 000, 45 000 and 25 000 M_r that are also associated with the parasite plasma membrane (A. G. Hernández & A. El-Homsi, unpublished). All except the 47 000 M_r component bind to a Sepharose–concanavalin A column. This component has been purified by phenol extraction (A. G. Hernández et al, unpublished). It is important to note that a glycoprotein with a similar M_r also binds to Sepharose–concanavalin A. These antigens are probably similar but, owing to glycoprotein microheterogeneity, they react differently with the lectins, as they also do with the antibodies (Hernández et al 1981).

The most likely explanation for these results is that differences in the leishmanial excreted products are due to the particular biological activity of each strain. This conclusion is supported by the report of Decker & Janovy (1974) who showed that the amount of protein and RNA secreted by a leishmanial strain could be related to the clinical manifestation of the particular *Leishmania* species; i.e. a strain causing an internal infection was more stable and excreted less material than did a cutaneous strain when incubated at body temperature. We have also found that radioactively labelled excreted products of *L. tropica, L. donovani* and *L. braziliensis* differ when their progress is followed by double labelling with [^{14}C]glucosamine and [^{3}H]leucine (A. G. Hernández and G. M. Slutzky, unpublished).

Production of excreted factors and the leishmanial cell surface

Promastigote production of excreted factors and its cell surface

Hernández et al (1980) demonstrated that 10–25% of the total protein synthesized by actively growing promastigote cells is excreted and that the excreted proteins do not result from cell lysis. Labelling with [^{3}H]glucosamine and [^{3}H]leucine suggests that some of the released material is glycoprotein. Production of excreted factors is inhibited by certain drugs. Decker & Janovy (1974) showed that the anti-leishmanial drug Stibophen inhibits production of excreted factors, and Hernández et al (1980) found a similar effect when using cycloheximide (100 μg/ml) and puromycin (0.5 mM). The promastigotes seem to excrete by at least two mechanisms: (a) an exocytic process, similar to the one mentioned by Adler (1964) and Hernández et al (1981), evidence for which has been obtained mainly by electron microscope studies; and (b) shedding of membrane components. By electron microscope studies we have been able to demonstrate (F. Dagger et al, unpublished) the formation of vesicles at the level of the cell surface similar to those found in the parasite-free medium. The cell surface of the NR promastigotes can be iodinated with ^{125}I and the soluble products released into the incubation medium can then be compared by autoradiography with those associated with the plasma membrane. When the particulate fraction is obtained by differential centrifugation of the same medium, at least six identical glycoproteins are found in each fraction. The total amount of protein shed in 24 h is 15% of the total label associated with the NR cell surface. This demonstrates clearly that in the NR strain of *L. braziliensis*, some of the so-called excretion factors are localized at the cell surface and, moreover, that the product purified by us and tested for biological activity in macrophages is also derived from the parasitic plasma membrane. These compounds are likely to be associated with the cell coat that surrounds the promastigote. This coat appears to have a special function in the penetration and survival of *Leishmania* species in macrophages, as suggested by the following experiments. When the NR promastigotes are treated with tunicamycin at 2 μg/ml, mannose incorporation is inhibited by 64% and leucine incorporation by 35%. In these conditions the cell coat disappears and the living parasites are engulfed by macrophages about twice as fast as non-treated parasites, and further digested (A. G. Hernández et al, unpublished).

On the other hand, the LBY strain of *L. braziliensis* is poorly phagocytized, and the parasites that *are* phagocytized are digested in less than six hours. When purified excreted factors from the NR strain are added to the medium containing the LBY strain and incubated, binding and penetration of the parasite in the cell host is promoted, and the parasites remain there for at least three days. At this point it is convenient to recall the main differences we have found between the cell surfaces of the NR and LBY strains (Hernández et al 1981) and their possible relation to excreted factors. The promastigote form of NR has a greater number of concanavalin A receptors associated with a highly exposed negative charge, and the cells are readily agglutinated in the presence of concanavalin A and *Ricinus communis* agglutinin. On the other hand, the non-pathogenic LBY promastigotes are not agglutinated by *Ricinus* agglutinin, their concanavalin A receptors are present in small numbers and their cell surfaces lack a negative charge. More recently, Jacobson et al (1982) demonstrated small but significant differences in lectin reactivities of different strains as serotyped by excretion factors, and showed that some of these differences may be related to differences in parasite dissemination.

It seems probable that these products, when localized in the cell surface of the promastigotes, act as regulators of the penetration rate of the parasite, thus allowing for differentiation as one of the key factors in parasite survival (Lewis & Peters 1977). Once inside the macrophage, the presence of the parasite's excreted factors and their release may have other effects, which I shall mention below.

Amastigote production of excretion factors and its cell surface

Evidence of production of excretion factors by the amastigote form of *Leishmania* species is more indirect. Schnur et al (1972) showed that antigenic material can be obtained by short-term incubation *in vitro* of spleen and epididymes of infected hamsters. We obtained similar results when incubating footpads of infected hamsters and mice under similar conditions. Amastigotes, isolated from these lesions by using concanavalin A as described by Infante et al (1980) and observed under phase-contrast microscopy, showed a surrounding mesh-like matrix. This matrix, which can be removed but not totally eliminated by washing with phosphate-buffered saline, binds concanavalin A and anti-*Leishmania* serum. That antibodies to antigenic-active glycoproteins (excreted factors) are present in sera of infected hamsters was demonstrated by Decker-Jackson & Honigberg (1978), indicating that these substances are produced by the parasites inside their host. Slutzky & Greenblatt (1979) found, in macrophages late-infected with *L. tropica*, a compound that comigrates with the labelled excreted factors produced by *L. tropica* promastigotes. Thus, amastigotes retain the ability to synthesize excreted factors. In collaboration with Dr T. Dishon (The Hebrew University) we have detected the presence of excreted factors in the culture medium of J774G8 macrophages infected with *L. mexicana*. Electron microscope studies carried out by Scorza et al (1983) in Venezuela have shown a sequence of events that seem to involve secretion of material through the flagellar pocket (Fig. 1). This material fills the phagocytic vacuole, whereas the parasite remains attached to the vacuole membrane. Benchimol & De Souza (1981) have shown a similar structure of amastigote–vacuole attachment. Freeze-fracture replicas showed an array of intramembranous particles in some areas of the parasite plasma membrane that resembled a gap junction.

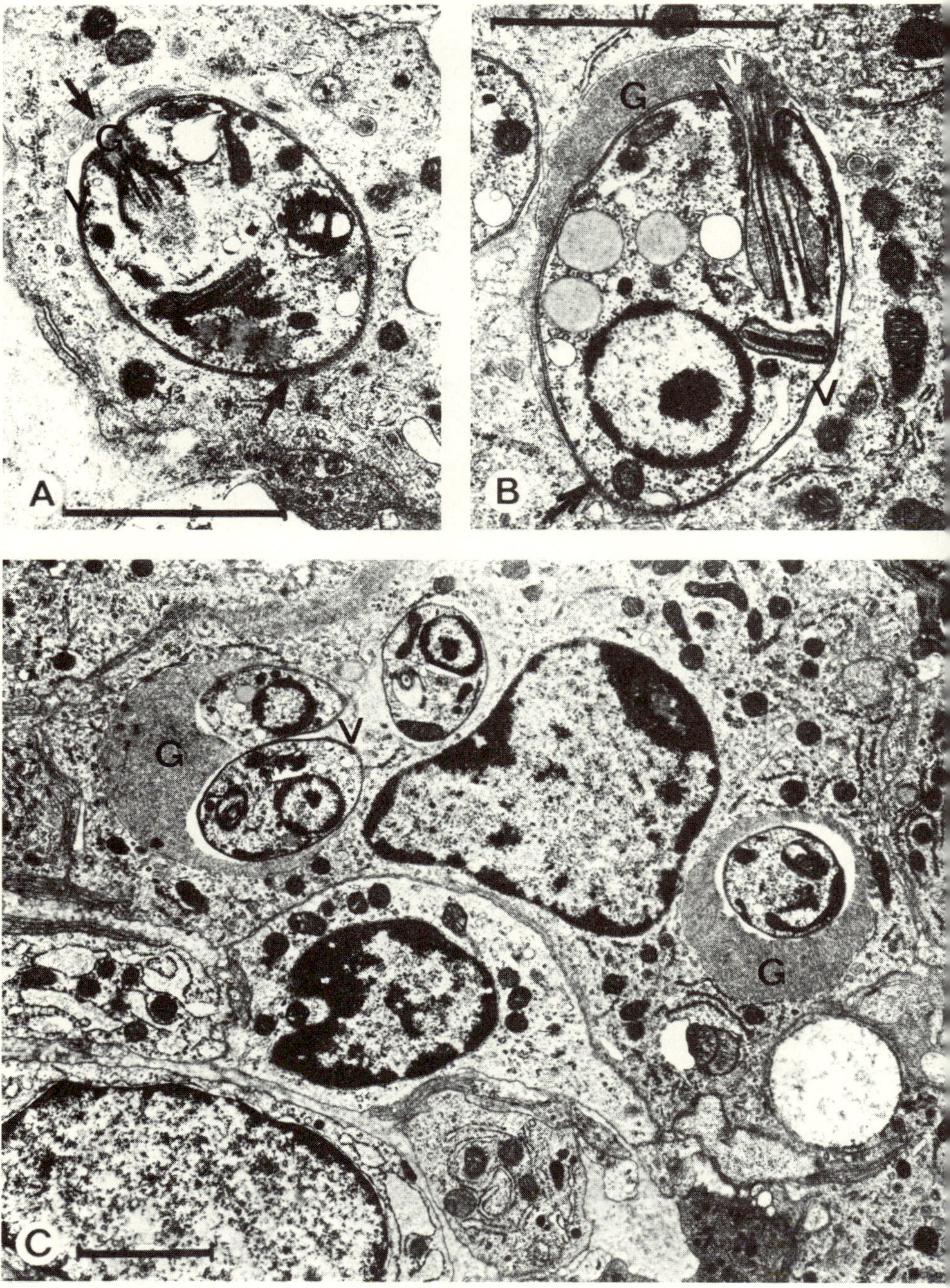
A
C
V
B
G
V
C
G
V
G

This adhesion may be important in the interaction between the leishmanial parasite and its host cell. In fact, Bhattacharya & Janovy (1975) have shown molecular exchanges between parasites and host cell.

In the process of transformation from promastigote to amastigote form, apparently through an endocytic process, we have detected a 50% reduction in the number of concanavalin A receptors, as well as a reduced number of exposed negative charges at the cell surface. Although the amastigotes bind concanavalin A, they are not agglutinated by it. This suggests profound changes in the dynamics of the cell surface, e.g. in membrane fluidity, when transformation occurs (Hernández et al 1977, 1981). However, they are still able to bind anti-*Leishmania* sera produced for excretion-factor serotyping.

Leishmania species in their different physiological forms thus release a certain amount of metabolic products into their surroundings. From the evidence presented, the materials released by the promastigote form cannot be considered experimental artifacts. Part of the excreted factors appear to be bound to the cell surface of the organism and they could be membrane or transient membrane components that are clearly related immunologically to permanent membrane structures. Their presence in the promastigote cell surface may act as a regulator of parasite penetration into the host cell, thus allowing differentiation to occur in the presence of a specific signal.

The substances released by the parasites appear to be able to reach the host-cell cytoplasm and plasma membrane, where they may produce important metabolic changes (see next section). The excretion occurs by exocytosis and by a shedding mechanism. Since the parasite devotes considerable amounts of energy to production and excretion of the factors, it can be assumed that they benefit the parasite in some way.

Possible biological role of leishmanial excreted products

Very little is known about the biological role of excreted factors. Suggestions about their action on macrophage activity or host immunological machinery are based on interpretations from different experimental designs, and almost every study using excreted substances has involved poorly characterized biochemical material. The following categories of excreted factor action on macrophages will be considered.

FIG. 1. Electron microscopy of thin sections of tissue infected with *L. garhami* n.sp., showing phagocytic vacuoles (V) that contain amastigotes. The upper arrows (in A and B) indicate, at the anterior end of the amastigotes, the flagellar pocket, and the presence of an evenly distributed granulation (G) suggestive of secretion through this structure. At the opposite end are the parasites attached to the wall of the vacuole (lower arrows). Bar = 2 μm. (Reproduced from Scorza et al (1983) with permission of the author and the publisher).

Excreted factors and clinical pathology of leishmaniasis

Decker & Janovy (1974) have associated clinical manifestations of disease with differences in production of excreted factors by *L. donovani* and *L. mexicana*. They showed that this production may be altered by environmental temperature and substrate in a species-specific manner. In the presence of glucose, *L. donovani* excreted mostly low M_r compounds and RNA. On the other hand, *L. mexicana* secreted (i.e. excreted) more of the higher M_r compounds whether glucose was present or not.

From these results, Decker & Janovy (1974) proposed that the clinical manifestations of infection with those parasites could be the result of blockade, by low M_r proteins, of T cell processing both of the antigen and, consequently, of any serum antibody with a very low binding specificity for the introduced hapten. Also, it has been postulated that the haemolytic anaemia characteristically observed in persons suffering from kala-azar is caused by an autoimmune response. The anaemia is said to result from enhanced engulfment and destruction of red cells by splenic phagocytes. These effects are possibly due to a response elicited by antigens common to parasite and host or by circulating antigens released by the living parasites and adsorbed onto the red cells (Decker-Jackson & Honigberg 1978).

Conditioning of growth medium

In medium conditioned with partially purified excreted factors from *L. donovani*, El-On et al (1979) observed a shortened lag phase of promastigotes. However, both conditioned and non-conditioned cultures produced equal numbers of promastigotes per unit volume by the end of growth. These workers proposed that excreted factors around the cell prevent early aggregation of parasites, thus allowing them a better access to the surrounding media. I believe there are other explanations. Early deposits of excreted factors on the parasite cell surface may help in bringing close to the parasite the growth factors needed for its development, such as albumin to which excreted factors bind (Slutzky et al 1979). Also, excreted factors could act as membrane stabilizers. We have noticed that cells treated with tunicamycin (2 μg/ml or 6 μg/ml) lack surface coat and display a great fragility, with the plasma membrane tending to form ruffles. Thus, the cells tend to lyse (F. Dagger et al, unpublished).

Lysosomal enzyme activity

Inhibition of acid phosphatase activity in macrophages infected with *L. mexicana mexicana* led Lewis & Peters (1977) to suggest that intracellular

Leishmania avoid digestion by interfering with the activity of lysosomal enzymes that are freely delivered to the parasitophorous vacuole. However, partially purified excreted factors from *L. donovani* did not affect acid phosphatase, β-glucuronidase and N-acetyl-β-glucosaminidase activities from lysed peritoneal exudates of mice strains C3H/He (resistant to the infection) and G57BL/10ScSn (susceptible). In both cases inhibition (72%) of β-galactosidase was demonstrated (El-On et al 1980). Although these results appear to conflict with each other they exemplify some of the problems that I mentioned in the introduction of this section. The factor(s) tested by El-On et al (1980) is probably one of the many secreted by *L. donovani* (Decker-Jackson & Honigberg 1978) and by *L. braziliensis* (Hernández et al 1980, 1981). Different excreted products may have different functions, and more knowledge is needed about the production and chemistry of the products.

Passive resistance

One of the biological functions in which the leishmanial cell surface has been implicated is protection of the parasite against hydrolytic degradation by lysosomal enzymes released into the phagocytic vacuole (Chang & Dwyer 1978). In the absence of any surface coat that might serve as a physical barrier to digestive enzymes it has been assumed that the resistance of amastigotes to lysosomal enzymes is due to a refractory property of the plasma membrane. However, I have two comments. First, it is possible that the same components shed by the amastigotes (Lewis & Peters 1977) are present as permanent or transient membrane components. Second, the suggestion that a 'shield' or 'cloud' of leishmanial material impermeable to potentially bactericidal chemicals does not exist comes from the lack of evidence for a physical barrier. However, I think that the idea cannot be discarded because, as we have seen, a great amount of material apparently excreted by the parasite surrounds the amastigote in the parasitophorous vacuole. In addition, amastigotes isolated by using mild conditions of rupture (Infante et al 1980) are immersed in a meshlike coat that, by washing, can be diminished but not totally eliminated (Hernández et al 1981).

Macrophage activity

It is possible that excreted factors go beyond mere resistance in their effect on macrophages. Handman & Greenblatt (1977) have shown that excreted factors allow parasites to grow in otherwise non-permissive macrophages. Further, infection with *Leishmania* species alters overall macrophage activity, because recently infected macrophages show an apparent shift in the synthetic pattern of high M_r components (Slutzky & Greenblatt 1979). Thus, parasites appear to affect the host cell's machinery of protein synthesis directly. Leishmanial infection also alters the pinocytic rate of the host cell, as shown by Chang (1980). Kutish & Janovy (1981) demonstrated that infective parasites could suppress macrophage digestive capacity, possibly through an active process in which communicator molecules, which inhibit specific functions, are released by intracellular amastigotes. Alternatively, they proposed that macrophage digestive capacity, in the period following initial lysosomal fusion with the parasitophorous vacuole, could be inhibited passively through depletion of the macrophage metabolic pool by the living intracellular amastigotes. Experiments from my laboratory support the first of these hypotheses: peritoneal macrophages and macrophages of the permanent cell line J774-G8, when treated with purified excreted factor from *L. braziliensis*, showed inhibition of the endocytic rate for [^{125}I]albumin and [^{14}C]sucrose (Fig. 2). Furthermore, digestion of albumin in treated macrophages took place in about double the time for that in the control. Material obtained from culture medium alone did not produce the above effects, which are not the result of an overload of material because the inhibition did not depend on the number of cells used in the assay. Neither does the inhibition appear to be due to the interaction of purified excreted factor with albumin at the level of the macrophage cell surface because macrophages previously treated with the purified material, and those that have removed it from the external face of the cell surface, retained inhibition of endocytic rate and showed almost no digestive capacity for albumin (N. Rodríguez et al 1983).

In conclusion, excreted material from *Leishmania* species may alter the macrophage membrane properties as well as other metabolic activities of these cells. It seems possible that leishmanial products convert the phagocytic and potentially bactericidal macrophage to a primarily 'metabolic cell', as proposed by Draper (1981) for macrophage infection with *Mycobacterium lepramurium*.

General comments

Parasite survival within the host may depend on the capacity of the organism to become intracellular and on its speed of transformation from the promastigote to the amastigote form. Substances located at the parasite cell surface, in contact with the host cell surface, may regulate entry and transformation of the organism. This transformation and the changes that accompany it may render the macrophage resistant to the attack of lysosomal enzymes. It is also

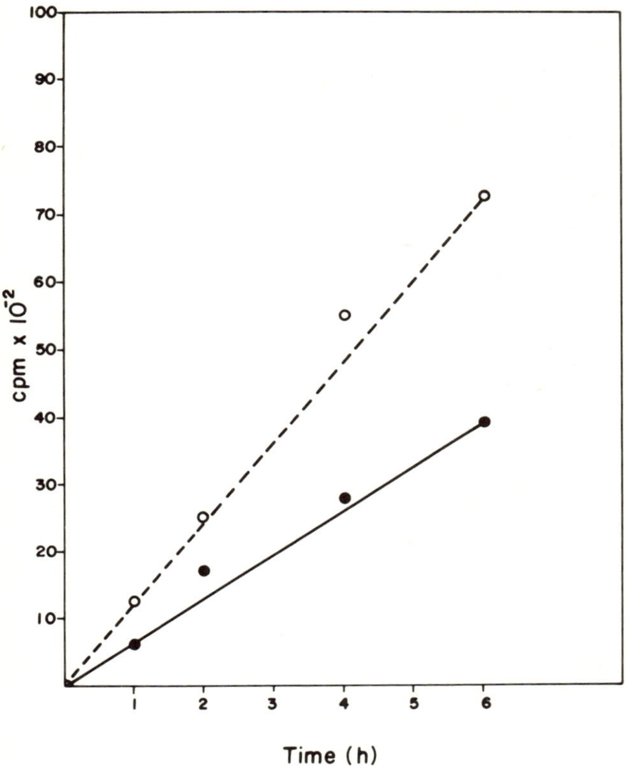

FIG. 2. Time course of fluid endocytosis by J774-G8 macrophages. [^{14}C]sucrose was used as a tracer of fluid endocytosis. Open circles, control cells; filled circles, cells treated with purified excreted factors.

conceivable that once transformation has occurred specific signals condition the excretion of different leishmanial products which protect the parasite itself from digestion in a 'passive' form (by forming a 'shield' or 'cloud' around the organism) or in an 'active' form (by inhibition of lysosomal enzymes or by altering macrophage metabolism). Excreted products may leave the parasitophorous vacuole and affect various macrophage activities such as function of its plasma membrane and its metabolic performance including protein synthesis and oxidative machineries. This would confirm (Mauel 1980) that whereas phagolysosome formation is a prerequisite for eventual digestion of intracellular microorganisms it may not be sufficient in itself to affect the parasite lethally, and the production of adequate metabolic response by the host cell may also be required.

Acknowledgements

This work was supported by grants CDCH C-01-1-79, C-01-5-81 and CONICIT DDCT-SALT 9. I wish to express my gratitude to my colleagues whose work is mentioned here as unpublished; their work forms the basis of several of the hypotheses presented herein. I am also grateful to Drs F. Dagger and K. Dawidowicz for reviewing the manuscript and to Mrs Lourdes Zerpa for invaluable help in preparation of the manuscript.

REFERENCES

Adler S 1964 *Leishmania*. Adv Parasitol 2:35-96

Benchimol M, De Souza W 1981 *Leishmania mexicana amazonensis*. Attachment to the membrane of the phagocytic vacuole of macrophages *in vivo*. Z Parasitenkd 66:25-29

Bhattacharya A, Janovy J Jr 1975 *Leishmania donovani*: autoradiographic evidence for molecular exchanges between parasites and host cells. Exp Parasitol 37:353-360

Chang KP 1980 Endocytosis of *Leishmania*-infected macrophages. Fluorometry of pinocytic rate, lysosome–phagosome fusion and intralysosomal pH. In: Van den Bossche H (ed) The host–invader interplay. Elsevier/North-Holland, Amsterdam, p 231-234

Chang KP, Dwyer D 1978 *Leishmania donovani*–hamster macrophage interactions *in vitro*: cell entry, intracellular survival and multiplication of amastigotes. J Exp Med 147:515-530

Dawidowicz K, Hernández AG, Infante RB, Convit J 1975 The surface membrane of *Leishmania*. The effects of lectins in different stages of *L. braziliensis*. J Parasitol 61:950-953

Decker JE, Janovy J Jr 1974 *Leishmania donovani* and *L. mexicana*: production of the excretion factor. Comp Biochem Physiol B Comp Biochem 49:513-523

Decker-Jackson JE, Honigberg BM 1978 Glycoproteins released by *Leishmania donovani*: immunologic relationships with host and bacterial antigens and preliminary biochemical analysis. J Protozool 25:514-525

Draper P 1981 Mycobacterial inhibition of intracellular killing. In: O'Grady F, Smith H (eds) Microbial perturbations of host defences (The Beecham Colloquia). Academic Press, London, p 143-164

El-On J, Schur LF, Greenblatt CL 1979 *Leishmania donovani*: physicochemical, immunological and biological characterization of excreted factors from promastigotes. Exp Parasitol 47:254-259

El-On J, Bradley DJ, Freeman JC 1980 *Leishmania donovani*: action of excreted factor on hydrolytic enzyme activity of macrophages from mice with genetically different resistance to infection. Exp Parasitol 49:167-174

Handman E, Greenblatt CL 1977 Promotion of leishmanial infections in non-permissive host macrophages by conditioned medium. Z Parasitenkd 53:143-147

Hernández AG, Infante RB, La Riva G, De Vera O, Dawidowicz K, Convit J 1977 The surface membrane of *Leishmania*. II: Energy-dependent agglutination of *L. braziliensis* by concanavalin A. Acta Cient Venez 28:380-384

Hernández AG, Rodríguez N, Dagger F, Greenblatt CL 1980 Production and secretion of *L. braziliensis* proteins. Mol Biochem Parasitol 1:143-149

Hernández AG, Argüello C, Ayesta C et al 1981 The surface membrane of *Leishmania*. In: Slutzky G (ed) The biochemistry of parasites. Pergamon Press, Oxford, p 47-65

Infante RB, Hernández AG, Riggione F, Dawidowicz K 1980 A new method for the partial purification of *Leishmania* amastigotes from cutaneous lesions. Parasitology 80:105-112

Jacobson RL, Slutzky GM, Greenblatt CL, Schnur LF 1982 Surface reaction of *Leishmania*. I: Lectin-mediated agglutination. Ann Trop Med Parasitol 76:45-52
Kutish GF, Janovy J Jr 1981 Inhibition of *in vitro* macrophage digestion capacity by infection with *Leishmania donovani*. J Parasitol 67:457-462
Lewis DH, Peters W 1977 The resistance of intracellular *Leishmania* parasites to digestion by lysosomal enzymes. Ann Trop Med Parasitol 71:295-312
Mauel J 1980 The biology of the macrophage–*Leishmania* interaction. In: Van den Bossche H (ed) The host–invader interplay. Elsevier/North-Holland, Amsterdam, p 165-177
Rodríguez N, Hernández AG, Merino F 1983 The effect of a purified excreted factor (EF) from *Leishmania braziliensis* on macrophage activity. Int Arch Allergy Appl Immunol, in press
Schnur LF, Zuckerman A 1977 Leishmanial excreted (EF) serotypes in Sudan, Kenya and Ethiopia. Ann Trop Med Parasitol 71:273-294
Schnur LF, Zuckerman A, Greenblatt CL 1972 Leishmanial serotypes as distinguished by the gel diffusion of factors excreted *in vitro* and *in vivo*. Isr J Med Sci 8:932-942
Scorza JV, Palacios-Pru E, Carnevalli M 1983 Relaciones Hospedador-parásito entre *Leishmania sp*. de Venezuela e histiocitos de lesiones dérmicas en hamsters. Acta Cient Venez, in press
Semprevivo LH, MacLeod ME 1981 Characterization of the exometabolite of *L. donovani* as a novel glycopeptidophospho-sphingolipid. Biochem Biophys Res Commun 103:1179-1185
Slutzky GM, Greenblatt CL 1977 Isolation of a carbohydrate-rich immunologically active factor from cultures of *L. tropica*. FEBS (Fed Eur Biochem Soc) Lett 80:401-404
Slutzky GM, Greenblatt CL 1979 Analysis by SDS–polyacrylamide gel electrophoresis of an immunologically active factor of *Leishmania tropica* from growth media, promastigotes and infected macrophages. Biochem Med 21:70-77
Slutzky GM, El-On J, Greenblatt CL 1979 Leishmanial excreted factor: protein bound and free forms from promastigote cultures of *Leishmania tropica* and *L. donovani*. Infect Immun 26:916-924

DISCUSSION

Warren: Several years ago the Hadassah group were working with leishmanial excretory factors. They *boiled* the supernatant from leishmanial cell cultures and obtained a white powder that seemed to do everything you mentioned (El-On et al 1979). Hamburger & Ben-Sasson (1981) also boiled whole schistosomula to see if it exposed other surface groups that might be useful for immunizing animals against schistosomiasis, but this did not work. How does their work fit in with your work?

Hernández: I became interested in this field after meeting Professor C.L. Greenblatt. Our results fit quite well with their results which I mentioned in my paper, but we have nevertheless developed our own procedure for purification of the factors. We cannot obtain any precipitate after boiling of the medium. However, the final product that we isolate is resistant to boiling in terms of the reaction with the antigen.

Nogueira: When you showed the cell-surface profile of the iodinated organisms you found a 63 K and a 50 K protein and a doublet of 23–25 K. This is nearly the same profile that we have obtained with *Leishmania donovani.* You have used a reduced gel in these results, but do you know what the profile looks like when you use an unreduced gel?

Hernández: No.

Nogueira: I'm asking this because we used to see a 65 K protein, a 50 K protein and a doublet at 20–25 K. The relationship between the amounts of 50 K and 65 K proteins was variable from experiment to experiment. However, when we used unreduced gels we found that all the 65 K protein disappeared and everything appeared as the 50 K protein. After immunoprecipitations we also found only the 50 K protein. But if we used reduced gels we saw both components, until we realized that the reducing agent in the sample buffer was old. Under fully reduced conditions we see only the 65 K. Do you see any variability in the proportions of 50 K and 63 K proteins? When you purified the excreted factors you mentioned only a 47 K component. Do you ever see the 63 K component after purifying?

Hernández: We haven't observed this with the 50 K protein, but it is probable that the 47 K component is a degradation product of the 63 K protein that we have seen. We tested the 47 K component in reduced and unreduced conditions and saw virtually no variation in the relative molecular mass (M_r). When we purify our fraction by concanavalin A–Sepharose we can obtain another product that binds to concanavalin A and is eluted by α-methylmannopyranoside which has the same M_r as the 47 K component but different affinity for the antisera. For example, the 47 K protein that is isolated as a non-binding protein reacts against serotype A, B and AB, whereas the other one, which binds to the concanavalin A–Sepharose, reacts only with the A and the AB but not with the B serotype. We have purified the 63 K protein already by using diethylaminoethyl cellulose and I think it is a different compound to the 54 K compound, which binds to the concanavalin A–Sepharose and is impossible to remove under normal conditions.

Nogueira: It would be interesting to do peptide mapping to investigate if they are related. Have you tested whether the leishmanial excreted factors affect lysosome–phagosome fusion in the macrophage? One could do this by using dextran of different sizes, and acridine orange, to see if the excreted factors enhance or inhibit fusion.

Hernández: I have done one experiment similar to that described by Edelson & Cohn (1974) using concanavalin A, labelled with fluorescein isothiocyanate. In the presence of excreted factors one can observe that the number of vesicles inside the macrophage is reduced, but that they remain there for a long time. Perhaps fusion is also diminished, but I am not sure.

Mirelman: I would like you to clarify something about the carbohydrate-binding property of the excreted factors. You mentioned that you can block the binding of excreted factors to the macrophage by galactose. Can you also block the binding of the parasite to the excreted factors when you coat the parasite with galactose?

Hernández: Yes. If we treat the parasite (LBY) with excreted factors and afterwards add the parasite in the presence of galactose, the binding is blocked. So the galactose seems also to be blocking the binding to the parasite.

Mirelman: Secondly, with regard to the binding of the excreted factor that you cannot elute back from the concanavalin A–Sepharose column, you could try two possible things. Perhaps the galactose-binding activity binds to the Sepharose which, as you know, is polygalactose, so that may explain why you cannot elute. In addition, you could try 50% ethylene glycol, which has been known to help remove hydrophobic binding as it occurs for instance in the purification of interferon. Furthermore, as you know, the commercial product tunicamycin contains a lot of protein-synthesis inhibitors; thus it is not only an *N*-glycosidic inhibitor. Duksin & Mahoney (1982) from our Institute have purified tunicamycin and separated it into different inhibitory activities. They now have obtained some very clean tunicamycin that will block only *N*-glycosidic activities. Have you ever tested whether your preparation has some protein-synthesis inhibitory properties?

Hernández: I agree that could be possible. However, we have seen a small inhibitory activity (≈35%) on protein synthesis in *Leishmania* species. In addition, we have also observed other effects in the parasite as a consequence of the presence of tunicamycin. For example, the transport of amino acids decreases by about 20%, so the incorporation of the precursor will be diminished. In addition, we have detected the dissociation of ribosomes from the rough endoplasmic reticulum in the presence of tunicamycin. We don't know if this happens because a protein-synthesis inhibitor is present or because of other effects that the tunicamycin induces in this parasite.

Warren: Are the parasites alive after you have treated them with tunicamycin?

Hernández: Yes. We have tested this. At 2 μg/ml of tunicamycin, 98% remain viable. At concentrations greater than 2 μg/ml the viability decreases.

Warren: So why do they not multiply within the macrophages; perhaps they are damaged?

Hernández: I agree. They do not have a cell coat and anything could happen to them.

Piras: Do you really need to use that much tunicamycin? If one uses a much smaller dose, as we do with *Trypanosoma cruzi* (50 ng/ml), we see no inhibition of protein synthesis, but we obtain the full inhibitory effect on parasite penetration. Perhaps with the high doses the side effects of a contaminant become apparent. Our source is from Dr G. Tamura in Japan. It is interesting that Dr Hernández found that tunicamycin stimulates both the adhesion and the interiorization of *Leishmania* species. Our results (this volume) showed that tunicamycin, while stimulating adhesion in *T. cruzi* slightly, does stop penetration completely. Although these are different parasites, I wonder whether the difference resides more on the target cell. We are using fibroblasts as host cells and Dr Hernández is using macrophages. Perhaps Dr Nogueira might comment on whether she has data on the blood forms and macrophages with tunicamycin. This would be important because it might show that the mechanism of penetration in the two cell types is completely different. Once a parasite attaches to the macrophage, which is a professional phagocytic cell, it will just be interiorized, but the situation would probably be quite different for fibroblastic cells.

Nogueira: No; I have never tried that.

Hernández: We tested the doses from 0.1 to 10.0 μg/ml and the optimal dose for these studies in *Leishmania* species was 2 μg/ml. The dose of tunicamycin that inhibits glycosylation varies in different systems.

Martinez-Palomo: These excreted factors have great biological significance. Recently Black et al (1982) have shown for *Trypanosoma brucei* that excreted factors represent components released from the cytoplasm of the cell and not from the surface. You have used terms such as exocytosis, secretion and excretion interchangeably, but these are completely different terms from the cell biological point of view. It is important to clarify this point, although I know this is difficult. For the time being I think that you can speak only about 'external factors'. I know that Carlos Argüello (unpublished observations), has recently demonstrated that *Leishmania braziliensis* is capable of secreting extracellular components that produce a fibrillar network that has some similarities to fibronectin. If this is so, it means that most of these components are *secreted*, and are *extracellular* components.

Hernández: Our last experiment suggests that shedding of material takes place from *Leishmania* species. We can also be sure that an exocytic mechanism is working in this parasite. We have also seen fusion of vesicles with flagellar pocket membrane, suggesting secretion. As you said, with Dr Argüello we have also observed fibrillar material around the parasite.

Andrade: How sure can you be, about these secretory/excretory products in culture, since some of the parasites may degenerate and some material may diffuse through the cell membrane?

Hernández: We have some direct and some indirect evidence. The proportion of material found in the medium is always constant, in proportion to the total labelled material associated with the parasite. If there were damage, one would expect to see peaks or irregularities all along the entire growth curve. We also labelled the parasite with [^{3}H]thymidine and [^{3}H]uridine, and the amount of labelled material did not follow the kinetics obtained when we labelled with [^{3}H]leucine or [^{3}H]glucosamine. If the parasite is disrupted one would expect that uridine-labelled compounds should accompany, in the same proportion, compounds labelled with [^{3}H]leucine, but this does not happen. Futhermore, when the secretion experiments are done in serum-free medium, one of the key points is to check viability. After two hours of incubation one may well detect the presence of products outside, when all the cells are apparently functioning well.

Klebanoff: A word of caution regarding surface-labelling of proteins with iodine: if one binds relatively few molecules of iodine, one can identify surface proteins without adversely affecting the cell. But if iodination is more extensive, the cell may be damaged or killed, and lysis may release proteins that are subsequently iodinated (Klebanoff & Clark 1975). So it is important to know precisely how the iodination is done, how much total iodine is being bound to the surface (not just radioactive iodine) and whether, as a consequence of this iodination, the microorganism or cell is damaged.

Hernández: We faced this problem when we first started our work with lactoperoxidase. We used to iodinate in the cold for 15 min and later check the viability. With Iodo-Gen we don't have this problem: we are using a small amount of iodine and we don't need to use peroxide. The cleanness of the autoradiography after gel electrophoresis suggests that the iodide is not penetrating; that is, the label does not get inside the parasite. We can also label the material in parallel, with glucosamine. So I don't think we have this problem, although I agree that we have to be very careful in each experiment.

Nussenzweig: You postulated that the excreted factors are important in the interaction of the parasite with the macrophage and the subsequent intracellular fate of *Leishmania* species. Can you distinguish the excreted factors from different leishmanial isolates by their different tropism for different cells? Is there any correlation?

Hernández: I wish we could do that! We can distinguish between isolates by the reaction between the excreted factors and a given antiserum. That is why we are interested in purifying the compound, so as to study the glycosidic composition of this portion of the molecule. We think that this could explain differences in tropism and differences in behaviour of a given strain when it confronts the macrophage.

Hudson: Although one would not doubt the biological occurrence of excreted factors, the difficulty is to establish their physiological relevance. Have you looked at the effect of these same factors on other cells or, alternatively, have you looked in patients to see whether your reported conversion of the macrophage to a primary metabolic cell is one of the hallmarks of the resultant disease?

Hernández: Decker-Jackson & Honigberg (1978) showed that experimentally prepared hyperimmune sera from mice react with promastigote antigens. This proved suitable for the detection of antigenic active glycoprotein, which I mentioned in my paper. But we have not tested what happens in macrophages in the lesion. We have not looked for any effects on unrelated cells.

REFERENCES

Black SJ, Hewett RS, Sendashonga CN 1982 *Trypanosoma brucei* variable surface antigen is released by degenerating parasites but not by actively dividing parasites. Parasite Immunol (Oxf) 4:233-244

Decker-Jackson JE, Honigberg BM 1978 Glycoproteins released by *Leishmania donovani*: immunologic relationships with host and bacterial antigens and preliminary biochemical analysis. J Protozool 25:514-525

Duksin D, Mahoney WC 1982 Relationship of the structure and biological activity of the natural homologues of tunicamycin. J Biol Chem 257:3105-3109

Edelson PJ, Cohn ZA 1974 Effects of concanavalin A on mouse peritoneal macrophages. J Exp Med 140:1364-1387

El-On J, Schnur LF, Greenblatt CL 1979 *Leishmania donovani*: physicochemical, immunological and biological characterization of excreted factor from promastigotes. Exp Parasitol 47:254-259

Hamburger J, Ben-Sasson SA 1981 Serobiological differentiation between antischistosomal (*Schistosoma mansoni*) antisera. Tropenmed Parasitol 32:43-47

Klebanoff SJ, Clark RA 1975 Hemolysis and iodination of erythrocyte components by a myeloperoxidase-mediated system. Blood 45:699-707

Factors influencing the host response to *Leishmania mexicana*

HILDA PÉREZ

Laboratorio de Inmunoparasitología, Centro de Microbiología y Biología Celular, Instituto Venezolano de Investigaciones Científicas, Apartado 1827, Caracas 1010A, Venezuela

Abstract The immune response of resistant and susceptible mice infected with *Leishmania mexicana* has been studied. In resistant mice infection was associated with the development of delayed hypersensitivity to parasite antigens and the development of specific antibodies, and protective immunity to a subsequent challenge infection with *L. mexicana* was demonstrable. After adoptive transfer of lymph node cells and peritoneal cells from immune donors, recipient mice showed an increased ability to control a challenge infection. T lymphocytes from recovering mice, transferred together with parasite antigens, mediated a specific delayed hypersensitivity. In a local cell-transfer assay, peritoneal cells from immune mice produced significant protection against a living inoculum. Immune serum enhanced the protection conferred by peritoneal cells, but immune serum alone was ineffective. It is postulated that immunity to *L. mexicana* is mediated by collaboration between T-cell activated macrophages and antibodies. In susceptible BALB/c mice, infection with *L. mexicana* led to the activation of specific and non-specific suppressor cells. The former are related to T cells whereas the latter belong to the splenic population of adherent cells. Non-specific suppression by these adherent cells was at least partially associated with the release of a suppressor factor that could inhibit the blastogenic response of normal spleen cells activated by mitogens. Both *in vitro* and *in vivo* studies suggested the participation of a high parasite load in the induction of non-specific suppressor cells and polyclonal lymphocyte activation.

1983 Cytopathology of parasitic disease. Pitman Books, London (Ciba Foundation symposium 99), p 157-173

American *Leishmania* are trypanosomatid flagellates with heteroxenous parasitic development involving sandfly vectors and wild mammalian reservoirs. The parasites appear as oval amastigotes in the mononuclear phagocytic cell of the vertebrate host and as promastigotes in the alimentary canal of sandflies and in cultures. Two complexes of American *Leishmania*, *L. mexicana* and *L. braziliensis*, are now recognized by biological, biochemical and immunological criteria (Lainson & Shaw 1978, Chance 1979).

In humans the diseases caused by parasites of the *L. mexicana* complex may vary from a relatively benign localized ulcer to a disseminated progressive disease, as manifested in diffuse cutaneous leishmaniasis (DCL). Different subspecies of *L. mexicana*, *L. mexicana pifanoi* (in Venezuela) and *L. mexicana amazonensis* (in Brazil) are thought to be responsible for the DCL (Lainson & Shaw 1978). However, some evidence indicates that the host response could also determine the clinical manifestations of American cutaneous leishmaniasis (ACL) (Convit et al 1972).

The study of *Leishmania* species in experimental models has provided an understanding of the host factors that regulate the course of infection with these parasites. It is now accepted that, at least in the mouse model, the susceptibility to *L. donovani*, *L. tropica* and *L. mexicana* is under genetic control (Bradley 1974, Kellina 1978, Howard et al 1980a, Pérez et al 1979a). Genetic factors seem to regulate both the innate susceptibility of the mononuclear phagocytic cell and the ability of the host to develop a successful immune response leading to elimination (or control) of the parasites (reviewed by Bradley 1980).

A satisfactory model for the mucocutaneous form of ACL caused by *L. braziliensis* has yet to be found. In this paper the discussion will be restricted to responses of some inbred mouse strains that have provided valuable models for both the spontaneously healing and the progressive forms of ACL caused by parasites of the *L. mexicana* type.

Experimental system

The study was done with a human isolate from patient AZV. This isolate is considered to be *L. mexicana*, from the following data. Parasites were isolated by the late Dr J. W. Torrealba from a Venezuelan patient who showed a localized ulcer on the left elbow and who manifested conspicuous delayed hypersensitivity in the leishmanin test. The ulcer resolved satisfactorily after therapy. This isolate of *Leishmania* produced fast-growing lesions when inoculated subcutaneously into hamsters, and multiplied readily in NNN medium and other conventional culture media (Pérez et al 1979a). The AZV isolate exhibited suprapylarial development in the gut of experimentally infected specimens of *Lutzomya towsendi* (J. Scorza, unpublished observations), and it was immunologically indistinguishable from other isolates of *L. mexicana*, but clearly different from isolates of *L. braziliensis* (Petralanda et al 1980). Enzymic profiles were compatible with *L. mexicana* (G. Grimaldi, personal communication), and ultrastructural examination showed a perinuclear kinetoplast, as observed by Shaw & Lainson (1976) for *L. mexicana*.

After subcutaneous inoculation of *L. mexicana* (AZV isolate) into the footpad or tail base of resistant mice strains C3H/He, CBA, C57BL/6 and AKR (Pérez et al 1979a and unpublished data), palpable nodes developed within 4–6 weeks. Thereafter, lesions progressively increased until weeks 10–12 of infection when they began to resolve. At this time ultrastructural examination showed a granuloma with numerous lymphocytes, plasma cells, some eosinophils and macrophages, containing undamaged and damaged parasites. Damaged parasites were frequently seen in phagocytic vacuoles loaded with electron-dense material, and unless a large inoculum (10^5–10^8 parasites) had been given, the granuloma progressively disappeared and the lesions resolved in 4–5 months, after which parasites were rarely found. These are the general characteristics of what we call a 'self-limiting' infection. In contrast, BALB/c and DBA/2 mice develop progressive lesions. The highest susceptibility was manifested by BALB/c mice. Lesions in these animals showed numerous heavily parasitized macrophages, plasma-like cells and eosinophils, and few, if any, lymphocytes. The infection disseminated gradually until, after several months, parasites could be found in the spleen and some animals died in a cachectic-like state. This is the classical picture of what we have termed a 'non-limiting' infection.

Immune responses in 'self-limiting' infections

Animal models of self-limiting cutaneous leishmaniasis provide a system for analysing the nature of the immune response that leads to subsequent protective immunity. T-lymphocyte-deprived and congenitally athymic (nu/nu) mice develop chronic progressive infections (Preston et al 1972, Handman et al 1979), which indicates that T cells play a primary part in recovery from infection. However, the precise mechanism by which T cells control the parasite population is still undefined. A direct interaction between sensitized lymphocytes and parasitized macrophages, leading to destruction of the infected cell, was suggested by Bray & Bryceson (1968) in their work on *L. enriettii* in guinea-pigs. The possibility that sensitized T cells operate through generating activated macrophages is supported by evidence that macrophages from immune mice do not maintain growth of parasites *in vitro* as well as do macrophages from uninfected mice (Miller & Twohy 1969, Handman & Spira 1977), and that soluble mediators released by specifically and non-specifically stimulated T cells activate macrophages, resulting in intracellular destruction of parasites (Mauel et al 1978, Louis et al 1979, Nacy et al 1981). The protective effect (against *L. mexicana*) conferred by the adoptive transfer of lymph node cells and peritoneal cells from recovering C57BL/6 mice into syngeneic normal recipients (H. Pérez, unpublished data) is probably related to the generation of activated macrophages *in vivo*.

Delayed hypersensitivity to parasite antigens is prominent in cutaneous leishmaniasis but its relationship to protective immunity has yet to be demonstrated. In C3H/He and C57BL/6 mice infected with *L. mexicana*, delayed hypersensitivity to leishmanial antigens appears at three weeks of infection, and a high level of both delayed hypersensitivity and protective immunity is present early (at 5 weeks) in the infection (Pérez et al 1981, M. Ortega & H. Pérez, unpublished data). The delayed hypersensitivity to leishmanial antigens persists long after animals have resolved their lesions. Recovered mice manifest strong protective immunity, and only a transient papule can be seen at the site of reinfection (Pérez et al 1979b). A large infiltration of lymphocytes and macrophages characterizes the delayed hypersensitivity, and it may be possible that delayed hypersensitivity provokes the recruitment and activation of macrophages at the site of reinfection, leading to elimination of parasites. There is evidence that inoculation of *L. enriettii* at the site of a delayed hypersensitivity response to chlorodinitrobenzene markedly suppressed the development of lesions at that site (Behin et al 1977). It is therefore possible that the localization of immune cells at the site of infection provides useful information about the effector mechanism of immunity to *Leishmania*. Peripheral lymph node cells and peritoneal cells from recovering animals, when injected together with parasite antigens, brought about a delayed hypersensitivity at 24 h (H. Pérez et al, unpublished data). When peritoneal cells were injected together with amastigotes in the footpad of syngeneic normal recipients, the size of the lesions was significantly reduced, compared to those developed by animals receiving peritoneal cells from normal donors. The protective activity of immune cells does not appear to be a non-specific effect, since peritoneal cells from normal mice had no effect on the course of lesions. Immune peritoneal cells depleted of the adherent-cell population showed a reduced ability to inhibit the development of lesions. Immune serum containing anti-*Leishmania* antibodies significantly enhanced the level of protection conferred by immune peritoneal cells, but immune serum alone did not modify the course of infection (Pérez 1980a). Further work demonstrated that the adherent cell population that was recovered after separation of immune peritoneal cells in plastic dishes provided a significant protection in the presence of immune serum (H. Pérez et al, unpublished data).

There is some controversy about the role of antibodies in immunity to *Leishmania* (Bryceson 1975, Rezai et al 1971). A synergistic mechanism involving cells and antibodies seems to operate in the immunity against *L. enriettii* (Poulter 1980). Other evidence indicates that serum from mice infected with *L. donovani* contains cytophilic antibodies and opsonins for both amastigotes and promastigotes (Herman 1980). Plasma cells are also present in the lesions of recovering mice. It is possible that the secretion of antibodies into the area surrounding parasites favours their phagocytosis by activated macrophages, thus resulting in an accelerated rate of intracellular killing. Poulter (1980) suggested that serum-mediated phagocytosis of parasites could be particularly efficient in the elimination of a primary infection.

A number of interactions involving mononuclear phagocytes, T cells and antibodies is probably required to produce effective destruction of *Leishmania* parasites.

Immunodepression in 'self-limiting' infections

An interesting aspect of the immune response of resistant C3H/He and C57BL/6 mice infected with *L. mexicana* is the depression of the immunoglobulin M–plaque-forming cell (IgM–PFC) response to sheep red blood cells (sheep RBC) and the depression of the lymphoproliferative responses to phytohaemagglutinin observed when the lesions reached their maximum size. This immunodepression was transient, because immunoresponsiveness was restored as the mice recovered from the infection (Pérez et al 1981 and unpublished data). It is noteworthy that during the period of immunodepression spleen cells from infected mice showed a reduced capacity to respond to the *in vitro* immunization with sheep RBC, and were capable of suppressing the primary antibody response of normal spleen cells (Pérez et al 1981). On the other hand, comparison of the delayed hypersensitivity responses induced by the subcutaneous and by the intravenous immunization of infected mice with sheep RBC revealed normal or enhanced reactions to the sheep RBC in the subcutaneously immunized mice. In contrast, intravenously immunized mice showed a transiently reduced ability to develop delayed hypersensitivity to sheep RBC, and this reduction coincided with the maximum development of lesions. Because infected mice showed an intense delayed hypersensitivity to leishmanial antigens, and displayed anti-parasitic antibodies and protective immunity to a challenge infection (Pérez et al 1981), it is likely that the immunodepression observed in resistant mice does not depend on depressed T-cell sensitization. The transient depression of the immune response observed in resistant mice infected with *L. mexicana* was probably restricted to the spleen. A depression of splenic (but not lymph-node) antibody responses to sheep RBC was observed in mice infected with *Plasmodium berghei yoelii* (Weindanz & Rank 1975). Trapping of parasite antigens in the spleen, when lesions reach maximum sizes, probably interferes with the ability of splenic macrophages to process newly introduced antigens. Macrophages treated *in vitro* with excreted *Leishmania* factors showed impairment of their ability to incorporate and to process [^{125}I] albumin (N. Rodríguez et al, unpublished observations). However, this explanation alone does not account for the suppressor effect shown by spleen cells from infected mice during the period of immunodepression (Pérez et al 1981). The contribution of suppressor macrophages, parasite products, or both, to the regulatory function of immune cells has yet to be examined. Recent work indicates depressed peripheral lymphoproliferative responses to phytohaemagglutinin in patients suffering from localized cutaneous leishmaniasis (Castes et al 1983). Whether such transient immunodepression compromises the host response to other infections is at present unknown.

Immune response in 'non-self-limiting' infections

A complex immunosuppression involving antigen-specific T suppressor cells, non-specific suppressor macrophages and polyclonal activation is generated during chronic infection of BALB/c mice with *L. mexicana*. Two different effects were observed throughout the course of infection. A transitory increase in the number of IgM–PFC to sheep RBC, and increased lymphoproliferative responses to T- and B-cell compartments, were seen at 4–8 weeks of infection. At the same time, infected mice were able to express delayed hypersensitivity to leishmanial antigens (Arredondo & Pérez 1979). As infection progressed, specific and non-specific immune responses gradually became suppressed. At 16 weeks of infection delayed hypersensitivity to parasite antigens, lymphoblastogenic responses to mitogens and the capacity to develop cellular and humoral responses to sheep RBC were markedly reduced. At 14–16 weeks, and thereafter, spleen cells from infected mice suppressed the response of normal spleen cells to T- and B-cell mitogens. Suppression was markedly increased at 20 weeks of infection and persisted through to terminal infection at 25–27 weeks. Peripheral lymph nodes remained free of suppression until the infection became terminal. Non-specific suppression was due to the generation, in spleens of infected mice, of a population of adherent macrophage-like cells (H. Pérez & J. Bolívar, unpublished results). A relatively small number of adherent cells was sufficient to suppress the mitogen-induced proliferation of normal spleen cells. Furthermore, supernatants obtained from the culture fluid of adherent cells showed suppressor activity. It has been suggested that immunoregulatory materials released by macrophages may exert suppressor effects via their interaction with other regulatory T cells (Stobo 1977). Our studies on the mode of action of the suppressor factor released by suppressor adherent cells have been inconclusive. Unfractionated cells, or T cells from the spleens of normal mice, precultured with suppressor supernatants and then washed and added to normal spleen cells did not manifest suppressor effects. Moreover, normal splenocytes that were precultured with suppressor supernatants and then washed showed excellent viability and responded normally to stimulation with T- and B-cell mitogens. As parasite antigens have been detected on the surface of infected cells (Handman et al 1979, Farah et al 1975, Berman & Dwyer 1981), a working hypothesis is that parasite products trapped by adherent cells and released into the cultured fluid exert suppressor activity via a direct interaction with proliferating cells. Suppressor supernatants were effective only at the start of lymphocyte activation (0–2 h) and not when added 24 h after stimulation. Binding of parasite products to the lymphocyte plasma membrane may interfere with the early events that are initiated in the plasma membrane and which finally result in lymphocyte proliferation (Northoff et al 1978). The possible participation of parasite products in the immunosuppression exerted by adherent spleen cells is reinforced by our observations that a crude preparation of parasite antigens induced significant suppressor cell activity in normal BALB/c spleen-cell cultures, as determined by inhibition of syngeneic cell responsiveness to phytohaemagglutinin. The suppression induced by parasite antigens was dose-dependent and was drastically reduced by removal of the adherent cells. Howard et al (1980b) reported the activation of specific T suppressor cells in the spleens of BALB/c mice infected with *L. tropica*. Non-adherent spleen cells from BALB/c mice chronically infected with *L. mexicana* responded normally to concanavalin A and failed to manifest non-specific suppressor activity *in vitro*. However, this cell population interfered with the early delayed hypersensitivity to leishmanial antigens induced by a live infection, without affecting the delayed hypersensitivity induced by sensitization with sheep RBC. Cells expressing specific suppression were sensitive to treatment with anti-theta antibody and were negative when tested for non-specific esterases. All this evidence suggests that a T suppressor cell also mediates the suppression of the delayed hypersensitivity to parasite antigens observed in BALB/c mice chronically infected with *L. mexicana*. Specific T suppressor cells could not be found before 12–14 weeks of infection and their appearance in the spleens of infected mice preceded that of non-specific suppressor cells. One may speculate that the suppression of cellular responses to parasite antigens, leading to uncontrolled proliferation of parasites, effectively activates non-specific suppressor mechanisms via the interaction of parasite products with regulatory cells. In addition, suppressor factors released by specifically activated T suppressor cells can be absorbed by macrophages, which then display non-specific suppressor effects (Tada & Okumura 1979).

The mechanism by which the circuit of immune responses is deviated towards parasite protection is an enigma. BALB/c, nu/nu mice, which develop severe disease after inoculation with *L. tropica*, can be protected by a minimal number of normal spleen cells, but this protection can be abrogated by spleen cells from chronically infected mice (Mitchell et al 1981). Cells involved in the abrogation of protection were apparently T cells, bearing the $Ly1^+$ phenotype (Mitchell et al 1981). These workers suggested that this type of T cell acts on other T cells involved in the expression of delayed hypersensitivity and macrophage activation. We have been unable to demonstrate facilitated development of lesions in normal BALB/c mice adoptively transferred with unfractionated cells or with T cells from spleens of chronically infected syngeneic donors. Surprisingly, in one of three experiments, spleen cells from chronically infected mice conferred a certain level of protection. Another unexpected finding was that chronically infected BALB/c mice manifested a certain level of protection to a challenge infection, as indicated by the inhibition of lesion development. However, reinfected mice showed increased mortality. Hence, it is difficult to determine whether we are dealing with true immunity or with an artifact resulting from the technique used to assess the course of infection. One could speculate that increased mortality of re-infected mice is due to a rapid visceralization of parasites as a consequence of a decreased ability to develop an inflammatory response at the site of re-infection. This would lead to a 'reduced' size of lesions. Numerous plasma cells can be observed in the lesions of BALB/c mice chronically infected with *L. mexicana*, which might suggest a role for B cells in the chronic nature of the infection. In the absence of activated macrophages, opsonization of parasites by antibodies may facilitate the access of parasites to a highly permissive intracellular environment. Our search for a role for antibodies in increasing the severity of disease has been inconclusive. Lesions developed by mice given serum from chronically infected mice and then inoculated with *L. mexicana* were greater (but not significantly so) than those of control mice receiving normal serum. There are obvious difficulties with the analysis of serum- and cell-transfer experiments in a long-term assay. Another consequence of the chronic infection produced by *L. mexicana* in BALB/c mice is the stimulation of the heterophil antibodies. Preliminary observations indicate that inoculation of BALB/c mice with a large inoculum of *L. mexicana* is followed by a rapid increase in the basal number of plaque-forming cells to sheep RBC that are coated with trinitrophenyl (A. Jorquera & H. Pérez, unpublished results). Whether polyclonal activation induced by parasite antigens leads to alterations in regulatory T cells (Lagrange et al 1975, Lagrange & Mackaness 1975, Louis & Lambert 1979) has yet to be established.

It is noteworthy that malnutrition (Pérez et al 1979c) or inoculation of resistant hosts with a high number of parasites (Pérez 1980b) leads to chronic infections, accompanied by a reduced capacity to express delayed hypersensitivity to parasite antigens. In these cases, we have been unable to demonstrate the activation of specific T suppressor cells, and different mechanisms may thus be involved in the depression of delayed hypersensitivity to parasite antigens observed in chronic leishmaniasis. However, the analysis of the immune responses of experimental hosts to one isolate of a parasite is an over-simplification of the problem. Little attention has been given to the heterogeneity of *Leishmania* parasites, which could be particularly relevant to American *Leishmania* species. An interesting observation made in our laboratory is that C3H/He mice, which are very resistant to the *L. mexicana* isolate from patient AZV, were quite susceptible to an isolate of *L. mexicana amazonensis* obtained from a wild reservoir. In these circumstances C3H/He mice developed a chronic infection that was concomitant with a strong delayed hypersensitivity to parasite antigens.

Acknowledgements

This article results from work performed in this laboratory during the last four years in collaboration with J. W. Torrealba, B. Arredondo, I. Malavé, R. Machado, J. Bolívar, M. Ortega, M. De La Rosa and A. Jorquera. I am also indebted to those colleagues who allowed me to refer to their unpublished work.

REFERENCES

Arredondo B, Pérez H 1979 Alterations of the immune response associated with chronic experimental leishmaniasis. Infect Immun 25:16-22

Behin R, Mauel J, Rowe DS 1977 Mechanism of protective immunity in experimental cutaneous leishmaniasis in the guinea-pig by delayed hypersensitivity reactions to unrelated antigens. Clin Exp Immunol 29:320-325

Berman JD, Dwyer DM 1981 Expression of *Leishmania* antigens on the surface membrane of infected human macrophages *in vitro*. Clin Exp Immunol 44:342-348

Bradley DJ 1974 Genetic control of natural resistance to *Leishmania donovani* infection. Nature (Lond) 283:72-73

Bradley DJ 1980 Genetic control of resistance to protozoal infections. In: Skamene E et al (eds) Genetic control of natural resistance to infection and malignancy. (Perspect Immunol Ser) Academic Press, New York, p 9-25

Bray RS, Bryceson ADM 1968 Cutaneous leishmaniasis in the guinea-pig. Action of sensitized lymphocytes on infected macrophages. Lancet 2:898-899

Bryceson ADM 1975 Mechanism of disease in leishmaniasis. In: Taylor AER, Muller R (eds) Pathogenic processes in parasitic infections. Blackwell Scientific Publications, Oxford, p 85-100

Castes M, Agnelli A, Verde D, Rondón AJ 1983 Characterization of the cellular immune response in American cutaneous leishmaniasis. Immunol Immunopathol, in press

Chance ML 1979 The identification of *Leishmania*. In: Taylor AER, Muller R (eds) Problems in the identification of parasites and their vectors. Blackwell Scientific Publications, Oxford, p 55-74

Convit J, Pinardi ME, Rondón AJ 1972 Diffuse cutaneous leishmaniasis: a disease due to an immunological defect of the host. Trans R Soc Trop Med Hyg 66:603-610

Farah FS, Samra SA, Nuwayri-Salti N 1975 The role of macrophages in cutaneous leishmaniasis. Immunology 29:755-764

Handman E, Spira DT 1977 Growth of *Leishmania* amastigotes in macrophages from immune and normal mice. Z Parasitenkd 53:75-81

Handman E, Ceredig R, Mitchell G 1979 Murine cutaneous leishmaniasis: disease patterns in intact and nude mice of various genotypes and examination of some differences between normal and immune macrophages. Aust J Exp Biol Med Sci 57:9-29

Herman R 1980 Cytophilic and opsonic antibodies in visceral leishmaniasis in mice. Infect Immun 28:585-593

Howard JG, Hale C, Chan-Liew WL 1980a Immunological regulation of experimental cutaneous leishmaniasis. I: Immunogenetic aspects of suceptibility to *Leishmania tropica* in mice. Parasite Immunol (Oxf) 2:303-314

Howard JG, Hale C, Liew FY 1980b Immunological regulation of experimental cutaneous leishmaniasis. III: The nature and significance of the specific suppression of cell mediated immunity in mice highly susceptible to *Leishmania tropica*. J Exp Med 152:594-607

Kellina OI 1973 Differences of susceptibility of inbred mice of different strains to *Leishmania tropica major*. [Russian] Med Parazitol Parazit Bolezni 42:279-285

Lagrange PH, Mackaness GB 1975 Effects of bacterial lipopolysaccharide on the induction and expression of cell-mediated immunity. II: Stimulation of efferent arc. J Immunol 114:447-451

Lagrange PH, Mackaness GB, Miller T, Pardon P 1975 Effect of bacterial lipopolysaccharide on the induction and expression of cell-mediated immunity. I: Depression of afferent arc. J Immunol 114:442-446

Lainson R, Shaw JJ 1978 Epidemiology and ecology of leishmaniasis in Latin-America. Nature (Lond) 273:595-600

Louis J, Lambert PH 1979 Lipopolysaccharides: from immunostimulation to autoimmunity. Springer Semin Immunopathol 2:215-228

Louis J, Moedder E, Behin R, Howard E 1979 Recognition of protozoan parasite antigens by murine T lymphocytes. I: Induction of specific T lymphocyte-dependent poliferative responses to *L. tropica*. Eur J Immunol 9:841-847

Mauel J, Büchmüller Y, Behin R 1978 Studies on the mechanisms of macrophage activation. I: Destruction of intracellular *Leishmania enriettii* in macrophage activated by cocultivation with stimulated lymphocytes. J Exp Med 148:393-407

Miller HC, Twohy D 1969 Cellular immunity to *Leishmania donovani* in macrophages in culture. J Parasitol 55:200-207

Mitchell GF, Curtis JM, Scollay RG, Handman E 1981 Resistance and abrogation of resistance to cutaneous leishmaniasis in reconstituted BALB/c nude mice. Aust J Exp Biol Med Sci 59:539-554

Nacy CA, Meltzer MS, Leonard EJ, Wyler DJ 1981 Intracellular replication and lymphokine-induced destruction in C3H/HeN mouse macrophages. J Immunol 127:2381-2386

Northoff H, Dörken B, Resch K 1978 Ligand dependent modulation of membrane phopholipid in metabolism in Con A stimulated macrophages. Exp Cell Res 113:189-195

Pérez H 1980a Macrophages as mediators of immunity to *Leishmania mexicana*. In: Van den Bossche (ed) The host–invader interplay. Elsevier/North-Holland, Amsterdam, p 475-478

Pérez H 1980b La infección experimental del ratón con *Leishmania mexicana*: efecto del número de parásitos inoculados sobre el curso de la infección. Acta Cient Venez 31:174-179

Pérez H, Labrador F, Torrealba JW 1979a Variations in the response of five strains of mice to *Leishmania mexicana*. Int J Parasitol 9:27-32

Pérez H, Arrendondo B, Machado R 1979b *Leishmania mexicana* and *L. tropica*: cross immunity in C57BL/6 mice. Exp Parasitol 48:9-14

Pérez H, Malavé I, Arrendondo B 1979c The effect of protein calorie-malnutrition on the course of *Leishmania mexicana* infection in C57BL/6 mice. Clin Exp Immunol 38:453-460

Pérez H, Pocino M, Malavé I 1981 Nonspecific immunodepression and protective immunity in mice infected with *Leishmania mexicana*. Infect Immun 32:415-419

Petralanda I, Arango M, Lugo E, Yarzabal L 1980 Estudios immunoquímicos de leishmanias americanas. Inmunol Clin 3:7-26

Preston PM, Carter RL, Leuchars E, Davies AJS, Dumonde DC 1972 Experimental cutaneous leishmaniasis. III: Effects of thymectomy on the course of infection of CBA mice with *Leishmania tropica*. Clin Exp Immunol 10:337-357

Poulter LW 1980 Mechanism of immunity to leishmaniasis. I: Evidence for a changing basis of protection in self-limiting disease. Clin Exp Immunol 39:14-26

Rezai H, Gettner S, Behforouz N 1971 Anti-leishmanial activity of immune guinea-pig serum. J Med Microbiol 5:371-375

Shaw JJ, Lainson R 1976 Leishmaniasis in Brazil. XI: Observations of the morphology of *Leishmania* of the *braziliensis* and *mexicana* complexes. J Trop Med Hyg 79:9-13

Stobo J 1977 Immunosuppression in man: suppression by macrophages can be mediated by interactions with regulatory T cells. J Immunol 119:918-924

Tada T, Okumura K 1979 The role of antigen-specific T cell factors in the immune response. Adv Immunol 28:1-87

Weindanz WP, Rank RG 1975 Regional immunosuppression induced by *Plasmodium berghei yoelii*. Infect Immun 11:211-212

DISCUSSION

Chang: Howard et al (1982) have been using intravenously administered *Leishmania tropica* promastigotes for immunization of mice. This procedure seems also to protect the mice from infection by the South American species of *Leishmania*. Have you tried the same thing?

Pérez: There is cross immunity between *Leishmania mexicana* and *L. tropica major*. However, mice that are immune to *L. tropica* do not display the same level of protection to a challenge with *L. mexicana*. We have tried the immunization experiments very carefully and, under certain conditions, immunized animals will develop cellular responses and antibodies to parasite antigens. Immunized genetically susceptible mice show protection to a challenge infection, in the sense that lesions appear later and are smaller than those of control animals. However, in our hands, once infection is established in immunized susceptible mice, they will not regress.

Hudson: The regulation of suppression, which you described as being probably a B cell phenomenon rather than a T cell phenomenon, suggests that regulation via an anti-idiotype mechanism might be a real possibility in Chagas' disease. Can you transfer the regulation by supernatants and, secondly, does an anti-immunoglobulin column deplete that transfer?

Pérez: We are running that experiment now. Under our experimental conditions suppressor B cells do not appear in DBA/2 mice until the 20th week of infection. We now have to wait for the right time after infection to continue the work on fractionation of the cell involved in the suppression. Regarding the regulatory effect of supernatant, we have not looked for its effect on suppression.

Pfefferkorn: In your experiments with mice immune to *L. mexicana* you showed both a smaller lesion and a lesion that *disappeared* more rapidly. Initially these lesions also increased in diameter more rapidly. Does this suggest that the immune response plays a role in the pathogenesis? And what about the role of the immune response in the pathogenesis of the lesion in the chronic diseased mouse?

Pérez: What we see during the first days after re-infection is probably an accelerated cellular reaction to inoculation by the re-infecting living parasite. The lesion growth itself seems to be accelerated.

Sharma: In your suppression studies where you used macrophages from spleens did you find that peritoneal macrophages from the same susceptible mice can also suppress the response?

Pérez: No. We have not looked for suppressor macrophages in the peritoneal cavity of susceptible mice.

O'Daly: With *Trypanosoma cruzi* we have been working (J.A. O'Daly et al, unpublished work) on the suppression and protection problem in C3H/He and C57 BL/6 mice. We have studied the progressive immunological responses to concanavalin A (Con A), phytohaemagglutinin (PHA), lipopolysaccharide (LPS) and dextran sulphate (DS) in mice inoculated with 500 trypanosomes of the Y strain of *T. cruzi*. We demonstrated, as did Kierszenbaum & Hayes (1980) in CBA mice, the recovery of the response to all four mitogens, more so to the T cell mitogens (Con A and PHA) than to the B cell mitogens (LPS and DS). There is also total suppression to low and high molecular weight antigens of *T. cruzi* at 17 days after infection; the spleen grows 5–6 times the normal size and then decreases. There are significant differences between the strains of mice that we used. The suppression is more evident when one takes the antigens from *T. cruzi* cultured at 34 and 37 °C. We have also found, by using immunofluorescence, a very large peak of IgG- and IgM-bearing cells in both the spleen and the lymph nodes at the time of maximum suppression. The supernatant from cultured cells at 17 days post-infection contains a 36 000 M_r protein that can induce suppression in normal cells. By doing co-culture experiments of T cells from spleen isolated by Sephadex G-10 columns, and of macrophages obtained by adherence to plastic, we could demonstrate that T cells are not suppressive. The suppression seems to be located in macrophages when they are co-cultured with a population of normal cells. There is also a change in the agglutinability of B cells taken at 17 days post-infection when we use an antibody produced against live (but not with one produced against dead) parasites in rabbits. We have not found a significant correlation between parasite load and suppression in our work.

Hudson: Dr O'Daly, in the conditions in which you observed a diminished T cell response but a vastly increased IgM and IgG response, did you look at the clonal spectrotype to see if it is either polyclonal or restricted?

O'Daly: No. We used only the IgG polyclonal. I might add that we also studied in those mice, by serial sections of the heart and skeletal muscle, the presence of amastigotes and inflammatory infiltrates in the recovery period, to see if we could identify parasites (J.A. O'Daly et al, unpublished work). We found neither amastigotes nor inflammatory nodes. The peak in parasite numbers and inflammation in the muscle and heart cells is exactly coincident with the suppression and with the peaks of IgG and IgM in spleen and lymph nodes. When we removed the cover slides and did cryostatic sections, we tried to stain with anti-IgG and anti-IgM the cells from inflammatory foci in the heart, and they did not stain. So perhaps they are cytotoxic or other kinds of cells. Proliferation in the lymph nodes is one thing and proliferation in the tissues is another. We also tried re-infection of animals in the recovery period and they did not re-infect or show the suppression that was shown on first infection; neither did they show the peaks of IgG and IgM.

Sher: I am very interested in your finding, Dr Pérez, of an *L. mexicana amazonensis* strain that produces a chronic infection in resistant mice. As I shall be discussing (this volume) we have found what seems to be a dichotomy between different cutaneous *Leishmania* strains in terms of their ability to produce self-healing or chronic infections in normally non-susceptible mice. Have you been able to relate this behaviour to the origin of the strain in terms of the disease produced in the original patient? Do the two isolates come from patients with different disease manifestations—i.e. one from a self-healing lesion and the other from a persistent chronic lesion? Secondly, have you been able to establish a good model of *Leishmania braziliensis* infection in mice?

Pérez: The isolate of *L. mexicana* was obtained from a human case (patient AZV) of localized cutaneous leishmaniasis. The other strain—*L. mexicana amazonensis*—was, as I mentioned at the end of my paper, obtained from a wild reservoir. Our own experience with *L. braziliensis* in mice leads us to believe that mice are not very good models for *L. braziliensis* infection. We have an isolate of *L. braziliensis* from a mucocutaneous case of American cutaneous leishmaniasis and we found that this isolate produced very small lesions in mice. Although some mice may recover, there is a big increase in mortality in mice infected with *L. braziliensis*. Mice recovering from infection with *L. braziliensis* will show some immunity to a challenge with *L. mexicana*, but the opposite does not occur. This confirms the results found by Lainson & Shaw (1977) in the rhesus monkey. The results are important because they indicate that a future vaccine against American cutaneous leishmaniasis should be polyvalent.

Sher: Have you ever seen a chronic infection, of the type you described for *L. mexicana amazonensis*, in a resistant mouse after inoculation with *L. braziliensis*?

Pérez: Not in terms of a lesion, but I do wonder about the visceralization of *L. braziliensis* in mice.

Warren: Have you used any of the new monoclonal antibodies, produced by McMahon Pratt & David (1981) to differentiate between the species that you are using? The infecting agent that produces the pathological effects in schistosomiasis does not multiply, but with leishmaniasis one finds, in contrast, a combination of a multiplying organism and a host response. It is necessary to identify the aetiology of the lesion: could it be caused by over-multiplication of parasites, such as lesions found in lepromatous leprosy; or could it be caused by a high degree of delayed hypersensitivity responses, as in tuberculoid leprosy?

Pérez: This is interesting because we have no satisfactory means of following the course of the infection in cutaneous leishmaniasis. However, if we take pieces of the lesion in culture medium and follow the progress of the parasite population by comparing it with the size of lesion, we can see that the parasites disappear first, and then the lesion resolves. This sort of study is very expensive and time-consuming.

Wyler: If genetic recombination occurs naturally among parasite subpopulations in the sandfly, then the kinds of things that we are studying in the laboratory might miss some important aspects of the disease. By the same token, our use of inbred mice may hide the expression of a genetic restriction of certain leishmanial antigens, responses to which might be critical with respect to pathogenesis or protection. So even if we were to resolve the controversy about what constitutes a leishmanial species, I'm not sure we could readily answer the question of why the course of infection differs for different isolates and in different hosts.

Sher: In terms of the study of leishmanial infection in experimental models, I feel that the most important consideration is not the species or sub-species of parasite but the nature of the disease produced by the organism both in the original patient and in the laboratory host. This is not to say that parasite speciation is not important in the classification of leishmanial infections. However, variations in both the host and the parasite species may play a more crucial role in determining disease pathogenesis.

Warren: I agree. We have used a similar strategy in studies of schistosomiasis. It is also important to use animal models that mimic the specific disease of interest in the human host.

Pérez: We have to be cautious about that because, if you remember, we tried to see the effect of an isolated parasite obtained from a case of diffuse cutaneous leishmaniasis. We compared it with the course of infection in resistant and susceptible mice, and found that the isolated strain induced a self-limiting pattern of infection in resistant mice and a chronic infection in BALB/c mice.

Andrade: We have just recently completed a histological comparative study of the lesions in BALB/c mice and A/J mice infected in the footpad with *L. mexicana amazonensis* (Z.A. Andrade et al, unpublished work). In the first four days one cannot distinguish between the two because there is a non-specific acute inflammatory reaction in both. From 6–7 days one sees a real difference. The BALB/c mice develop a monomorphic reaction with vacuolated macrophages, whereas the A/J mice will develop a mixed cell reaction, with lymphocytes, macrophages, and fibroblastic proliferation. Do you have any histological results on the immunized mice indicating whether this non-specific reaction is present?

Pérez: We have studied the ultrastructure of lesions through the course of infection in resistant and susceptible mice. Lesions of chronically infected BALB/c mice are heavily infiltrated with infected macrophages, making it difficult to see the limits between the plasma membranes of infected cells. Plasma cells and eosinophils are also present. In resistant mice recovering from a primary infection, lesions are infiltrated with lymphocytes, plasma cells and many infected and non-infected macrophages. Many of the intracellular parasites seem to be degenerating inside vacuoles loaded with electron-dense material.

Martinez-Palomo: One of the basic problems in leishmaniasis, as in other protozoan diseases, is to define precise taxonomic criteria to characterize the differences between strains. Very recently we have been able to collaborate with P. Sargeaunt in order to define species differences between pathogenic and non-pathogenic strains of *Entamoeba histolytica* by the use of the isoenzyme method. The results are very promising. Others have also tried monoclonal antibodies, which seem to be too specific for this type of work. Have similar isoenzyme methods been used in the study of *Leishmania* species?

Pérez: Yes. Buoyant density of DNA, isoenzymes and morphological characteristics have all been applied but I don't think any of these methods on their own can give useful information about the taxonomy of the parasites. Perhaps the best way to approach the problem is to use monoclonal antibodies.

Warren: The work of Wirth & McMahon Pratt (1982) on DNA hybridization may also differentiate between strains.

Hernández: I agree that attempts to characterize the pathogenic and non-pathogenic strains of *Leishmania* by the isoenzyme technique do not seem to be useful. We have done tests with six different isoenzymes, using six different strains, and each one differed from the others in at least one isoenzyme.

Mirelman: In the studies of isoenzymes in *Entamoeba* by Dr Sargeaunt, the first step is to take a parasite from a patient's faeces and to deduce from the type of lesion produced, e.g. a liver abscess, whether the parasite is pathogenic. The second step is the sub-cultivation of this parasite before doing the isoenzyme assay. This has been done in polyxenic cultures, and it is still rather unclear whether different flora may contribute to the isoenzyme pattern. Furthermore, the enzymic activities currently chosen for the isoenzyme characterization are not relevant for the pathogenic pathway of the parasite. So it seems to me that results from the isoenzyme method should be taken with caution in attempts to correlate pathogenic properties with the isoenzyme patterns.

Warren: Dr Martinez-Palomo has also been taking human strains of *E. histolytica* and doing repeated studies, including examination of the bowel of patients to make sure that there are no pathological lesions. This has clearly differentiated human non-pathogenic strains from human pathogenic strains.

Pérez: In culturing *Leishmania* parasites we may be forced to select a parasite that is well adapted to *in vitro* conditions. We are now trying to isolate the parasite from the patient and to cryopreserve the parasite so that we can work with material that has had few *in vivo* or *in vitro* passages.

Nussenzweig: Examination of restriction enzyme maps of the kinetoplast DNA allows for a good discrimination between different strains of *T. cruzi*, and yields very reproducible results (Morel et al 1980). Similar techniques are being applied to distinguish different *Leishmania* species, but this work is in its preliminary stages.

Pérez: I agree. Perhaps the activation of different suppressor cells in animals may also be related to the genetic capability of the host to recognize some given antigens of the parasite.

REFERENCES

Howard JG, Nicklin S, Hale C, Liew FY 1982 Prophylactic immunization against experimental leishmaniasis. I: Protection induced in mice genetically vulnerable to fatal *Leishmania tropica* infection. J Immunol 129:2206-2212

Kierszenbaum F, Hayes MM 1980 Evaluation of lymphocyte response to polyclonal activators during acute and chronic experimental *Trypanosoma cruzi* infection. Am J Trop Med Hyg 29:708-710

Lainson R, Shaw JJ 1977 Leishmaniasis in Brazil. 12: Observations on cross immunity in monkeys and man infected with *Leishmania mexicana mexicana*, *L. m. amazonensis*, *L. braziliensis braziliensis*, *L. b. guyanensis* and *L. b. panamensis*. J Trop Med Hyg 80:29-35

McMahon Pratt D, David JR 1981 Monoclonal antibodies that distinguish between New World species of *Leishmania*. Nature (Lond) 291:581-583

Morel C, Chiari E, Plessmann Camargo E, Mattei D, Romanha M, Simpson L 1980 Strains and clones of *Trypanosoma cruzi* can be characterized by pattern of restriction endonuclease products of kinetoplast DNA minicircles. Proc Natl Acad Sci USA 77:6810-6814

Wirth DF, McMahon Pratt D 1982 Rapid identification of *Leishmania* species by specific hybridization of kinetoplast DNA in cutaneous lesions. Proc Natl Acad Sci USA 79:6999-7003

Host and parasite factors influencing the expression of cutaneous leishmaniasis

ALAN SHER, DAVID L. SACKS and PHILLIP A. SCOTT

Immunology and Cell Biology Section, Laboratory of Parasitic Diseases, National Institute of Allergy and Infectious Diseases, National Institutes of Health, Bethesda, Maryland 20205, USA

Abstract Host and parasite factors influencing the expression of cutaneous leishmaniasis were investigated in two murine models of different leishmanial diseases. The role of B lymphocytes in the uncontrolled disease manifested by BALB/c mice infected with cutaneous leishmaniasis was investigated in animals of this inbred strain depleted of B cells by neonatal administration of anti-mouse μ-chain antisera. Whereas non-depleted control mice developed chronic metastatic infections with both *Leishmania tropica* and *Leishmania mexicana* and showed depressed delayed-type hypersensitivity when skin-tested with leishmanial antigens, the μ-suppressed mice controlled their initial lesions while displaying strong antigen-specific delayed-type hypersensitivity. These findings reveal an inverse relationship between humoral and cell-mediated immunity in the expression of chronic leishmaniasis and suggest that B lymphocytes or their products regulate the delayed-type hypersensitivity response to leishmanial infection. In a separate study, healing and chronic strains of *Leishmania* were compared for their susceptibility to killing by lymphokine-activated mouse peritoneal macrophages. Whereas amastigotes of the healing strains were readily destroyed by these macrophages, amastigotes of two *Leishmania* strains, previously shown to produce chronic infections in mice, were resistant to killing by the same cells. These findings suggest that the ability of certain leishmanial strains to induce chronic disease may result from their capacity to evade intracellular destruction by activated macrophages.

1983 Cytopathology of parasitic disease. Pitman Books, London (Ciba Foundation symposium 99), p 174-189

Leishmaniasis is a protozoan disease with a spectrum of clinical manifestations that can be related both to the species or strain of infecting parasite and to the nature of the immune response mounted by the host (Turk & Bryceson 1971, Mauel et al 1974, Belehu et al 1980). Cutaneous leishmanial infections are either self-healing or chronic and occur either in the presence or absence of delayed-type hypersensitivity (DTH) to leishmanial antigen preparations (Table 1). The self-healing form of the disease, which can be caused by *Leishmania tropica*, *Leishmania mexicana* and *Leishmania braziliensis*, is

TABLE 1. Variable clinical and immunological manifestations of cutaneous leishmaniasis[a]

Type of infection	*Disease*	*Major parasite complex(es)*	*Delayed-type hypersensitivity*
Self-healing	Oriental sore	*L. tropica*	+[b]
	Skin ulcer	*L. mexicana*, *L. braziliensis*	+[c]
Chronic	Recidivans	*L. tropica*	+[d]
	Mucocutaneous (espundia)	*L. braziliensis* (*L. mexicana*)	+[e]
	Diffuse cutaneous leishmaniasis	*L. tropica*, *L. mexicana*	–[f]

[a]Adapted from Mauel et al (1974). [b]Dostrovsky & Sagher (1946). [c]Tremonti & Walton (1970) and Lainson et al (1973). [d]Turk & Bryceson (1971). [e]Adler (1964) and Maekelt (1972). [f]Convit et al (1972).

characterized by localized (as opposed to metastatic) lesions and is accompanied by strong delayed-type skin test reactions. It is thus analogous in its immunopathology to tuberculoid leprosy.

Chronic cutaneous leishmaniasis has multiple forms and is caused by a variety of different *Leishmania* species. For the purposes of this paper, it is appropriate to classify these different disease manifestations on the basis of the immunological responses that accompany them. Thus, most chronic leishmanial diseases are associated with persistent DTH. The classical example of this type of infection is American mucocutaneous leishmaniasis (MCL), which is typically caused by parasites of the *L. braziliensis* complex. The mucocutaneous disease (also known as *espundia*) usually begins as a skin lesion which, months or years later, metastasizes to the oronasopharyngeal mucosa. A second form of chronic cutaneous infection associated with persistent cell-mediated immunity is leishmaniasis recidivans. This disease is characterized by the development of recrudescing lupoid nodules which form around primary lesions that have apparently healed.

Chronic cutaneous leishmaniasis can also occur in the absence of cell-mediated immunity. Thus, in diffuse cutaneous leishmaniasis (DCL), a primary nodule forms which later metastasizes to other parts of the skin. Classically, patients with DCL are negative in the Montenegro test but respond normally to tuberculin and other antigens. In both the human species and the BALB/c mouse model (see below) DCL has been attributed to host anergy resulting from the generation of suppressor cells (Petersen et al 1982, Howard et al 1980, Scott & Farrell 1981).

Thus, the outcome of cutaneous leishmanial infection is dictated both by the species or strain of organism and by the nature of the host's immunological response to the parasite. We have been attempting to delineate these host and parasite factors that underly the variable pathogenesis of cutaneous leishmaniasis in murine models of two different chronic leishmanial diseases. In our first model, a host factor, the BALB/c genotype, determines the pathogenesis of a persistent, disseminating infection analogous to DCL. DTH responses to the parasite become suppressed in these animals. In contrast, in the second model, the use of a particular parasite strain determines the generation of a chronic disease which, like MCL, persists in the face of strong host cell-mediated immunity. Our studies of these models reveal B lymphocyte responsiveness and resistance to macrophage-mediated killing as important host and parasite factors that influence the pathogenesis of chronic cutaneous leishmaniasis.

B Lymphocytes and the pathogenesis of chronic cutaneous leishmaniasis in BALB/c mice

The BALB/c mouse strain is highly and uniquely susceptible to infection with cutaneous strains of *Leishmania* (Kellina 1973, Pérez et al 1978). The primary lesion fails to heal, as it typically does in most other inbred mouse strains, and it disseminates and visceralizes, leading to death of the host. The dissemination of the disease occurs in the absence of DTH to leishmanial antigens, a state that is analogous to human DCL.

The classic studies of Howard et al (1980, 1981) on leishmaniasis in the BALB/c mouse have suggested that these animals, while capable of mounting a curative cell-mediated immunity against the parasite, are prevented from developing this response by the generation of *Leishmania*-specific suppressor T cells. There have been no data that directly support the earlier hypothesis (Garnham & Humphrey 1969, Bryceson et al 1972) that suppression of DTH and susceptibility to disease might be related to the blocking effect of humoral antibodies which are present during dissemination of the infection. Nevertheless, several recent observations have prompted us to re-examine this question. Whereas suppressor T lymphocytes usually express the $Ly1^-2^+$ phenotype and helper T cells (for the induction of antibody and DTH responses) express $Ly1^+,2^-$ phenotype (Cantor & Boyse 1977), the cells responsible for suppression of DTH and induction of disease in the *Leishmania*-infected BALB/c mouse have been shown by Liew et al (1982) to be $Ly1^+2^-$. Similarly, Mitchell et al (1981) demonstrated that the resistance to infection of minimally reconstituted BALB/c nude mice could be abrogated by the injection of small numbers of syngeneic $Ly2^-$ lymphocytes from chronically infected donors or, less consistently, by the transfer of immune serum from the same animals. These findings raise the possibility that $Ly1^+2^-$ T cells might contribute to the pathogenesis of chronic disease in the BALB/c model by cooperating with B cells in the production of antibodies that block the potentially curative cell-mediated response to the infection. Prompted by these data, we decided to assess directly the role of B lymphocytes and antibody in chronic BALB/c leishmanial infection by following the course of the disease in B-cell-depleted, μ-suppressed mice (D. L. Sacks et al, unpublished results).

BALB/c mice were μ-suppressed by injection from birth with goat anti-μ chain antisera using a standard protocol developed by Dr Richard Asofsky at the National Institutes of Health (Lawton et al 1972). These animals lacked detectable circulating immunoglobulin M (IgM) and were depleted (by 85–95%) of IgM-bearing splenic lymphocytes as determined by fluorescence-activated cell-sorter (FACS) analysis. In contrast, the level of Thy-1^+ T lymphocytes in the spleens of the mice was unaltered by the μ-suppression. The majority of the μ-suppressed mice failed to produce detectable anti-leishmanial antibodies (as measured by indirect immunofluorescence on fixed promastigotes) for as long as eight weeks after infection, although by 12 weeks low levels of antibody could be detected in many of the animals.

The susceptibility of these mice to infection with two different species of *Leishmania*, *L. tropica major* and *L. mexicana amazonensis*, was assessed. Promastigotes (10^6/animal) were injected subcutaneously at the base of the tail, and the size of the resulting lesions was measured with a vernier caliper. As shown in Fig. 1, normal BALB/c mice infected with either *L. tropica* or *L. mexicana* developed lesions that increased in an uncontrolled manner, eventually disseminating to the footpads and visceralizing to the liver and spleen. By 12 weeks after infection, over a third of these animals had died. The development of lesions in μ-suppressed mice was indistinguishable from that in controls until week 4, when progression was arrested in all μ-suppressed mice infected with either strain. Control of the primary lesion persisted in 14 of 15 *L. mexicana*-infected mice and 13 of 15 *L. tropica*-infected mice until termination of the experiment at 12 weeks. Significantly, the few anti-μ-treated mice that failed to control their lesions (data not shown) were those that had been only partially suppressed in terms of their anti-leishmanial antibody responses.

The animals in these experiments were tested for their DTH reactivity to a promastigote antigen preparation (Fig. 2). Whereas infected control mice responded with minimal-delayed footpad swelling at four and eight weeks after infection, the μ-suppressed animals displayed strong DTH reactions at both times. Thus, the ability of μ-suppressed mice to control their lesions correlated with their development of cell-mediated immunity to the parasite.

These experiments suggest that the inability of BALB/c mice to heal cutaneous leishmanial infection depends on B lymphocytes and possibly on their antibody products. Anti-μ-treated mice that were able to control their cutaneous lesions lacked detectable anti-leishmanial antibodies but displayed

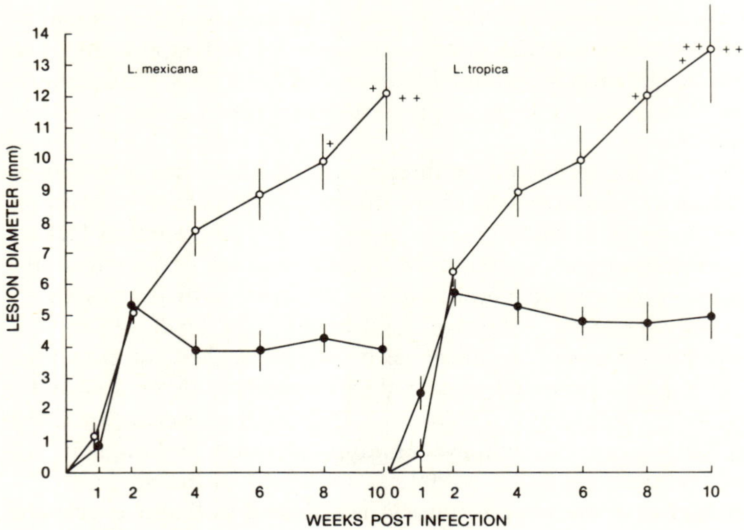

FIG. 1. The course of *L. tropica* and *L. mexicana* infection in anti-μ-treated (solid circles) and untreated, control (open circles) BALB/c mice. The mean lesion size ± 1 SEM(n = 15) is shown (+ shows deaths due to infection); (D. L. Sacks et al, unpublished results).

persistent DTH to leishmanial antigen. These findings are thus consistent with the inverse relationship between cell-mediated immunity and humoral immunity noted in previous immunological studies (e.g. Crowle & Hu 1965, Hellstrom & Hellstrom 1970). The exact mechanism by which the expression of leishmanial infection is governed by these opposing B-cell and T-cell functions is not clear.

Perhaps the simplest explanation of the above observations is that antibodies stimulated by *Leishmania* infection block the induction or expression of parasite-specific DTH by interfering with the recognition of antigen by T lymphocytes. Given the negative or inconsistent results obtained previously by investigators attempting to transfer suppression of healing passively in the BALB/c model with B cells or antibody (J. G. Howard, personal communication, Mitchell et al 1981), this hypothesis seems over-simplistic. Rather, given the strong evidence for the function of T suppressor lymphocytes in the induction of chronic disease in the model, the data are more consistent with a role for B lymphocytes in the generation of suppressor cells which in turn regulate the DTH response to leishmanial infection. This immunoregulatory function could be mediated by B cells directly, or possibly by circulating antibodies or immune complexes.

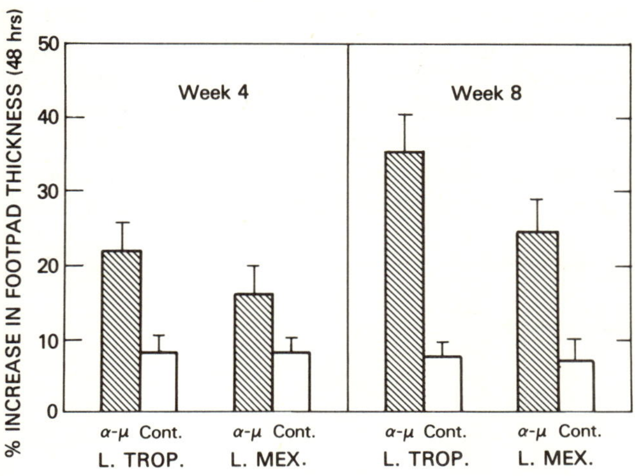

FIG. 2. Delayed footpad swelling (hypersensitivity) responses to promastigote antigen of μ-suppressed and control *Leishmania*-infected BALB/c mice. Animals were injected in the left hind-footpad with 25 μg of *Leishmania* in saline (prepared from *L. tropica* or *L. mexicana* promastigotes) and in the right-footpad with saline. Footpad thickness was measured at 48 h, and delayed-type hypersensitivity responses were expressed as the percentage increase in footpad thickness [(left − right/right) × 100]. The data shown are the mean ±1 SEM of individual readings on five mice per group. Similar results were obtained when footpad thickness was measured at 24 h instead of 48 h (D. L. Sacks et al, unpublished results).

The above evidence that B cells and/or humoral antibodies may be involved in the evolution of suppressed DTH and disease susceptibility in BALB/c mice may have important implications for the pathogenesis of chronic leishmaniasis in humans.

Resistance to macrophage-mediated killing as a parasite factor influencing the pathogenesis of chronic cutaneous leishmaniasis

As noted already, in certain forms of cutaneous leishmaniasis, such as MCL and recidivans, disease persists despite the induction by the host of strong cell-mediated immunity to the infecting parasites. Thus, the pathogenesis of disease in these circumstances appears to depend more on the nature of the parasite than on the responsiveness of the host to infection. Furthermore, the occurrence of chronic leishmanial infection in the face of heightened cellular immunity implies that the parasites involved may have developed specific mechanisms for escaping effector responses in the host.

We have been investigating the factors responsible for the survival of leishmanial parasites in the responsive host in a second murine model of chronic leishmaniasis. Mice of the C57BL/6 strain are normally resistant to infection by cutaneous species of *Leishmania* (Detolla et al 1981). However, a strain of *L. mexicana amazonensis* derived from a patient with MCL has been shown recently to produce chronic disease in these inbred animals (Barral et al 1983). As shown in Fig. 3, after infection with this strain (Maria-NIH),

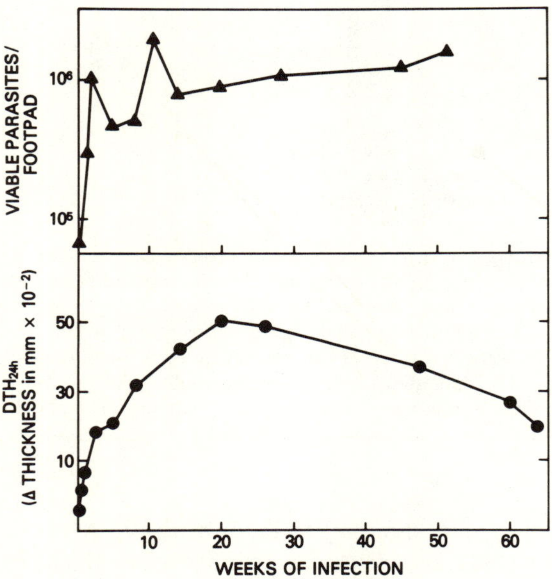

FIG. 3. Parasite levels and delayed-type hypersensitivity (DTH) in C57BL/6 mice infected with Maria-NIH strain (*L. mexicana amazonensis*). The animals were infected with 10^5 amastigotes in the left hind-footpad. Viable organisms in the lesions were counted by the method of Poulter (1979). DTH was measured 24 h after the injection of 50 μg of Maria strain promastigote antigen into the right hind-footpad. Each datum point is the mean of five or more individual assays. (Graph adapted from Barral et al 1982.)

C57BL/6 mice develop cutaneous lesions that persist despite the concomitant induction of strong DTH to the infection. Thus the murine disease induced by Maria-NIH is analogous to human MCL in its chronic nature and its immunological behaviour.

Because *Leishmania* are obligate intracellular parasites of macrophages, one explanation for the chronic lesions observed in Maria strain-infected mice might be the inability of infected macrophages to eliminate the parasite following activation by lymphokine (LK). For this reason, we (Scott et al 1983) decided to compare the survival of Maria strain amastigotes in activated C57BL/6 peritoneal macrophages with that of *L. tropica* strains which, typically, produce healing infections in the same mice.

As shown in Fig. 4, amastigotes of the Maria strain and a representative *L. tropica* strain replicate efficiently inside normal resident C57BL/6

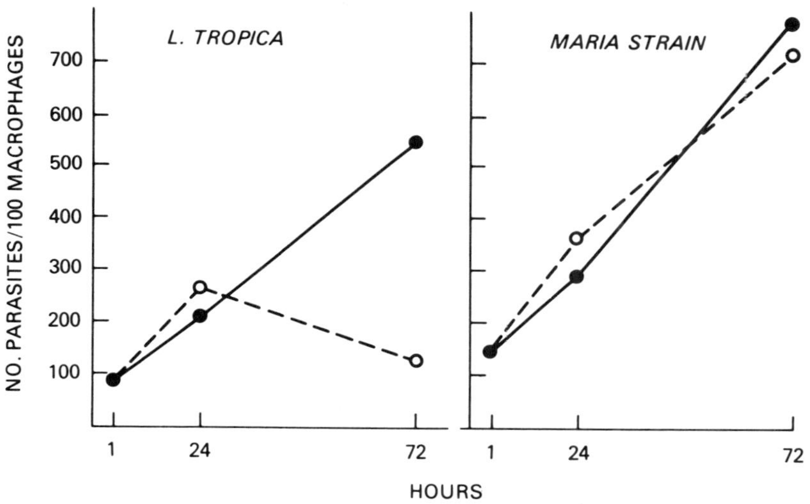

FIG. 4. Effect of lymphokine on *L. tropica* and Maria strain amastigote multiplication in C57BL/6 resident peritoneal macrophages. Cultured macrophage suspensions either received lymphokine (from BCG-primed lymphocytes challenged with purified protein derivative) 1 h after infection (dotted lines) or received no lymphokine (solid lines). The methods were adapted from Nacy et al (1981). Each datum point is the mean of four observations on duplicate cultures (a total of 1000 macrophages were scored). (Scott et al 1983.)

macrophages at 35 °C, the pre-established optimal temperature for intracellular growth. However, if the macrophages are activated by treatment with LK (generated by challenge, with purified protein derivative, of lymphocytes from BCG*-primed mice), the intracellular growth of the *L. tropica* strain is arrested and significant microbicidal activity is observed. In contrast, no microbicidal activity is observed against Maria strain amastigotes in

---

*Bacille Calmette-Guérin vaccine

macrophages treated with LK under identical conditions. The resistance of the Maria strain to macrophage microbicidal activity observed in this experiment is a consistent finding. The same result is obtained by using different doses and regimens of LK, homologous LK generated by antigen challenge of lymphocytes from Maria-strain-infected mice, as well as with different infecting amastigote : macrophage ratios.

The survival of Maria strain parasites in LK-treated macrophages does not appear to be due to an inhibition of activation by the organism. Thus, Maria-infected, LK-stimulated macrophages show unimpaired cytotoxic activity against tumour-cell targets. Furthermore, when simultaneously infected with Maria leishmanial parasites and *Toxoplasma gondii*, LK-treated macrophages exhibit microbicidal activity against *T. gondii* but not against the Maria amastigotes.

That resistance to macrophage-mediated killing may be a general property of parasites that induce chronic leishmaniasis is suggested by recent findings with Isabel-NIH, a leishmanial strain derived from a patient with DCL from the Dominican Republic (Petersen et al 1982). Isabel-NIH, like the Maria strain, produces persistent lesions in C57BL/6 mice (E. Petersen, personal communication) and in our experiments is not killed by activated macrophages. On the other hand, two *L. tropica* strains, each known to produce healing infections in C57BL/6 mice, were found to be readily destroyed by LK-treated macrophages. Further screening of strains derived from chronic and healing lesions is necessary to establish the generality of the above findings. Finally, it should be emphasized that the relationship which we have observed between chronicity of infection and resistance to macrophage microbicidal activity applies only to murine leishmaniasis. Studies of the behaviour of chronic and healing strains in activated human macrophages will be required before our findings can be extrapolated to human leishmaniasis.

Concluding comments

Our experimental findings summarized here emphasize the complex interplay between host and parasite factors in the expression of leishmanial disease. They also underline the importance of the genetic constitution of both host and parasite in the aetiology of cutaneous leishmaniasis. Although there is abundant evidence in the mouse about the influence of host genotype on responsiveness to leishmanial infection, there is a dearth of information about the genetic control of disease susceptibility in humans, which clearly provides an important area for future investigation.

Similarly, the study of genetic variations in *Leishmania* parasites that influence their virulence and immunological behaviour is also in its infancy.

The investigation of this problem should be greatly facilitated by the advent of monoclonal antibody and recombinant DNA probes for identifying *Leishmania* species and strains (Wirth & McMahon Pratt 1982). It is only with this fundamental understanding of parasite virulence and host responsiveness that the basis of the most intriguing aspect of leishmaniasis—its variable pathogenesis—will be revealed.

Acknowledgements

We are grateful to Drs F. A. Neva, J. G. Howard, C. A. Nacy and E. A. Petersen for their helpful advice and encouragement and thank A. Barral for permission to reproduce the data shown in Fig. 3.

REFERENCES

Adler S 1964 *Leishmania*. Adv Parasitol 2:35-96

Barral A, Petersen EA, Sacks DL, Neva FA 1983 Late metastatic leishmaniasis in the mouse. A possible model for mucocutaneous disease. Am J Trop Med Hyg, in press

Belehu A, Louis JA, Pugin P, Miescher PA 1980 Immunopathological aspects of leishmaniasis. Springer Semin Immunopathol 2:399-415

Bryceson ADM, Preston PM, Bray RS, Domonde DC 1972 Experimental cutaneous leishmaniasis. II: Effects of immunosuppression and antigenic competition on the course of infection with *Leishmania enriettii* in the guinea pig. Clin Exp Immunol 10:305-312

Cantor H, Boyse EA 1977 Regulation of cellular and humoral immunity by T-cell subclasses. In: Origins of lymphocyte diversity. Cold Spring Harbor Symp Quant Biol 41:23-29

Convit J, Pinardi ME, Rondon AJ 1972 Diffuse cutaneous leishmaniasis: a disease due to an immunological defect of the host. Trans R Soc Trop Med Hyg 66:603-610

Crowle AJ, Hu CC 1965 Inhibition of the development of delayed hypersensitivity by treatment with antiserum. J Immunol 94:553-562

Detolla LJ, Scott PA, Farrell JP 1981 Single gene control of resistance to cutaneous leishmaniasis in mice. Immunogenetics 14:29-39

Dostrovsky A, Sagher F 1946 The intracutaneous test in cutaneous leishmaniasis. Ann Trop Med Parasitol 40:265-269

Garnham PC, Humphrey JH 1969 Problems in leishmaniasis related to immunology. Curr Top Microbiol Immunol 48:29-40

Hellstrom KE, Hellstrom I 1970 Immunological enhancement as studied by cell culture techniques. Annu Rev Microbiol 24:373-394

Howard JG, Hale C, Liew FY 1980 Immunological regulation of experimental cutaneous leishmaniasis. III: Nature and significance of specific suppression of cell-mediated immunity in mice highly susceptible to *Leishmania tropica*. J Exp Med 152:594-601

Howard JG, Hale C, Liew FY 1981 Immunological regulation of experimental cutaneous leishmaniasis. IV: Prophylactic effect of sublethal irradiation as a result of abrogation of suppressor T cell generation in mice genetically susceptible to *Leishmania tropica*. J Exp Med 153:557-563

Kellina OI 1973 Differences of susceptibility of inbred mice of different strains to *Leishmania tropica major*. [Russian] Med Parazitol Parazit Bolezni 42:279-285

Lainson R, Shaw JJ, Ward RD, Fraiha H 1973 Leishmaniasis in Brazil. IX: Considerations on the *Leishmania braziliensis* complex: importance of sandflies of the genus Psychodopygus in the transmission of *L. braziliensis braziliensis* in North Brazil. Trans R Soc Trop Med Hyg 67:184-196

Lawton AR, Asofsky R, Hylton MB, Cooper MD 1972 Suppression of immunoglobulin class synthesis in mice. I: Effects of treatment with antibody to μ-chain. J Exp Med 135:277-285

Liew FY, Hale C, Howard JG 1982 Immunologic regulation of experimental cutaneous leishmaniasis. V: Characterization of effector and specific suppressor T cells. J Immunol 128:1917-1923

Maekelt GA 1972 Immune response to intracellular parasites. I: *Leishmania*. In: Soulsby EJL (ed) Immunity to animal parasites. Academic Press, New York, p 343-363

Mauel J, Behin R, Noerjasin B, Doyle JJ 1974 Survival and death of *Leishmania* in macrophages. In: Parasites in the immunized host: mechanisms of survival. Associated Scientific Publishers, Amsterdam (Ciba Found Symp 25) p 225-242

Mitchell GF, Curtis JM, Scollay RG, Handman EA 1981 Resistance and abrogation of resistance to cutaneous leishmaniasis in reconstituted BALB/c nude mice. Aust J Exp Biol Med Sci 59:539-554

Nacy CA, Meltzer MS, Leonard EJ, Wyler DJ 1981 Intracellular replication and lymphokine-induced destruction of *Leishmania tropica* in C3H/HeN mouse macrophages. J Immunol 127:2381-2389

Pérez H, Arredondo B, Mercedes G 1978 Comparative study of American cutaneous leishmaniasis and diffuse cutaneous leishmaniasis in two strains of inbred mice. Infect Immun 22:301-310

Petersen EA, Neva FA, Oster CN, Dias HB 1982 Specific inhibition of lymphocyte-proliferation responses by adherent suppressor cells in diffuse cutaneous leishmaniasis. N Engl J Med 306:387-391

Poulter LW 1979 The quantification of viable *Leishmania enriettii* from infected guinea pig tissues. Clin Exp Immunol 36:24-29

Scott PA, Farrell JP 1981 Experimental cutaneous leishmaniasis. I: Nonspecific immunodepression in BALB/c mice with *Leishmania tropica*. J Immunol 127:2395-2400

Scott PA, Sacks DL, Sher A 1983 Resistance to macrophage-mediated killing as a factor influencing the pathogenesis of chronic cutaneous leishmaniasis. J Immunol, in press

Tremonti L, Walton BC 1970 Blast transformation and migration–inhibition in toxoplasmosis and leishmaniasis. Am J Trop Med Hyg 19:49-56

Turk JL, Bryceson ADM 1971 Immunological phenomena in leprosy and related diseases. Adv Immunol 13:209-266

Wirth DF, McMahon Pratt D 1982 Rapid identification of *Leishmania* species by specific hybridization of kinetoplast DNA in cutaneous lesions. Proc Natl Acad Sci USA 79:6999-7003

DISCUSSION

Nogueira: Did you test the capability of the resistant strains of *Leishmania* to induce a phagocytic burst in the cells?

Sher: No. Dr Klebanoff has also suggested that we do this experiment.

Nogueira: One could just do a reduction with nitroblue tetrazolium to give an immediate answer. This might indicate which strains have specific surface components to induce the burst.

Pérez: You treated your BALB/c mice with anti-μ serum, but we should remember that in BALB/c mice infection with *Leishmania mexicana* (and perhaps *Leishmania tropica* as well) will be followed by polyclonal activation of B cells. Parasite antigens and the induction of polyclonal activation do not seem to be related to a living infection. Perhaps you are interfering with the phenomenon of polyclonal activation by treating your animals with the anti-μ serum.

Sher: Since μ-suppressed mice are B-cell depleted, they should not show polyclonal B cell activation after infection.

Nussenzweig: Could you tell us more about the immune mechanisms operating in the anti-μ experiments? You said that the absence of antibodies does not seem to be responsible for the resistance of μ-suppressed mice, so what seems to be the mechanism?

Sher: We can only speculate at this point. There is evidence from other laboratories that B cells and immune complexes are involved in the induction of suppressor T cells. For instance, Janeway & Gershon observed that μ-suppressed mice are defective in their ability to generate idiotype specific T-suppressor cells (R. Gershon, personal communication). We have been attempting to demonstrate an effect of μ-suppression on the generation of *Leishmania*-specific suppressors by means of cell-transfer experiments. This work is still in progress.

Nussenzweig: Working with a cloned parasite population, at least in experimental animals, would simplify the observed phenomena and facilitate the identification of different populations of suppressor cells. In addition, different parasite fractions containing distinct antigens are likely to be responsible for these multiple effects. Therefore, one must separate these factors in order to understand the basic phenomena.

Pérez: Polyclonal activation is also related to the alteration in regulatory T cells that we see in BALB/c mice chronically infected with *L. mexicana*. Have you looked at the generation time for multiplication in *L. mexicana amazonensis* and compared it to that for other strains of *Leishmania?*

Sher: The multiplication rates of the Maria strain and our *L. tropica* strain are very similar.

Pérez: To look at the multiplication of the leishmanial parasite only by counting promastigotes is not sufficient.

Sher: I'm talking about the multiplication of the parasites in macrophages, whereas you apparently were referring to their growth in culture. In fact the growth rates of the two strains in liquid culture are also very similar.

Pérez: The strain of *L. mexicana amazonensis* that we have been using has a smaller generation time than *L. mexicana*. We think that there is rapid accumulation of parasite antigens in the intracellular environment, which may lead to the changes we are observing.

Warren: I believe that the work of McMahon Pratt & David (1981) was originally designed to differentiate *L. mexicana* from *Leishmania braziliensis*, the latter being the cause of espundia (mucocutaneous leishmaniasis) and the former being the cause of a sore-like lesion. Is the *L. mexicana amazonensis* a true strain of *L. mexicana*? It seems to be more of an espundia-like organism.

Sher: There have been reports of mucocutaneous leishmaniasis caused by *L. mexicana*, as well as by *L. braziliensis* (e.g. Barral et al 1983). This is one of the reasons why one may want to consider the disease as being more important than the species (p 169).

Warren: What will the work with monoclonal antibodies eventually do to help in diagnosis? Is this work capable of telling us whether particular organisms are more or less likely to cause espundia or not?

Pérez: I would like to comment on that. We must be aware of the situation in endemic areas, where a patient could be infected with more than one parasite. I would be very cautious about saying that *L. mexicana amazonensis* will produce the mucocutaneous form of American cutaneous leishmaniasis. We have found, in mucocutaneous leishmaniasis, a small number of parasites, and we know that lesions caused by *L. mexicana amazonensis* are very rich in parasites.

Sher: We are now trying to find isolates that come directly from mucocutaneous lesions. Most of the isolates available tend to come from peripheral lesions, and there is no way that one can be sure that the same organisms are responsible for the mucocutaneous disease in the same patient.

Wyler: One of the features of *L. mexicana amazonensis*, as Dr Chang's paper showed (this volume) is that several amastigotes are present within a very large vacuole. This is a feature less frequently observed with *L. tropica* or *Leishmania donovani* infections. Could this biological difference explain your findings?

Sher: We certainly have observed the same phenomenon with the Maria strain and also with the *L. mexicana amazonensis* that was susceptible to killing. The Isabel strain (from the patient with diffuse cutaneous leishmaniasis) also produces multiple amastigotes within a single vacuole and, as I mentioned, is resistant to intracellular killing.

Wyler: Antibody might function in an additional manner in this disease. We have found that macrophages pretreated *in vitro* with lymphokine have a reduced capacity to take up amastigotes *in vitro*. Similarly, macrophages isolated from infected animals also ingest the parasites less readily than macrophages from uninfected mice (C.B. Panosian & D.J. Wyler, unpublished work). On the other hand, IgG-sensitized sheep red blood cells are taken up at normal rates by these macrophages. It is therefore possible that if antibody coats the amastigotes it may facilitate their entry into these macrophages which would otherwise be defective in their ability to ingest the parasites.

Nogueira: Have you tried immune serum on this resistant Maria strain? By analogy with *Toxoplasma gondii*, if resistance has anything to do with the induction of a phagocytic burst, you may induce one with immune serum.

Sher: In preliminary experiments, there is no effect of immune serum on the killing of either *L. tropica* or Maria strain amastigotes by activated macrophages.

Pfefferkorn: You specified that the killing assays were done at 35 °C. What happens if you move the temperature up to core body temperature?

Sher: The first thing that one observes is that the growth of the Maria strain in normal macrophages is absent. At 37 °C intracellular killing of the parasites is also observed. Nevertheless, the point remains that 37 °C is neither the optimum temperature for growth of the parasites intracellularly nor the temperature at which the parasite exists in the body. Indeed, Frank Neva at the NIH has been treating cutaneous leishmaniasis by local application of heat (unpublished). This treatment is based on the idea that the parasite does not survive at temperatures higher than 35 °C.

Chang: The number of amastigotes in each vacuole is not very consistent. In your infection experiments, you used amastigotes to study the lymphokine-activated killing of the parasites. Have you tried using promastigotes?

Sher: Our results with promastigotes, though pointing to the same conclusion, are less consistent. Promastigotes, in general, are more sensitive than amastigotes to intracellular killing and, whereas Maria-strain amastigotes are resistant at 35 °C, Maria promastigotes do appear to be susceptible to killing in certain experiments. Since leishmanial infections are maintained by amastigotes, and not by promastigotes, this observation does not refute our hypothesis that the Maria strain can produce chronic infection because of its ability to survive in activated macrophages.

Hernández: I would like to stress Dr Chang's remarks about the number of parasites per vacuole. In a diffuse cutaneous leishmaniasis strain adapted to mouse macrophages the number of parasites that we have measured, using the same system that Dr Chang uses, is very sparse, although the parasites are definitely there; we have never seen more than 8 or 9 up to the 6th day of culture. The *L. mexicana amazonensis* strain that Dr Chang used, however, was present as 100 per macrophage after only three days. I also have a comment in relation to excreted factors. The problem of their characterization is not in the species but in the particular strain. You mentioned two strains of *L. mexicana amazonensis*, only one of which survived, so it is not a problem of the species but of the particular isolate that you are working with.

Sher: I agree.

Hernández: One can distinguish between isolates from parasites that are believed to belong to the same species by using excreted factors. Kutish & Janovy (1981) infected macrophages with *L. donovani* and used, as a control, a non-pathogenic *L. donovani* strain. Then they infected the macrophage with *Leptomonas costoris*, and although this organism survived in the macrophage infected with the pathogenic *Leishmania* species it did not when the macrophage was loaded with a non-pathogenic strain. They concluded that infection by *L. donovani* induces important changes in the macrophage, making it unable to digest the *L. costoris*. So a metabolic product from the leishmanial parasite may induce changes in the macrophage. I gather that promastigotes of the strain from the Dominican Republic, unlike other isolated strains, do not grow at higher temperatures.

Dr L.F. Schnur et al (personal communication; see also Petersen et al 1982) concluded that this strain shows characteristics of *L. mexicana* and *L. braziliensis*. Nevertheless, in the *L. mexicana* strain the promastigote culture can be established at 28 or 25 °C, but it seems that the Dominican Republic strain has to be cultured at 18 to 20 °C for optimal growth of the parasite.

Sher: We maintain the strain at 26 °C, the same temperature at which we grow promastigotes of most of our other strains. This isolate from the Dominican Republic strain is clearly a different strain, nevertheless, because it has not been definitively typed by using routine methods for speciation of *Leishmania*.

Butterworth: It sounds as though you are all dealing with isolates from individual patients which show genetically stable differences on transmission to a variety of experimental hosts. One could think of two ways in which these differences might arise. First, they may be strain differences that have been cyclically transmitted through the insect vector and the mammalian host over many generations. Secondly, they might have emerged by mutation of individual parasites within the particular host from which one has isolated the organism. Of the two possibilities, particularly in the case of espundia, the latter would seem more probable: the parasites associated with espundia would have little chance of transmission through the insect vector, because of the lack of organisms in the lesion. Therefore one may be dealing with genetically stable mutants that have happened to emerge in the later stages of infection of particular patients. Theoretically, it should be possible, in your self-healing strains of mice, to reproduce this situation by recovering organisms *late* in chronic infections (just before the animal heals). In this way, you may select for mutant organisms that are resistant to macrophage killing. One could then compare these mutants with the original isolate used to initiate the lesion. This might indicate the mechanism whereby the mutant population would be resistant to macrophage killing.

Sher: I agree entirely. I suspect that parasites obtained from cutaneous sores are quite different from those that metastasize to mucocutaneous sites and cause espundia. It would be fascinating if isolates from these two different types of lesions obtained from the same patient differed in their susceptibility to intracellular killing by macrophages.

REFERENCES

Barral A, Petersen EA, Sacks DL, Neva FA 1983 Late metastatic leishmaniasis in the mouse. A possible model for mucocutaneous disease. Am J Trop Med Hyg, in press

Kutish GF, Janovy J Jr 1981 Inhibition of *in vitro* macrophage digestion capacity by infection with *Leishmania donovani*. J Parasitol 67:457-462

McMahon Pratt D, David JR 1981 Monoclonal antibodies that distinguish between New World species of *Leishmania*. Nature (Lond) 291:581-583

Petersen EA, Neva FA, Oster CN, Dias HB 1982 Specific inhibition of lymphocyte-proliferation responses by adherent suppressor cells in diffuse cutaneous leishmaniasis. N Engl J Med 306:387-391

Regulation of fibroblast functions by products of schistosomal egg granulomas: potential role in the pathogenesis of hepatic fibrosis

DAVID J. WYLER

Division of Geographic Medicine, Department of Medicine, Tufts University School of Medicine, 136 Harrison Avenue, Boston, Massachusetts 02111, USA

Abstract Recent observations suggest a molecular link between granuloma formation and hepatic fibrosis in schistosomiasis. Egg granulomas isolated from *Schistosoma mansoni*-infected mice, when cultured in serum-free medium, produce a variety of biologically active molecules that affect fibroblast function. One group of molecules—proteins with an estimated relative molecular mass (M_r) of 30 000—stimulate fibroblast proliferation *in vitro*. These molecules have interleukin (IL)-1-like activity when assayed in thymocyte cultures but are biochemically distinct from previously characterized murine IL-1. Fibroblast mitogenic activity is also produced by macrophages isolated from granulomas and by extracts of *S. mansoni* eggs. The egg-derived activity is distinct from the granuloma cell-derived material on the basis of M_r and isoelectric point determinations. Egg extracts also contain concanavalin A-binding substances which are not directly mitogenic for fibroblasts but can stimulate spleen cells from infected mice to produce fibroblast mitogenic activity *in vitro*. A large chemoattractant molecule (>200 000 M_r) for fibroblasts has also been identified in supernatants from granuloma cultures and in supernatants from macrophages isolated from granulomas. This activity is abolished by treatment with anti-fibronectin antibody, suggesting that it is fibronectin or a cleavage product thereof. Molecules similar to or identical with the fibroblast mitogenic factors from the granulomas have been identified, and they inhibit the contraction of fibroblast-populated collagen lattices. These activities may be important in the pathogenesis of hepatic fibrosis in schistosomiasis, and pharmacological modification of their production or of their effects on target fibroblasts might theoretically prevent hepatic fibrosis in this disease.

1983 Cytopathology of parasitic disease. Pitman Books, London (Ciba Foundation symposium 99) p 190-206

A striking feature of the pathogenesis of schistosomiasis is that the host response, rather than the invasiveness of the parasite, underlies most of the observed morbidity and mortality. The pathological hallmark of the disease is the egg granuloma, a collection of inflammatory cells that surround eggs deposited in the mesenteric, hepatic portal, pelvic or 'ectopic' (e.g. central nervous system) venous beds. In the last two decades, investigators have begun to define the immunological mechanisms involved in formation of egg granulomas, substantial progress being facilitated by the murine model of schistosomiasis mansoni (Warren & DeWitt 1958). Extensive observations confirm that at least in this model—and probably in human schistosomiasis as well—the granuloma forms as a result of a delayed-type hypersensitivity response to egg antigens (Warren et al 1967, Boros 1978, Warren 1982). Furthermore, adoptive cell-transfer studies with enriched T-lymphocyte populations from mice sensitized to egg antigen suggest that granuloma *formation* is under the control of helper T cells, while the subsequent spontaneous *regression* of the granulomas appears to be modulated by subpopulations of suppressor T cells. Recruitment from the circulation to the developing granuloma of inflammatory cells such as eosinophils (James & Colley 1975, Lewis et al 1977) and mononuclear phagocytes (Lewis et al 1977, Boros et al 1973) may be mediated by soluble products of activated T lymphocytes (lymphokines). These remarkable findings have served not only to enhance our understanding of the pathogenesis of schistosomiasis specifically but have also provided the first clear understanding of the immunopathogenesis of hypersensitivity granulomas generally.

Granuloma formation in the livers of individuals infected with *Schistosoma mansoni* and *Schistosoma japonicum* precedes the subsequent periportal fibrosis that underlies the clinically important complications of the infection, namely gastrointestinal haemorrhage due to portal hypertension. Characteristic of this fibrosis is its perivascular distribution, with sparing of the lobular architecture. Furthermore, hepatocellular function remains preserved until very late in the disease (Rodriguez et al 1955). This feature distinguishes *Schistosoma*-induced hepatic fibrosis from cirrhosis due to a variety of aetiological agents such as viral infection, toxins and nutritional deficiencies. Furthermore, it defines the clinical important pathology as essentially a 'plumbing' problem. The periportal fibrosis results in portal hypertension, increased blood flow through the collateral circulation (such as the gastric and oesophageal veins), the formation of varices and their subsequent rupture leading to gastrointestinal haemorrhage. It is reasonable to conclude therefore that in the absence of the portal obstruction due to fibrosis, infection with *S. mansoni* and *S. japonicum* would probably result in a relatively benign disease.

Unfortunately, as for pathological fibrosis generally, little is known about the pathogenesis of hepatic fibrosis in schistosomiasis. Since chronic inflammation frequently results in tissue fibrosis at many sites including liver, lung, skin and joint spaces, an appropriate hypothesis is that the egg granuloma may somehow initiate or control the subsequent hepatic fibrogenesis. This review will summarize evidence supporting the hypothesis of molecular links between the cells that comprise the egg granuloma and the hepatic fibrogenesis in *S. mansoni* infections. *In vitro* experiments have shown that egg granulomas, macrophages from granulomas and the egg themselves contain and produce biologically active molecules that can promote, in fibroblasts, chemotaxis, proliferation, collagen synthesis and prostaglandin secretion, and can inhibit contraction of fibroblast-populated collagen matrices. In addition to shedding light on pathogenesis in schistosomiasis specifically, this model may also be ideally suited for investigations of the interface between the immunoregulation of chronic inflammation and the subsequent fibrosis generally.

Materials and methods

Outbred (NIH) or inbred (C57B1/6) female mice (18–20 g) were infected intraperitoneally with 50–150 cercariae of *S. mansoni* (Puerto Rican strain) and sacrificed eight weeks later. Granulomas were isolated by a simple technique (Pellegrino & Brener 1956) of homogenizing livers in a Waring blender and sequentially sedimenting the granulomas at 1 ***g*** in Hanks' buffer (HBSS). Hepatic cell debris remained suspended in the supernatant and the pellet contained granulomas virtually free of hepatocytes. For some experiments, the isolated granulomas were then dissociated into a suspension of their constituent cells by incubation (37 °C) with collagenase (500 U/ml) in HBSS. After the first 30 min of incubation in collagenase, granulomas were resuspended in fresh collagenase solution and further incubated for 30 min. The cell suspensions derived from the two treatments were pooled, washed extensively with HBSS, treated with Tris-NH_4Cl to lyse the erythrocytes, rewashed in HBSS, and suspended in supplemented culture medium RPMI 1640 which contained antibiotics and 10% heat-inactivated fetal bovine serum.

Intact granulomas were suspended in serum-free supplemented medium RPMI 1640 at a 10% (vol/vol) density and were incubated in 75 cm^2 tissue-culture flasks for 24–72 h in a humid 5% CO_2–95% air atmosphere. Culture supernatants were retrieved after centrifugation (200 ***g*** × 10 min) and were subjected to one of three treatments: (1) dialysis against medium; (2) ultrafiltration; or (3) lyophilization following dialysis against 0.15 M $NH_4(CO_3)_2$. These processed culture supernatants were then tested directly in fibroblast cultures or were first fractionated by a variety of techniques before testing (see below).

Cultures highly enriched for granuloma-derived macrophages (95–99%

latex-ingesting adherent cells; 95% Fc receptor-bearing) were prepared by plating suspensions of dissociated granuloma cells (10^7/3 ml) in 60 mm-diameter polystyrene culture dishes and incubating (at 37 °C in an atmosphere of 5% CO_2–95% air) for 2 h. Non-adherent cells were removed by washing with warm HBSS, and adherent cells were further incubated in serum-free supplemented medium. Culture supernatants were retrieved, centrifuged and processed as described above for granuloma supernatants.

Soluble egg antigens (SEA) of *S. mansoni* were prepared as previously described (Boros & Warren 1970). For some experiments these antigens were fractionated into a glycoprotein fraction, containing an important antigen MSA-1 (Pelley & Pelley 1976), by chromatography on a concanavalin A affinity column as previously described (Pelley & Pelley 1976).

Diploid dermal fibroblast cultures were established from abdominal wall skin of guinea-pigs and mice and from human foreskins by methods previously described (Wyler et al 1981). These cells were not transformed, they exhibited contact inhibition and they synthesized collagen. For proliferation assays, fibroblasts were plated in serum-containing medium at a density of 5×10^4–10^5 cells per 16 mm-diameter well, in 24-well culture plates. After overnight incubation at 37 °C, cells were extensively washed free of serum with HBSS and were further incubated for 24 h in 1 ml serum-free medium. The relevant samples (diluted in medium) to be tested for fibroblast mitogenic activity were then added in a volume of 100 μl and cultures were incubated for 24–72 h before addition of [^{3}H]thymidine (0.5 μCi/well; specific activity 6.7 Ci/mM) for the final 4 h of incubation. Cells were trypsinized and harvested onto glass-fibre filters with a multi-sample automatic harvester before their radionucleotide incorporation was assessed in a β-scintillation counter.

Methods have previously been described for assessing the presence of fibroblast chemotactic activity (Postlethwaite et al 1976), the synthesis of collagen (Peterkofsky & Diegelmann 1977), the secretion of prostaglandin (Wahl et al 1977), the intracellular concentrations of 3′–5′ cyclic adenosine monophosphate (cAMP) (McCarthy et al 1980) and the contraction of collagen lattices (Bell et al 1979).

Results

Granuloma-derived fibroblast-stimulating activity

Dialysed supernatants from granuloma cultures stimulated the uptake of [^{3}H] thymidine by quiescent dermal fibroblasts of guinea-pig, mouse and human origin (Wyler et al 1981). The uptake and incorporation of radionucleotide into trichloroacetic acid (TCA)-precipitable material was shown truly to reflect cell proliferation as determined by cell enumeration (Wyler et al 1981). Net uptake of tritiated thymidine began as early as 24 h after addition of granuloma supernatants to fibroblast cultures and continued for 72 h. The supernatant had to be present for at least 18 h for the mitogenic effect to be observed; brief (2–12 h) exposures of fibroblasts to the supernatants followed by washing did not elicit this response upon further incubation for up to 48 h. High concentrations of supernatant failed to stimulate the uptake of [^{3}H]thymidine and were, in fact, inhibitory (Fig. 1).

In addition to stimulating proliferation of fibroblasts, supernatants from granuloma cultures stimulated secretion of prostaglandin E_2 and increased the intracellular concentrations of cAMP (Fig. 1, Wyler et al 1981). Fur-

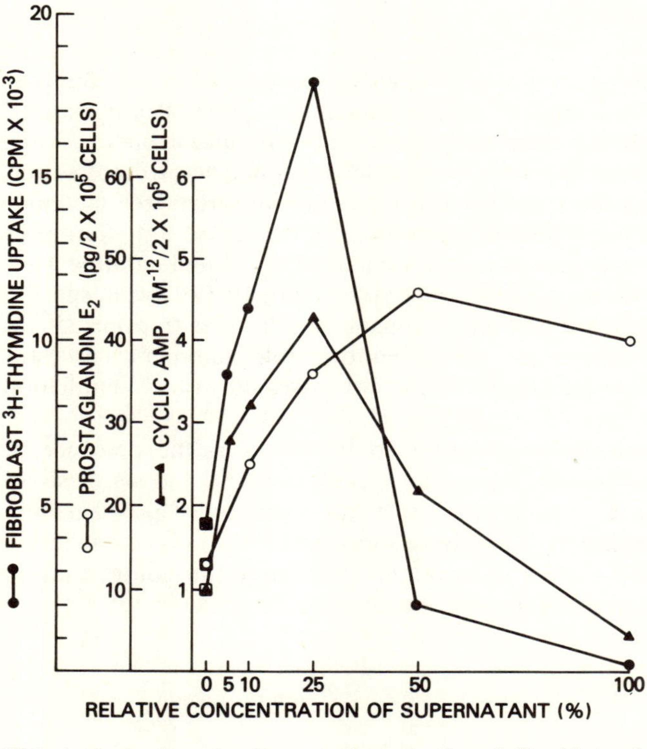

FIG. 1. Activation of quiescent guinea-pig dermal fibroblast cultures *in vitro* by dialysed supernatants from egg granuloma cultures. Responses, measured as uptake of [^{3}H]thymidine, PGE_2 secretion and intracellular cAMP activity, are shown as mean of triplicate determinations (SEM 10% of the mean), for a representative granuloma supernatant preparation. (Reprinted from Wyler et al (1981) by permission of The University of Chicago © 1981 by The University of Chicago.)

TABLE 1 *In vitro* synthesis of collagen by guinea-pig fibroblasts stimulated with crude granuloma supernatant

Additive to fibroblast culture	*Incorporation (c.p.m.) of [^{3}H]proline into:*					
	Total TCA-precipitable material			*Collagenase-sensitive material*		
	Supernatant[a]	*Cells*[b]	*Total*	*Supernatant*	*Cells*	*Total*
Medium	5 867	16 319	22 186	4 106	1 603	5 709
Granuloma Supernatant A[c]	10 296	32 463	42 759	7 527	3 993	11 522
Granuloma Supernatant B[c]	9 955	36 045	46 000	7 159	3 779	10 938

[a]Incorporation (counts per min, c.p.m) was measured in fibroblast culture supernatant after precipitation with trichloroacetic acid (TCA) and dialysis (to remove unincorporated [^{3}H]proline). [b]c.p.m. in washed fibroblasts. [c]Dialysed granuloma supernatant tested at 1 : 10 final dilution.

thermore, these supernatants stimulated net synthesis of collagen by fibroblasts (Table 1; assay kindly performed by Dr Larry Wahl, National Institutes of Health). This net synthesis was not due to increased numbers of fibroblasts since the assay was done before the stimulated cells began to proliferate.

The release of fibroblast-stimulating activities into supernatants from granuloma cultures was apparently not caused by death of the granuloma cells, since the granulomas continued to synthesize proteins at increased levels during incubation for up to 72 h (Wyler et al 1981). On the other hand, since cytosol extracts of freshly isolated granulomas also contained activity that was mitogenic for fibroblasts (Wyler et al 1978), it was apparent that the factor(s) were already present in the granuloma cells.

Properties of granuloma-derived fibroblast mitogenic activity

To define the characteristics of the molecule(s) responsible for inducing fibroblast proliferation *in vitro*, unfractionated or partially purified granuloma supernatants were subjected to gel filtration, preparative isoelectric focusing and ion-exchange chromatography (Wyler & Rosenwasser 1982). On the basis of Sephadex G-200 column chromatography, peak fibroblast mitogenic activity could be resolved in fractions with estimated relative molecular mass (M_r) of about 30 000. When the column-purified material was subjected to isoelectric focusing in granular gel (at pH 3–9), activity was discerned in two fractions. Major activity was present in fractions with isoelectric point (pI) of 5–7, with peak activity at pI 6. Minor activity was also present in fractions with pI of 4.0–4.5. Ion-exchange chromatography (DEAE Sephadex A50), run with a linear gradient from 0–2 M NaCl, confirmed the heterogeneity of the active molecules contained in the gel filtration peak (M_r, 30 000). Major activity eluted from the ion exchange column with 0.4–0.7 M NaCl; minor activity was present in fractions that were eluted with 1.5–1.8 M NaCl. Furthermore, trypsin treatment of partially purified material (gel filtration) abolished the biological activity, as did heating to 100 °C for 10 min. Heating for 30 min at 56 °C, however, did not significantly alter the activity. Addition to fibroblast cultures of the inhibitor of serine esterase, phenylmethylsulphonylfluoride (PMSF), at 10^{-5} or 10^{-4} M concentrations did not alter the proliferative responses to the granuloma-derived factor(s).

To determine whether the activity was specific for fibroblasts, granuloma culture-derived material was added to cultures of bovine aortic smooth-muscle cells, bovine aortic endothelial cells and murine thymocytes in a conventional assay (Oppenheim et al 1976) used for detection of lymphocyte-activating factor (now called interleukin 1, IL-1). Crude supernatants stimulated proliferation of all three cell types. This activity was also present in some of the partially purified fractions. Specifically, thymocyte-stimulating and smooth-muscle-stimulating activity was present only in the fraction of approximately 30 000 M_r obtained by gel filtration. Thymocyte-stimulating activity was also present in fractions with pI of about 4.5, and minor activity was found in fractions with pI of about 5.5, obtained by preparative isoelectric focusing. Responses of endothelial cells to fractionated material were not tested.

These findings indicated that fibroblast-stimulating activity produced by the granulomas derived from at least two proteins with estimated M_r of 30 000 which lacked an intrinsic serine esterase activity that could explain their biological effects. Furthermore, these molecules seem to have mitogenic activity for other cells of mesenchymal origin and might be *functionally* related specifically to IL-1, although the molecular characteristics are distinct from *bona fide* murine IL-1 (Mizel & Mizel 1981).

Macrophages as a source of activity

Since the chronic egg granuloma is composed of a variety of cell types, including eosinophils, lymphocytes, macrophages and fibroblasts, as well as eggs containing viable embryos, any or all of these could be a source of the fibrogenic molecules. To define the source(s), we attempted to fractionate the suspensions of dissociated granuloma cells into populations highly enriched for one cell type. So far, using techniques of adherence to plastic and separation on density gradients, we have been only partially successful. Populations highly enriched for macrophages could be easily obtained by adherence to plastic culture dishes (see above), but lymphocytes and eosinophils invariably co-purified on density gradients, perhaps because the eosinophils were degranulated and thereby altered in their buoyant densities.

Supernatants from isolated granuloma macrophages contained activity that stimulated proliferation of fibroblasts and smooth muscle and endothelial cells *in vitro*. The activity also stimulated thymocyte proliferation in the IL-1 assay. We are now determining whether this activity resides in molecules with the same characteristics as those present in supernatants from cultures of intact granulomas. Of particular interest is the evidence that the isolated granuloma macrophages have phenotypic and functional characteristics of 'activated' macrophages (D. J. Wyler & M. Stadecker, unpublished observations). Specifically, this cell population has reduced 5′-nucleotidase activity (Karnovsky & Lazdins 1978) and ingested C3b-coated sheep erythrocytes (Bianco et al 1975) at higher rates than those achieved by resident peritoneal macrophages of uninfected mice (controls). Control macrophages failed to release spontaneously any fibroblast mitogenic activity. Thus, granuloma macrophages seem to be activated *in vivo* and can consequently elaborate constitutively a molecule(s) *in vitro* that is mitogenic for fibroblasts and other cells of mesenchymal origin.

Direct and indirect effects of soluble extracts of eggs on fibroblast proliferation

To investigate whether soluble products contained in (and possibly secreted by) the eggs could theoretically also participate in hepatic fibrogenesis, we tested aqueous extracts of *S. mansoni* eggs in fibroblast cultures for their ability to stimulate proliferation (Wyler & Tracy 1982). Mitogenic activity was present in crude extracts as well as in partially purified fractions. By using gel-filtration chromatography (Sephacryl S-200) we found that peak activity was present in fractions with an estimated M_r of 12 500, or slightly less, and with a pI of about 8, as revealed by preparative flat-bed isoelectric focusing in granular gel. Furthermore, when subjected to concanavalin A–Sepharose affinity chromatography, the extract could be fractionated into two components. The column fall-through (the non-binding fraction) had direct mitogenic activity for fibroblasts, whereas the bound fraction, when eluted from the column with α-methyl-D-mannoside lacked this activity. On the other hand, the bound fraction was able to induce sensitized spleen cells from *S. mansoni*-infected mice to release fibroblast-stimulating activity into their culture supernatants. Since resident peritoneal macrophages (from uninfected mice) that were co-cultured with the concanavalin A-binding fraction failed to secrete fibrogenic activity, the elaboration of such activity by mixed spleen-cell cultures was probably lymphocyte-dependent rather than being caused by direct stimulation of macrophages.

S. mansoni eggs thus appear to contain substances that can stimulate fibroblasts directly as well as ones that can do so indirectly, presumably through activating lymphocytes and perhaps by stimulating lymphokine release. The directly active material is distinct from that released into culture supernatants by intact granulomas in its estimated M_r, its pI and its lack of thymocyte-stimulating activity.

Fibroblast chemotactic activity from granulomas

In addition to containing biologically active molecules that can stimulate fibroblast proliferation and collagen synthesis, granuloma culture supernatants contain activity that promotes the directional (but not random) migration of fibroblasts in modified Boyden chambers (Wyler & Postlethwaite 1983). This chemoattractant was also present in culture supernatants of isolated granuloma macrophages, but not from those of resident peritoneal cells of uninfected or *S. mansoni*-infected mice. The chemoattractant had an estimated M_r of over 200 000 (on Sephadex G-200 gel filtration) and a pI of about 4.5 (by preparative flat-bed isoelectric focusing); it was trypsin-sensitive and heat-stable (at 56 °C for 45 min). Rabbit anti-human fibronectin antibody abolished the chemotactic activity in granuloma and macrophage supernatants, partially purified on Sephadex G-200, but did not do so when tested on a positive control chemoattractant, chick-skin collagen. These observations suggest that the granulomas, and specifically their constituent macrophages, produce fibronectin or a cleavage product thereof, which has chemotactic activity for fibroblasts.

Inhibition of contraction of fibroblast-populated collagen lattices in vitro *by soluble products of granulomas*

Gradual contraction of the fibrotic mass is a characteristic of normal wound healing and a feature of some types of pathological tissue fibrosis. The precise mechanisms involved are unknown, but a recently described assay (Bell et al 1979) may represent an *in vitro* correlate of this process and may permit detailed investigation of the cellular basis of contraction. Briefly, if fibroblasts are incorporated into collagen lattices prepared in Petri dishes and incubated in the presence of serum, the lattice undergoes progressive and uniform reduction in volume over a period of 3–4 days. The addition of microtubule inhibitors blocks this contraction, indicating the participation of cytoskeletal elements.

When crude or partially purified granuloma supernatants were added to the fibroblast-populated lattices, contraction was inhibited (D. J. Wyler & H. P. Ehrlich, unpublished observations). Only the (same) partially purified fractions that had induced fibroblast proliferation were able to inhibit contraction, but they did so without increasing fibroblast numbers in the lattices. The addition of indomethacin to granuloma supernatant-containing lattices prevented the inhibitory effect (i.e., contraction proceeded normally) but indomethacin alone had no effect. If prostaglandin E_1 was added alone, or in the presence of granuloma supernatants plus indomethacin, contraction was again inhibited. Since the granuloma supernatants were dialysed and contained undetectable amounts of prostaglandin E_2, this suggested that the granuloma-derived factor was stimulating the secretion of prostaglandins by fibroblasts (see Fig. 1) and that prostaglandins, in turn, acted back on the cell to inhibit contraction.

Discussion

The developing concept of how tissue fibrosis complicates chronic inflammation is that activated lymphocytes and macrophages produce biologically active soluble mediators that can recruit fibroblasts, stimulate their proliferation, and enhance their synthesis and secretion of collagen and other matrix substances (reviewed by Wahl & Wahl 1981). In addition, increased secretion of collagenase by fibroblast-like cells seems to be under the control of a macrophage product (monokine) similar to or identical with IL-1 (Krane et al 1982). Since collagenase from this source, as well as from macrophages (Wahl et al 1977), is likely to be produced during fibrosis at inflammatory sites, both the synthesis *and* the degradation of collagen are components of the process. In the specific case of the murine model of schistosomiasis mansoni, both the synthesis of collagen (Dunn et al 1977) and the secretion of collagenase (Takahashi et al 1980) by isolated granulomas have been documented. The egg granuloma is, thus, an ideal model for studying various aspects of the relationship between chronic inflammation and fibrosis. The fact that immunoregulation of granuloma formation and regression is so well defined makes this model particularly attractive.

From the findings reviewed here, the following hypothesis can be proposed about the pathogenesis of hepatic fibrosis in schistosomiasis mansoni (Fig. 2). Egg antigens sensitize T cells, which become activated to release a variety of lymphokines including macrophage-activating factor. This lymphokine, in turn, activates macrophages to secrete a variety of biologically active

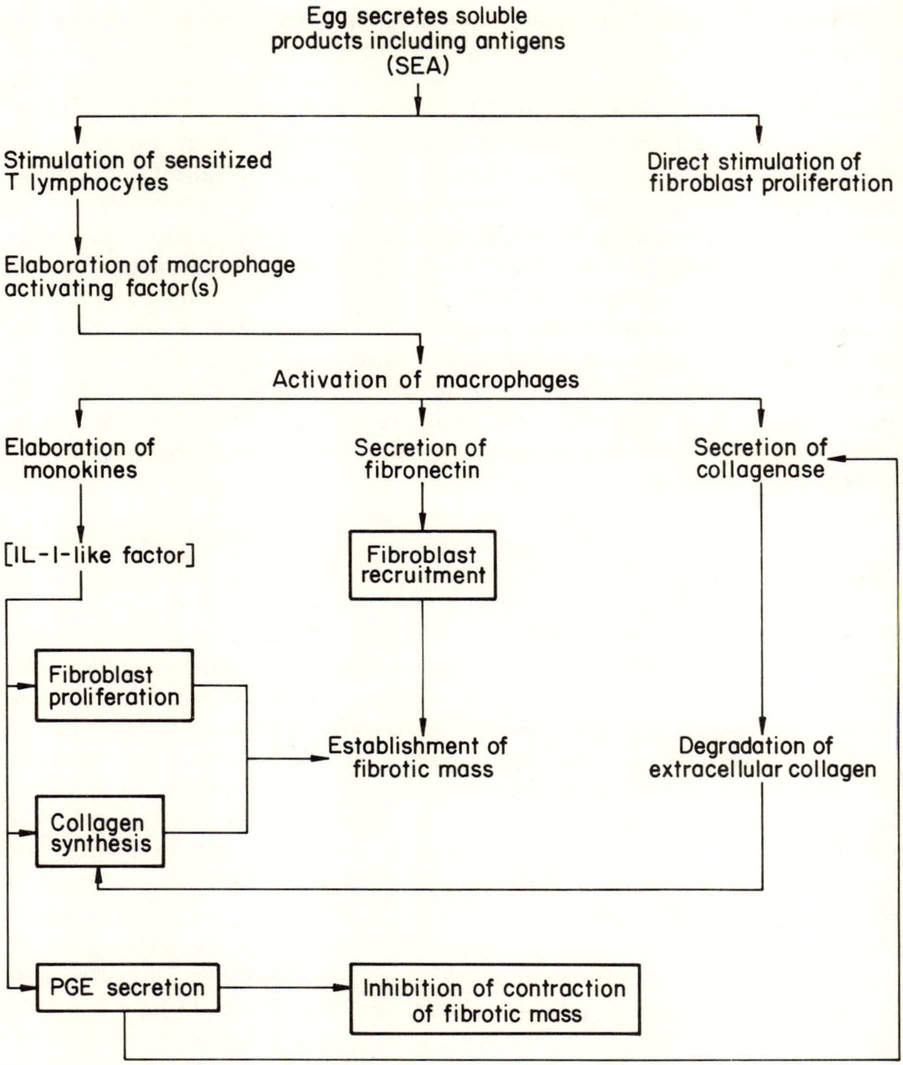

FIG. 2. Flow diagram of postulated mechanisms in pathogenesis of hepatic fibrosis in schistosomiasis mansoni.

substances, including fibronectin, IL-1 and growth factors that are mitogenic for fibroblasts (possibly similar to IL-1). Fibronectin participates in recruiting fibroblasts to the granuloma and may also serve as an adhesive molecule to hold the granuloma cells together. Other products promote the proliferation of fibroblasts and synthesis of collagen, and the secretion of prostaglandins and probably collagenase as well. Prostaglandins (of the E series) in turn may have a number of effects. They may promote collagenase secretion by the activated macrophages (Wahl et al 1977); they may serve as immunoregulatory molecules (Goodwin et al 1978); and they may feed back on the fibroblasts to inhibit contraction of the fibrotic mass. Since a characteristic feature of hepatic fibrosis in *S. mansoni* infection is preservation of the lobular architecture, it is reasonable to propose that contraction of the fibrotic mass does not occur. Possibly, products of the granuloma actively inhibit the contraction process.

The evidence presented suggests that molecular links exist between the egg granuloma inflammatory cells and fibroblasts. The properties of these activities are summarized in Table 2. However, it is difficult at present to test

TABLE 2. Properties of fibroblast-stimulating activities derived from *Schistosoma mansoni* egg granulomas

Fibroblast activity	*Source*	*M_r*[a]	*pI*[b]	*Heat-stability*[c]	*Trypsin-sensitivity*	*Other features*
Proliferation	Granuloma	≈30	6.0;4.5	+	+	IL-1 like[d]
	Macrophage	?	?	?	+	"
	Egg extract	≤12.5	8.0	+	+	no IL-1 activity
Collagen synthesis	Granuloma	?	?	?	?	
Chemotaxis	Granuloma	>200	4.5	+	+	Fibronectin-like[e]
	Macrophage	>200	4.5	+	+	"
Inhibition of contraction	Granuloma	≈30	6.0	+	+	PGE-mediated[f]
	Macrophage	?	?	?	?	
Prostaglandin secretion	Granuloma	?	?	?	?	

[a]Determined by gel filtration (Sephadex G-200 or Sephacryl S-200). [b]Determined by preparative flat-bed isoelectric focusing in granular gel. [c]Heated to 56 °C for 30–45 min. [d]Promotes thymocyte proliferation in IL-1 assay. [e]Activity lost by pretreatment with anti-fibronectin antibody. [f]Indomethacin interferes with effect; reproduced by addition of prostaglandin E_1 (PGE_1).

this hypothesis *in vivo*. Furthermore, the unique perivascular distribution of fibrosis in *S. mansoni* infection cannot be explained from these *in vitro* observations. One speculation which might unify the hypothesis with the characteristic anatomical distribution of fibrosis is that the biologically active molecules are transported from the granulomas to the perivascular tissue by lymphatics, and that they exert their effects there. Alternatively, the *in vitro* observations may prove to explain only the fibrosis of the granulomas; the perivascular fibrosis may result from entirely different mechanisms.

Many avenues remain to be explored before a cohesive and accurate concept of hepatic fibrosis in schistosomiasis can be developed. The role of granuloma cells other than macrophages in regulating fibroblast activities must be investigated. The potential participation of endothelial cells and vascular smooth-muscle cells in the fibrogenic process needs to be considered. Purification of the biologically active molecules has to be achieved to provide appropriate tools to probe the cellular biology and biochemistry of fibroblast activation. In addition, it may be fruitful to determine whether the immunoregulatory network, which apparently controls granuloma size during so-called 'modulation', also regulates elaboration of fibrogenic molecules. Finally, genetic determinants of the *degree* of hepatic fibrosis might be unravelled by use of the approaches described here with various inbred strains of mice.

Dissecting the molecular aspects of tissue fibrosis is more than an intellectual challenge. There is every reason to believe that such an approach could lead to the development of new chemotherapeutic agents or to the use of old ones for new purposes. While new antischistosomal agents such as praziquantel and water management undoubtedly improve prospects for the control of hepatosplenic schistosomiasis, there may be certain patients who could benefit from antifibrotic agents, if such were available.

Acknowledgement

This work was supported by U.S. Public Health Service grant AI 17615 from the National Institutes of Health.

REFERENCES

Bell E, Ivarsson B, Merrill C 1979 Production of a tissue-like structure by contraction of collagen lattices by human fibroblasts of different proliferative potential *in vitro*. Proc Natl Acad Sci USA 76:1273-1278

Bianco C, Griffin FM, Silverstein SC 1975 Studies of the macrophage complement receptor: alteration of receptor function upon macrophage activation. J Exp Med 141:1278-1290

Boros DL 1978 Granulomatous inflammations. Prog Allergy 24:183-267

Boros DL, Warren KS 1970 Delayed hypersensitivity-type granuloma formation and dermal reaction induced and elicited by a soluble factor isolated from *Schistosoma mansoni* eggs. J Exp Med 132:488-507

Boros DL, Warren KS, Pelley RP 1973 The secretion of migration inhibitory factor by intact schistosome egg granulomas maintained *in vitro*. Nature (Lond) 246:224-226

Dunn MA, Rojkind M, Warren KS, Hiatt PK, Rifas L, Seifter S 1977 Liver collagen synthesis in murine schistosomiasis. J Clin Invest 59:666-674

Goodwin JS, Messner RP, Peake GT 1978 Prostaglandin suppression of mitogen-stimulated lymphocytes *in vitro*: changes with mitogen dose and preincubation. J Clin Invest 62:753-760

James SL, Colley DG 1975 Eosinophils and immune mechanisms: production of the lymphokine eosinophil promotor (ESP) *in vitro* by isolated intact granulomas. J Reticuloendothel Soc 18:283-293

Karnovsky ML, Lazdins JK 1978 Biochemical criteria for activated macrophages. J Immunol 121:809-813

Krane SM, Goldring SR, Dayer JM 1982 Interactions among lymphocytes, monocytes, and other synovial cells in the rheumatoid synovium. Lymphokines 7:75-136

Lewis FA, Carter CE, Colley DG 1977 Eosinophils and immune mechanisms. V: Demonstration of mouse spleen cell-derived chemotactic activities for eosinophils and mononuclear cells and comparisons with eosinophil stimulation promoter. Cell Immunol 32:86-96

McCarthy JB, Wahl SM, Rees JC, Olsen CE, Sandberg AL, Wahl LM 1980 Mediation of macrophage collagenase production by 3′–5′ cyclic adenosine monophosphate. J Immunol 124:2405-2409

Mizel SB, Mizel D 1981 Purification to apparent homogeneity of murine interleukin 1. J Immunol 126:834-837

Oppenheim JJ, Shneyour A, Kook AI 1976 Enhancement of DNA synthesis and cAMP content of mouse thymocytes by mediator(s) derived from adherent cells. J Immunol 116:1466-1472

Pellegrino J, Brener L 1956 Method of isolating schistosome granulomas from mouse liver. J Parasitol 42:564

Pelley RP, Pelley RJ 1976 *S. mansoni* soluble egg antigens. IV: Biochemistry and immunochemistry of major serological antigens with particular emphasis on MSA_1. In: Van de Bosche H (ed) Biochemistry of parasites and host–parasite relationships. Elsevier/North-Holland Biomedical Press, Amsterdam, p 283-290

Peterkofsky B, Diegelmann 1977 Use of a mixture of proteinase-free collagenases for the specific assay of radioactive collagen in the presence of other proteins. Biochemistry 10:988-994

Postlethwaite AE, Synderman R, Kang AH 1976 The chemotactic attraction of human fibroblasts to a lymphocyte-derived factor. J Exp Med 144:1188-1203

Rodriguez HF, Garcia-Palmieri MR, Rivera JV, Rodriguez-Molina RA 1955 A comparative study of portal and bilharzial cirrhosis. Gastroenterology 29:235-246

Takahashi S, Dunn MA, Seifter S 1980 Liver collagenase in murine schistosomiasis. Gastroenterology 78:1425-1431

Wahl SM, Wahl LM 1981 Modulation of fibroblast growth and function by monokines and lymphokines. Lymphokines 2:179-201

Wahl LM, Olsen CE, Sandberg AL, Mergenhagen SE 1977 Prostaglandin regulation of macrophage collagenase production. Proc Natl Acad Sci USA 74:4955-4958

Warren KS 1982 The secret of the immunopathogenesis of schistosomiasis: *in vivo* models. Immunol Rev 61:189-213

Warren KS, DeWitt WB 1958 Production of portal hypertension and esophageal varices in the mouse. Proc Soc Exp Biol Med 98:99-101

Warren KS, Domingo EO, Cowan RBT 1967 Granuloma formation around schistosome eggs as a manifestation of delayed hypersensitivity. Am J Pathol 51:735-756

Wyler DJ, Rosenwasser LJ 1982 Fibroblast stimulation in schistosomiasis. II: Functional and biochemical characteristics of egg granuloma-derived fibroblast-stimulating factor. J Immunol 129:1706-1710

Wyler DJ, Tracy JW 1982 Direct and indirect effects of soluble extracts of *Schistosoma mansoni* eggs on fibroblast proliferation *in vitro*. Infect Immun 38:103-108

Wyler DJ, Postlethwaite AE 1983 Fibroblast stimulation in schistosomiasis. IV: Isolated egg granulomas elaborate a fibroblast chemoattractant *in vitro*. J Immunol 130:1371-1375

Wyler DJ, Wahl SM, Wahl LM 1978 Hepatic fibrosis in schistosomiasis: egg granulomas secrete fibroblast-stimulating factor *in vitro*. Science (Wash DC) 202:438-440

Wyler DJ, Wahl SM, Cheever AW, Wahl LM 1981 Fibroblast stimulation in schistosomiasis. I: Stimulation *in vitro* of fibroblasts by soluble products of egg granulomas. J Infect Dis 144:254-262

DISCUSSION

Nogueira: You saw the sensitization in mice infected with *Schistosoma mansoni* after eight weeks. Presumably you saw a relationship between the appearance of the sensitivity and the development of granulomas. Is your hypothesis that collagen degradation would sensitize them?

Wyler: We studied the mice at eight weeks of infection since this is when the granuloma size is at its peak. Whether there is any relationship between collagen hypersensitivity and granulomatous inflammation is uncertain. We are more interested in its relationship to amplification of the fibrotic response.

Andrade: The development of the periovular granuloma is essentially a fibrosing reaction. Sometimes one sees more fibroblasts than macrophages in the granuloma. Under electron microscopy one sees that the fibroblasts have secretory vesicles and abundant collagen fibres deposited, forming a loose framework which eventually becomes quite dense. Your work provides a major step in the understanding of the schistosomal periovular granuloma. However, when you imply that the diffuse portal fibrosis results from the same mechanism, I have some doubts. When we see a fibrosis, it is the end stage of something that began much earlier. When many eggs are present, one sees portal inflammation, proliferation of endothelial cells, destruction of blood vessels, as well as proliferation of bile ducts, perineural fibrosis, and fibrosis of the intima of the arteries (as also seen in cases of peptic ulcer or tuberculosis). These changes result from several stimuli: chemical mediators of inflammation, immunological factors, and so on. All of these stimulate fibroblasts, and most of the changes will eventually disappear, but the fibrosis will remain. Because collagen is an insoluble protein it will stay there longer. So it is difficult to correlate diffuse portal fibrosis with schistosomiasis in the way you have done.

Wyler: You are absolutely right in drawing attention to the fact that perivascular fibrosis is a complex process which may not arise simply as a consequence of elaboration of growth and other stimulating factors from granuloma cells. The proliferation of the intima and the vascular smooth muscle may however also depend on granuloma-derived factors. We have found that granulomas elaborate factors that stimulate proliferation of endothelial and vascular smooth muscle cells as well as fibroblasts (D.J. Wyler, unpublished observations). Yet I do not know how to account for differences in patterns of hepatic fibrosis in different animals infected with *S. mansoni*. Perhaps our new approach will stimulate others to search for these answers.

Butterworth: Looking at the very marked species differences in susceptibility to developing periportal fibrosis, particularly in primates, may indeed be a valuable approach. For example, the baboon develops no periportal fibrosis whereas the chimpanzee does (von Lichtenberg & Sadun 1968, Erickson et al 1971). The effects on autologous fibroblasts of granuloma products in these two species should, perhaps, be compared.

Warren: At the recent meeting of the American Association for the Study of Liver Diseases (1982, Chicago), schistosomiasis appeared to have become the most important model for studying liver fibrosis. (The only previously available model involved chronic carbon tetrachloride intoxication.) Dunn et al (1979) are doing this work in humans with schistosomiasis in Egypt, and Muñoz et al (1982) are studying amoebiasis in Mexico. As well as the differences in fibrogenesis among different experimental animals, there are differences in fibrogenesis in different organs of the body. Michael Dunn's group have shown that granulomas in the liver and in certain parts of the gut will develop fibrosis while other parts of the gut will not. Takahashi et al (1980) have also studied the balance between the *formation* of collagen and its *destruction* by collagenases. It seems that at any given time collagen production and its breakdown by collagenase are occurring simultaneously. If one sees a net production of collagen it is due to a greater rate of production than breakdown.

Butterworth: Can I further question your interpretation of the granuloma activity as being stimulated by interleukin-1 (IL-1)? Although the granuloma products appear to have IL-1-like activity in the thymocyte assay, an entirely separate molecule may be responsible for this effect, or may be inducing IL-1 production within the thymocyte assay itself. The fibroblast-stimulating activity differs markedly from IL-1 in relative molecular mass. Do you know anything about the heat stability and pH stability of the molecule?

Wyler: The activity is stable at 56 °C but destroyed at 100 °C. I believe that the fibroblast-stimulating molecules are not *bona fide* IL-1, although they act in a biologically similar manner *in vitro*. The thymocyte assay lacks macrophages, so it is doubtful that Il-1 is being generated during culture of these cells.

Butterworth: Monica Veith has recently been studying mononuclear cells recovered from patients with eosinophilia and high eosinophil killing activity (Veith et al 1983, M.C. Veith & A.E. Butterworth, unpublished observations). Such mononuclear cells, in the absence of stimulation with antigen or mitogen, produce an activity that markedly enhances the capacity of normal eosinophils to kill schistosomula. The activity, which is produced by an adherent, esterase-positive cell that is resistant to killing by a lytic antilymphocyte monoclonal antibody and complement, has a similar apparent molecular mass (35–45 K) to the one that you have described, and is heat-stable and trypsin-resistant.

Sharma: IL-1 tends to aggregate in serum-containing medium and often one does find this high-M_r IL-1. Do you work in serum-free conditions?

Wyler: Yes; all our work is with serum-free material. Nonetheless, it is certainly possible that our material contains aggregates.

Martinez-Palomo: In general, the use of modern techniques to understand host–parasite interactions has been applied mainly at the cellular and molecular level. But, as we have heard, the tissue level is also very important. Except for malaria and schistosomiasis, we know little about the pathology in both human diseases and animal models. There has been a recent revolution in the techniques available for studying pathology because the preservation of tissues and the sectioning and embedding methods available have greatly improved. In my experience, for amoebiasis, Chagas' disease, and onchocerciasis, the whole field of disease pathogenesis in humans remains to be re-described with these new tools. Many other parasitic diseases can also now be approached with these modern techniques for studying both classical pathology and experimental pathology, as we have just heard from Dr Wyler.

Warren: The granuloma is a combination of different cells, and we should certainly be careful not to overlook what is going on in the whole organism just because we are concerned sometimes only with individual cells.

REFERENCES

Dunn MA, Kamel R, Kamel IA et al 1979 Liver collagen synthesis in schistosomiasis mansoni. Gastroenterology 76:978-982

Erickson DG, Sadun EH, Lucia HL, von Lichtenberg F, Cheever AW 1971 *Schistosoma haematobium*: infections in five species of primates. Exp Parasitol 29:126-140

Muñoz ML, Calderón J, Rojkind M 1982 The collagenase of *Entamoeba histolytica*. J Exp Med 155:42-51

Takahashi S, Dunn MA, Seifter S 1980 Liver collagenase in murine schistosomiasis. Gastroenterology 78:1425-1431

Veith MC, Butterworth AE, Boylston AW 1983 The enhancement of eosinophil-mediated killing of schistosomula of *Schistosoma mansoni* by mononuclear cell products. In: Yoshida TY, Torisu M (eds) Immunobiology of the eosinophil. Elsevier/North-Holland, Amsterdam, in press

von Lichtenberg F, Sadun EH 1968 Experimental production of bilharzial pipe-stem fibrosis in the chimpanzee. Exp Parasitol 22:264-278

General discussion

Entry of sporozoites of *Theileria* into bovine lymphocytes (D. W. Fawcett)

Fawcett: One of the missions of the International Laboratory for Research on Animal Diseases (ILRAD) is to develop preventive measures against East Coast fever (theileriasis), a parasitic disease of great economic importance in the developing countries of East and Central Africa where it kills half a million cattle a year.

The arthropod vector of the disease is the brown ear-tick—*Rhipicephalus appendiculatus*. The infectious stage of the *Theileria parva* parasite, the sporozoite, develops in the tick salivary gland. This complex gland contains nine or more secretory cell types and secretes a cement-like substance involved in attachment to the host; a tanning agent, to harden the cement; one or more anticoagulants, to keep the blood meal flowing; and various enzymes and other biologically active substances yet to be characterized. A 10 mg tick may take in 3 ml blood during nine days of feeding. To solve the problem created by ingestion of this large volume of fluid, the tick has evolved the ingenious stratagem of transforming certain salivary glandular cells, which secrete only in the initial stages of feeding, into cells specialized for fluid transport (Fawcett et al 1981). This enables the tick to secrete a copious saliva which is pumped back into the host in the course of the blood meal. In this way, the burden of disposal of the excess water is passed on to the cow. It is in this transfer of saliva that the sporozoites of *Theileria parva* are introduced to the subcutaneous tissue of the mammalian host, where they enter lymphocytes mobilized at the site of tick attachment. Since lymphocytes are not phagocytic we have been interested in the mechanism of their invasion by the sporozoites of *Theileria parva*.

Sporozoites recovered from homogenates of infected ticks are exposed *in vitro* to a fraction of bovine peripheral blood leucocytes enriched in mononuclear cells (Stagg et al 1981). Sporozoites first adhere loosely to the surface of lymphocytes, with the sparse surface coat on the parasite apparently involved in the recognition phase. A very close contact is then established between the membranes of the sporozoite and the lymphocyte at the site of adherence, with no resolvable interspace between the two. As this close membrane apposition spreads laterally the sporozoite occupies a progressively deepening recess in

1983 Cytopathology of parasitic disease. Pitman Books, London (Ciba Foundation symposium 99) p 207-213

the lymphocyte surface (Fig. 1). When this 'zipping up' of the membranes has progressed around the entire circumference of the sporozoite, the rim of the invaginated lymphocyte membrane fuses over the parasite, which is then intracellular but enclosed in a tightly-applied, enveloping host-cell membrane acquired during its interiorization. Endocytosis is rapid, some sporozoites being found within lymphocytes as early as 10 min after being introduced. Entry may actually take less time but it took us about 10 min to spin and fix a coherent centrifugal pellet for electron microscopic examination.

The lymphocyte appears to be passive in the process. No mobilization of actin filaments was detected in the cytoplasm beneath the entering sporoblast and no encircling pseudopodia were formed. This suggests that, given a small (1 μm) spherical parasite and a malleable host-cell surface, 'zipping up' the membranes by ligand–receptor binding may cause the sporozoite to sink into the cell without significant expenditure of energy by the lymphocyte. To explore this possibility further we repeated the experiment at 2 °C and found that a significant number of sporozoites entered at this temperature and apparently about as rapidly as at 37 °C (Fawcett et al 1982). No data were gathered on the relative numbers entering per unit time at the two temperatures. The sporozoites are believed to enter only a subpopulation of lymphocytes. Even if all cells in the pellet were entered, the 1 μm parasite would be included in the plane of section, by chance, in only about one cell in ten. Therefore electron microscopy does not lend itself to quantitation in these experiments.

If endocytosis depends on binding of complementary molecules on the two cells, one would expect some slowing of the process at 2 °C due to lowered lateral mobility of ligands and receptors within the membranes (Lewis et al 1980). The finding of intracellular sporozoites, in any number, from 10 min onward even at this temperature seems to justify the conclusion that the entry of sporozoites of *Theileria parva* into bovine lymphocytes requires little or no energy. This contrasts with ingestion by 'professional' phagocytes, for which the attachment phase is independent of temperature but the interiorization does not occur below 18 °C (Griffin et al 1975).

In this *in vitro* system, when using a high ratio of sporozoites to cells, one observes that multiple entry is common, but it is probably rare *in vivo*. Sporozoites occasionally invade eosinophils. It is not clear whether they do so by passive endocytosis or by phagocytosis. Since the eosinophils are end stages, incapable of proliferation, their uptake of sporozoites is probably of little significance in the systemic dissemination of the parasites.

Members of the subphylum Apicomplexa typically possess a well defined apical end containing a conoid and two kinds of electron-dense organelles, the rhoptries and the micronemes. Entry of the sporozoites of this protozoan

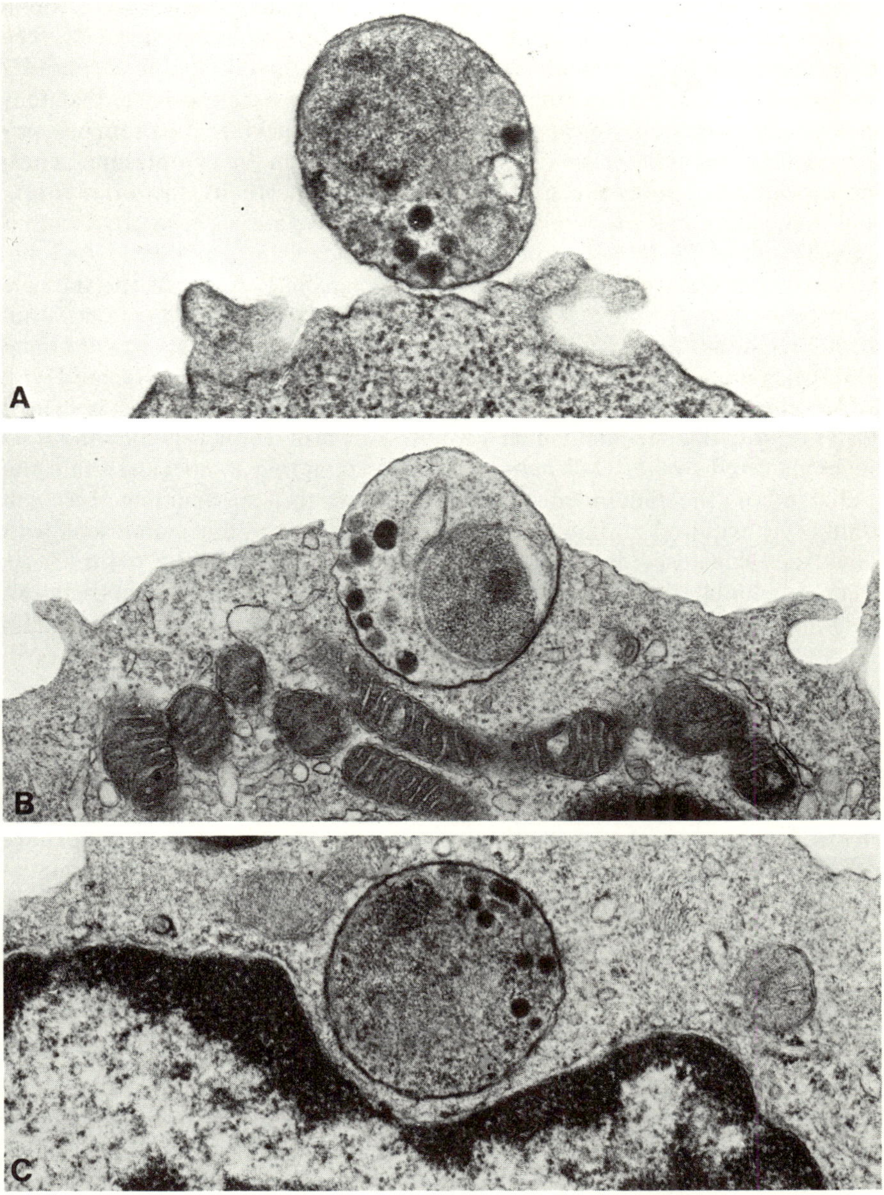

FIG. 1. (*Fawcett*) Successive stages in the entry of sporozoites of *Theileria parva* into bovine lymphocytes. Noteworthy is the absence of pseudopod formation by the lymphocyte and the very close apposition of its membrane to that of the parasite.

taxa into their host cells is generally believed to occur only when the membrane overlying the apical complex makes contact with the host cell. The rhoptries and micronemes are thought to play an essential role in parasite invasion. The spherical sporozoites of *Theileria* are exceptional in that they do not have an obvious apical complex. A conoid is lacking; the rhoptries may be associated with the plasma membrane anywhere in the cytoplasmic hemisphere; and the sporozoite can enter the lymphocyte in any orientation. Micronemes are still present in interiorized sporozoites. These observations suggest that, in *Theileria*, rhoptries and micronemes may not be involved in the entry process. Instead, they may participate in defence of the parasite against the phagolysosomal system of the host cell. The lymphocyte does not normally contain lysosomes but, when examined 24 h after sporozoite invasion, it has numerous small, membrane-limited dense bodies associated with the Golgi complex which are interpreted as newly formed lysosomes. These cluster around the parasite, which now does not contain micronemes and is no longer invested by host-cell membrane. It is tempting to speculate that the discharge of the micronemes may disperse the surrounding host-cell membrane acquired during entry. In the absence of the membrane with which they can fuse, the lysosomes are unable to destroy the parasite. As infected tick material becomes available we intend to study the gap between entry and 24 h in an effort to establish a temporal correlation between exocytosis of micronemes and dissolution of the surrounding host-cell membrane.

Chang: You mentioned that the *Theileria parva* parasites can enter the eosinophil. How well do they survive? Have you looked at whether they survive in the neutrophil?

Fawcett: Our preparations of peripheral blood leucocytes are intentionally enriched in mononuclear cells. There are very few granulocytes. We have seen no invaded neutrophils, but I cannot exclude the possibility that these cells would phagocytize sporozoites. Those seen within eosinophils had a tight-fitting investment of host-cell membrane, suggesting that they entered by passive endocytosis as in lymphocytes.

Nogueira: You mentioned ligand–receptor interaction. Did you pursue that more closely? Is the uptake mediated by Fc receptors, and can you modify the uptake by trypsinizing the parasite or the cell?

Fawcett: Such experiments are planned when adequate numbers of highly infected ticks become available. We have no observations yet as to whether Fc receptors are involved. In our efforts to modify the lymphocyte surface, the preliminary observations on cells pretreated with neuraminidase indicate that removal of sialic acid residues has no effect on sporozoite entry. We have started experiments with proteases in collaboration with Dr Ole MoiYoi but we do not yet have any results.

Nogueira: Can you recover and grow parasites from the infected lymphocytes after they are transformed, so as to use them as a source of re-infection?

Fawcett: In vivo the sporozoites that have entered lymphocytes go on to form multinucleate macroschizonts, which are partitioned to the daughter cells as the transformed lymphocytes proliferate and are then disseminated throughout the host. The macroschizonts ultimately undergo schizogony to produce many merozoites which then enter erythrocytes. *In vitro* the sporozoites develop into macroschizonts and the transformed cell lines can be carried indefinitely with all cells parasitized but, unfortunately, the macroschizonts rarely, if ever, go on to form merozoites in culture. Several groups at ILRAD are studying such cell lines.

Warren: One of the fascinating things about this organism is that it expresses parasite antigens on the surface of the lymphocyte but the response of the host is histocompatibility restricted. This means that if you want to immunize a cow by using its own lymphocytes you need only a small number of cells. If you immunize another cow, on the other hand, you need millions of lymphocytes.

Martinez-Palomo: This very interesting entry process resembles part of the interaction between liposomes and mammalian cells in the sense that there is apparently a non-active merging of lipid layers with the lipid bilayer of the plasma membrane. This process can be followed by freeze-fracture; have you tried this yourselves?

Fawcett: We do not have the equipment for freeze-fracturing. The entry does not involve actual fusion of membranes, but extremely close apposition of the two membranes back-to-back, as in a gap-junction. Nevertheless, it would be of interest to see the entry in freeze-fracture and to compare it to the so-called 'moving junction' described by Aikawa et al (1978) in the entry of merozoites of *Plasmodium* into erythrocytes.

Nogueira: It looks very much like *Trypanosoma cruzi* entry.

Martinez-Palomo: You describe the parasite membrane as surrounded by an array of dense spots that could, perhaps, be either actin or microtubules.

Fawcett: The dense, membrane-bounded bodies we see around the parasite 24 h after entry are small lysosomes formed in response to parasitism. They are not cytoskeletal elements. Indeed, the absence of actin filaments and microtubules in the host-cell cytoplasm adjacent to the parasite is one basis for our argument that the entry process is passive.

Hudson: In the lymphoid cell lines that you obtain by transformation through the macroschizonts, can you cure the lines of the infection, and do they still retain the transformed phenotype?

Fawcett: This is an interesting question. Two of my colleagues at ILRAD have treated cell lines with appropriate drugs and observed that the macroschizonts are destroyed. The host cells survive for four or five days and then die. This suggests that the transformed state is not a once-only differentiation that endures indefinitely, but one that must be maintained by the continuing presence of the intracellular parasite.

Hudson: Are transformed cells specific for parasite antigens? Alternatively, can the parasite enter a lymphocyte of any antigenic specificity?

Fawcett: It has been thought that the sporozoites are probably selective for a subpopulation of lymphocytes. Drs P. Lalor and S. Black in our immunology laboratory have recently separated several subpopulations of bovine lymphocytes and find that the sporozoites are less selctive than is commonly supposed.

Nussenzweig: The difficulty in analysing the sporozoite–host cell interaction is that until recently there was no good *in vitro* system available to examine it. You mentioned the polarity of malarial parasites in relation to host–cell interaction. While it is certainly true that *merozoites* have this polarity, this has not been shown for *sporozoites,* and I doubt that this will turn out to be the case. Another point is that interaction of sporozoites with macrophages involves not only phagocytosis but also active penetration of the parasites into these host cells (Danforth et al 1980). Thus, one can totally inhibit phagocytosis of other particles and still observe penetration of sporozoites into the macrophages. There is now a human hepatoma cell line available which has many of the biochemical characteristics of normal liver cells and many of the known hepatocyte receptors (Knowles et al 1980). Sporozoites of various malarial species do interact with this cloned hepatoma cell line; they enter and develop in these cells. Since we have characterized a parasite antigen that is distributed evenly over the surface (Aikawa et al 1980) we now intend to verify whether this antigen binds and interacts with a defined component of the hepatoma cell membrane, and to isolate the putative receptor.

Fawcett: Would you then expect sporozoites to enter in any orientation, as they do in *Theileria*, or would they still have to attach by the apex?

Nussenzweig: This question cannot yet be precisely answered since sporozoite–hepatoma cell interaction has not been examined at the ultrastructural level. When one treats sporozoites with a monoclonal antibody, which specifically reacts with a circumsporozoite protein that is present on the entire surface, one inhibits the attachment and penetration of the parasites (Hollingdale et al 1982). This effect is mediated not only by intact IgG but also by monovalent Fab fragments. Therefore, it is unlikely that inhibition of sporozoite infectivity is a secondary effect mediated by complement or by phagocytosis; it appears to be, rather, a direct effect of sporozoite–antibody interaction (Potocnjak et al 1980).

REFERENCES

Aikawa M, Miller LH, Johnson JG, Rabbege J 1978 Erythrocyte entry by malarial parasites: a moving junction between erythrocyte and parasite. J Cell Biol 77:72-82

Aikawa M, Yoshida N, Nussenzweig RS, Nussenzweig V 1980 The protective antigen of rodent malaria sporozoites (*Plasmodium berghei*) is a differentiation antigen. J Immunol 126:2494-2495

Danforth HD, Aikawa M, Cochrane AH, Nussenzweig RS 1980 Sporozoites of mammalian malaria: attachment to, interiorization and fate within macrophages. J Protozool 27:193-202

Fawcett DW, Doxsey S, Büscher G 1981 Salivary gland of the tick vector (*R. appendiculatus*) of East Coast fever. II: Cellular basis for fluid secretion in the type III acinus. Tissue Cell 13:231-253

Fawcett DW, Stagg DA, Doxsey S, Young A 1982 The entry of sporozoites of *Theileria parva* into bovine lymphocytes *in vitro*. Eur J Cell Biol 27:10-21

Griffin FM Jr, Griffin JA, Leider JE, Silverstein SC 1975 Studies on the mechanism of phagocytosis. I: Requirements for circumferential attachment of particle-bound ligands to specific receptors on the macrophage plasma membrane. J Exp Med 142:1263-1282

Hollingdale MR, Zavala F, Nussenzweig RS, Nussenzweig V 1982 Antibodies to the protective antigen of *Plasmodium berghei* sporozoites prevent entry into cultured cells. J Immunol 128:1929-1930

Knowles BB, Howe CC, Aden DP 1980 Human hepatocellular carcinoma cell lines secrete the major plasma proteins and Hepatitis B surface antigen. Science (Wash DC) 209:497

Lewis VT, Hafeman DG, McConnell HM 1980 Kinetics of antibody dependent binding of haptenated phospholipid vesicles to a macrophage related cell-line. Biochemistry 9:5376-5386

Potocnjak P, Yoshida N, Nussenzweig RS, Nussenzweig V 1980 Monovalent fragments (Fab) of monoclonal antibodies to a sporozoite surface antigen (Pb44) protect mice against malarial infection. J Exp Med 157:1504-1513

Stagg DA, Dolan TT, Leitch BL, Young AS 1981 The initial stages of infection of cattle cells with *Theileria parva* sporozoites in vitro. Parasitology 83:191-197

Mechanisms of myocardial damage in *Trypanosoma cruzi* infection

ZILTON A. ANDRADE

Gonçalo Moniz Research Center, Fundação Oswaldo Cruz, Federal University of Bahia Faculty of Medicine, Rua Valdemar Falcão, 121-Brotas, Salvador, BA 40.000, Bahia, Brazil

Abstract A study of pathological lesions caused by *Trypanosoma cruzi* in human and experimental hosts indicated that the main mechanisms of myocardial damage in Chagas' disease are the following. (1) During acute infection inflammatory lesions are related to parasite-induced destruction of myocardial cells, with probable participation of immune-complex reactions. When parasitism decreases, inflammation subsides and may disappear completely. (2) After recovery from acute infection the hosts remain infected but asymptomatic for a prolonged period of time. Focal fibrotic areas may be present in the myocardium, conducting tissue and autonomic nervous system, representing sequelae from the acute phase. Such sequelae may have or may acquire functional significance in some special circumstances. (3) Some patients with latent *T. cruzi* infection may progress to show a diffuse, active and fibrosing myocarditis without an apparent change in parasitological and immunological status from the asymptomatic phase. The microscopic changes in the heart are compatible with the presence of a delayed-type hypersensitivity process. An abolition of the suppressive factors of delayed hypersensitivity which are present during latent infection may be involved.

1983 Cytopathology of parasitic disease. Pitman Books, London (Ciba Foundation symposium 99), p 214-233

The mechanisms responsible for myocardial damage during the course of *Trypanosoma cruzi* infection are not completely understood. During acute infection when the parasites rapidly multiply within myocardial fibres, causing cellular destruction and inflammation, the mechanisms of myocardial damage are more evident. However, the chronic, diffuse and active myocarditis appearing in late infection is more complex, is not directly parasite-related, and its pathogenesis is still something of an enigma. Moreover, during the long interval between acute infection and late chronic manifestations, it is not yet established whether a latent, inactive infection or a slowly progressive pathological process is present.

This paper will attempt to interpret the pathogenesis of myocardial lesions in Chagas' disease from observations of autopsy materials both in humans and in experimental animals. I am well aware of the limitations of our methodology but on the other hand believe that its potentials have not yet been fully explored.

Since the mechanisms of myocardial damage seem to vary with the duration of infection, the three classical forms of clinical presentation of Chagas' disease—acute, indeterminate and chronic—will be considered separately.

Acute form of Chagas' disease

Vianna (1911), the first pathologist ever to observe a microscopic section of the heart infected with *T. cruzi*, noticed that this parasite multiplied within the cardiac fibres and that focal inflammation ensued only when the parasitized fibre ruptured. Indeed, *T. cruzi* amastigotes divide repeatedly by binary fission, pushing apart myofibrils, mitochondria and other organelles in the fibres without causing evident degenerative changes. A clear vacuole that was seen around the multiplying parasites by light microscopy seems to be an artifact, since it does not appear in well-fixed electron microscopic preparations. But when the parasites differentiate toward flagellate forms and pierce through and rupture the cell membrane, a focal leucocytic infiltration appears (Fig. 1). The earliest inflammatory responses observed in experimental animals consist of mononuclear cells, especially macrophages and lymphocytes. Coincident with the appearance of anti-*T. cruzi* antibodies in the serum, polymorphonuclear neutrophils begin to appear in increasing numbers around disintegrating parasitized fibres. At this time immunoglobulin, *T. cruzi* antigen(s) and complement can be demonstrated *in situ* by immunocytochemical methods.

Thus, the early myocardial damage caused by *T. cruzi* results in focal inflammation, and is directly related to parasite-induced cell destruction, which may release chemical mediators and perhaps induce *in situ* immune-complex reactions. A few days later in the infection, focal myocarditis tends to become diffuse. A predominantly lymphocytic infiltration, with many macrophages and a few plasma cells as well, cause dissociation of the muscle fibres. A moderate degree of interstitial oedema is also present. Some muscle fibres may exhibit isolated hyaline necrosis, and may soon undergo cellular and probably enzymic digestion.

What causes death of non-parasitized fibres is not clear, but anoxic damage resulting from interstitial myocarditis is one possible cause. Another is cell-membrane sensitization by parasitic antigens, followed by damage mediated by cellular and/or humoral immunological factors (Ribeiro dos Santos & Hudson 1980). With increasing parasitism and inflammation, the necrosis of

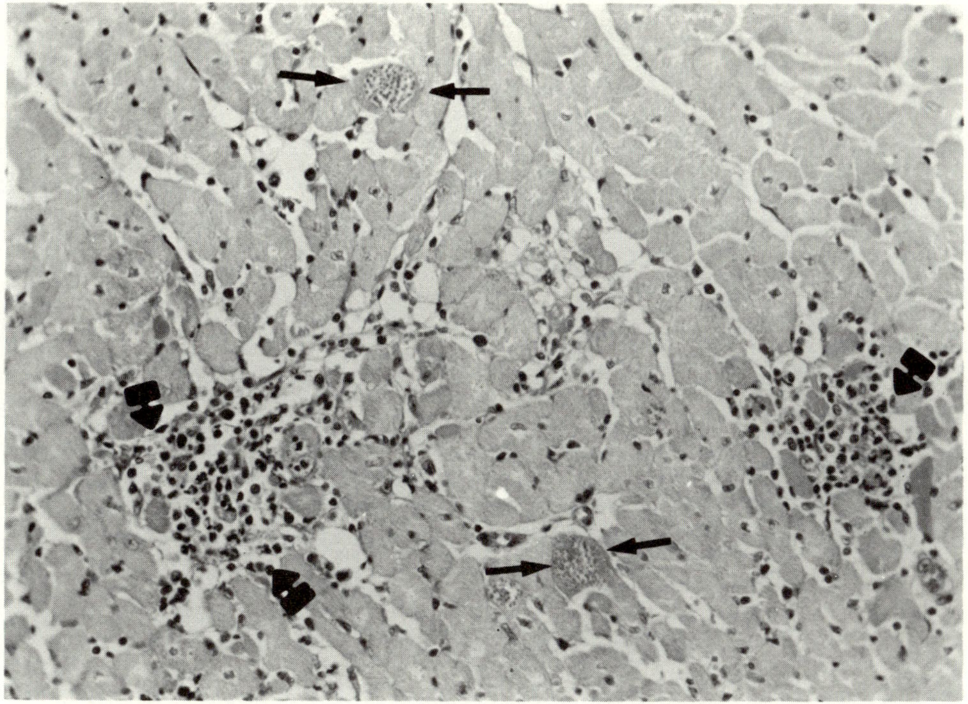

FIG. 1. Early changes in the myocardium of a young dog inoculated with *T. cruzi* 15 days previously. Long arrows point to intact parasitized fibres with no surrounding reaction. Shorter arrows point to focal inflammation after parasite-induced cell destruction. Haematoxylin and eosin staining; magnification × 150.

isolated fibres and of even larger focal areas in the myocardium become prominent features. This necrosis may lead to cardiac failure during acute Chagas' disease, and shows a good correlation with electrocardiographic (ECG) changes. Sometimes ECG tracings that suggest acute myocardial infarction and several types of cardiac block can be observed in the most severe cases (Andrade & Andrade 1980). It is important to emphasize that extensive cell destruction during acute *T. cruzi* infection occurs not only in the ordinary contractile myocardium but also in the conducting tissue. Damage may be seen in ganglionic neurons in the heart and elsewhere, especially in Auerbach's plexus of the digestive tract. All these reactions are related to the presence of intracellular parasites and local inflammation. During acute infection, although lesions usually predominate in the myocardium, parasites can disseminate and infect several cell types, such as skeletal and smooth muscles, macrophages, neural cells (glial, satellite, Schwann cells and even neurons), fibroblasts and, rarely, some epithelial cells. Wherever parasites induce cell destruction focal inflammation appears, which can be confluent and diffuse if the parasitism becomes more intense. All these inflammatory and degenerative changes subside when parasitism decreases either as a result of mounting host immunity or from the effects of chemotherapy. A direct relationship between parasites and tissue damage is thus clear for lesions found during the acute phase of Chagas' disease.

The introduction of *T. cruzi* into a previously uninfected human host is usually followed by acute infection, defined as the detection of trypomastigotes in peripheral blood by direct parasitological methods. However, this event may be accompanied by signs of acute disease (chagoma, Romaña's sign, fever or mild hepatosplenomegaly) or it may be asymptomatic. In both cases, evidence of immunodepression to *T. cruzi* antigens can be demonstrated.

The mortality rate in acute Chagas' disease is low in humans. Probably less than 10% of the patients will die, and those are usually children, who develop meningo-encephalitis, cardiac failure or non-specific bronchopneumonia. The majority survive although they continue to be infected. No spontaneous parasitological cure has been demonstrated in *T. cruzi* infection. However, the lesions disappear or become quiescent, and may reappear with a different morphological and pathogenic character in some patients after an interval of 5–10 years or more.

Chronic indeterminate form of Chagas' disease

Clinicians and investigators in Brazil are now realizing that this neglected stage of Chagas' disease seems to be the most important one. Conceptually, it was defined as asymptomatic chronic infection by *T. cruzi*. Evidence of infection can be obtained by xenodiagnosis (identification of the infected host) and/or immunological tests. Absence of manifestations should include a normal ECG and no changes in the digestive tract after radiological investigation. About three million people would fit these criteria in Brazil. They are usually young and are very often refused employment on the grounds that they are afflicted with Chagas' disease. Thus, legal and labour problems are connected with our poor understanding of what the indeterminate phase of Chagas' disease really means. Matters are aggravated because several individuals with chronic asymptomatic *T. cruzi* infection and a normal ECG may show abnormalities when examined with more refined and precise techniques. Pharmacological tests, mono- and bi-dimensional echocardiograms, electrograms of the bundle of His with or without artificial accelerations of cardiac rate, ventriculography, cine-angiocoronariography, and so on, may present abnormal results in such subjects (Amorim et al 1979, Acquatella et al 1980, Chiale et al 1982). This has usually been interpreted as the beginning of chronic symptomatic Chagas' myocarditis, which brings with it an ominous prognosis. However, insufficient pathological data exist to support the assumption that during the indeterminate phase of *T. cruzi* infection slowly progressing and relentless mechanisms of myocardial damage take place. During autopsies, in people without clinical cardiac disease but with positive serology and/or positive xenodiagnosis, the hearts are grossly normal, although some of them may show areas of myocardial thinning (atrophy) or even an apical aneurysm. Histologically, there may be focal fibrosis in the myocardium, a reduced number of neurons in atrial parasympathetic ganglia, and a few patchy areas of focal mononuclear infiltration. Signs of active inflammatory lesions are not regularly observed. During acute infection several structures that do not regenerate, such as muscle fibres in the myocardium and in the conducting tissues, as well as neurons, may be destroyed. Such lesions may give rise to minute foci of fibrous replacement that can be detected during later microscopic examination when all the changes of the acute phase have already disappeared (Fig. 2). Depending on the site or extent of such sequelae their functional significance may vary. The changes of the intermediate phase can be experimentally analysed with the canine model of Chagas' disease. *T. cruzi* infections in dogs can produce all three classical forms of the disease—acute, indeterminate and chronic. Recently (Andrade et al 1981) we studied the cardiac changes in nine dogs that survived acute infection. These animals presented ECG alterations compatible with acute myocarditis 20 to 30 days after inoculation. Three were treated with nifurtimox (Lampit) and the others recovered spontaneously. They were sacrificed 8 months to 3 years after infection. They presented positive serology (complement fixation test with titres ranging from 1 : 23 to

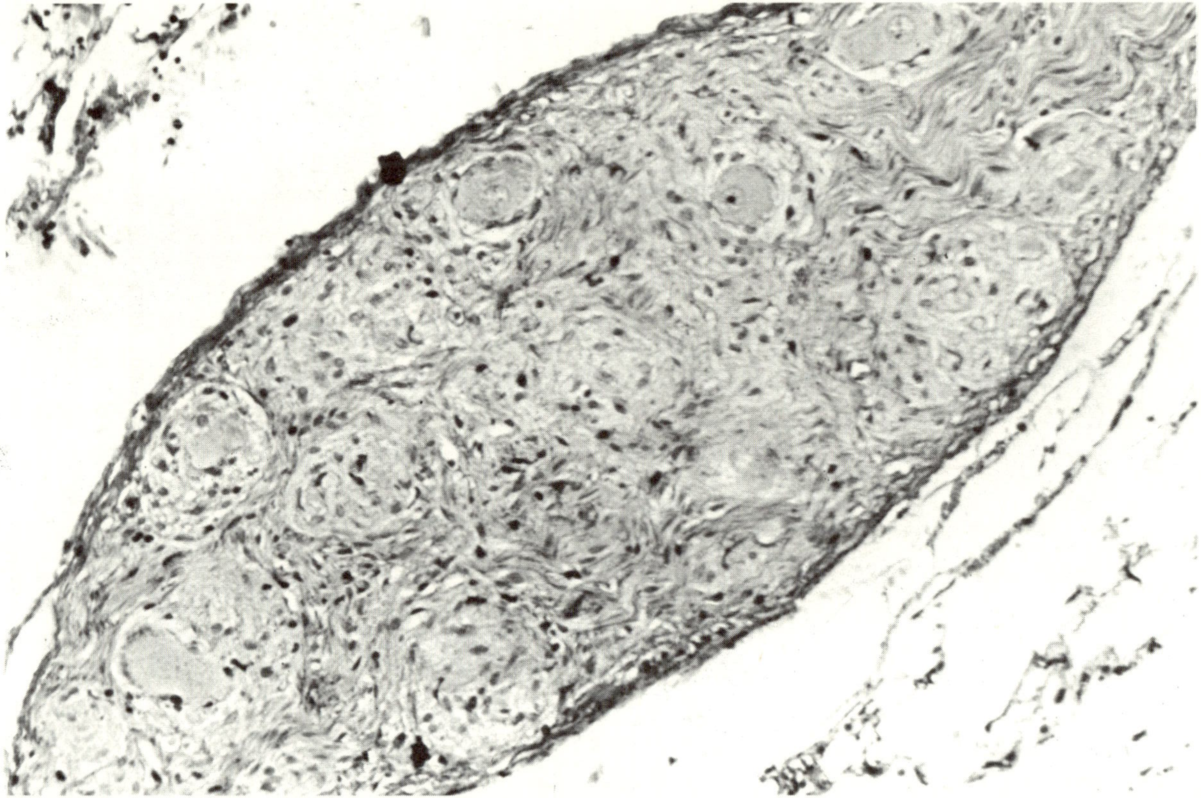

FIG. 2. Parasympathetic nervous ganglion in the epicardial fatty tissue of the right atrium in a human with chronic Chagas' disease. Almost total destruction of neurons and their replacement by fibrosis can be seen. Inflammatory cells are reduced to a few scattered lymphocytes. Masson trichrome staining; magnification × 150.

1 : 128) and no apparent signs of disease, and they repeatedly had an ECG within normal limits. Histological examination revealed no active inflammation, but patchy areas of focal cellular accumulation were occasionally seen in the myocardium. The main findings were fibrous replacement, sclero-atrophy, and fatty infiltration along the conducting tissue of the heart. It involved the sino-atrial node, the atrioventricular node, the main bundle of His and, especially, the right bundle branch (Fig. 3). Focal fibrosis was also found in the myocardium proper. There was considerable destruction and fibrosis of the autonomic nervous system in the heart, oesophagus and colon,

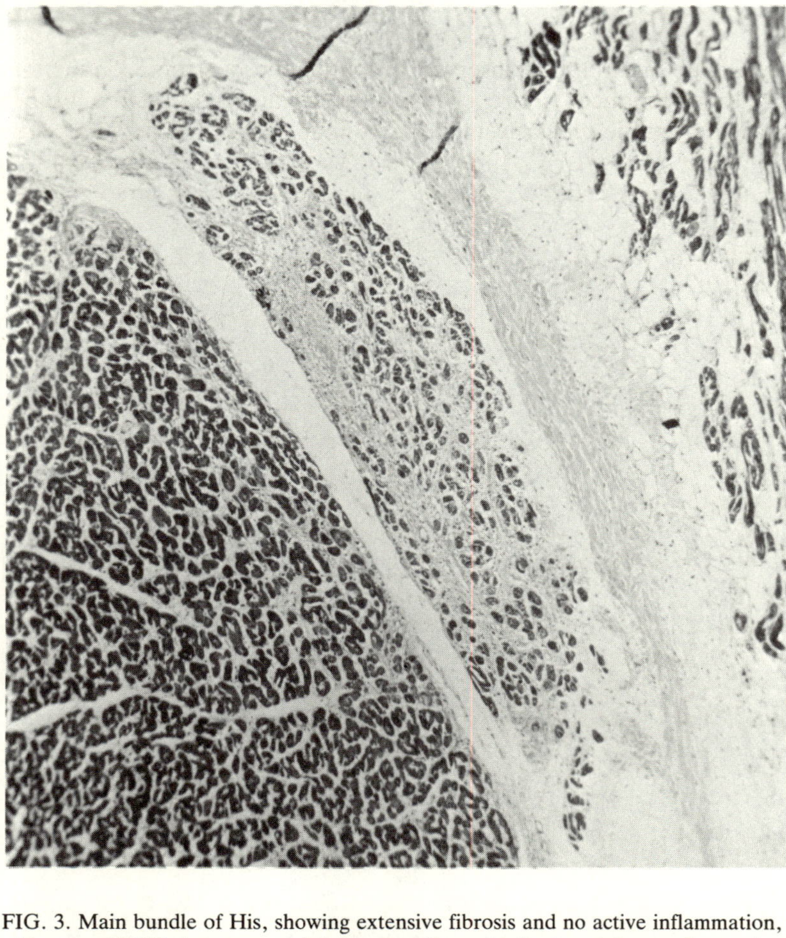

FIG. 3. Main bundle of His, showing extensive fibrosis and no active inflammation, from a dog with normal ECG that recovered from acute *T. cruzi* infection eight months previously. Masson trichrome staining; magnification × 50.

while inflammation was scanty or non-existent. These findings were suggestive of sequelae remaining from the acute phase of the infection, which is usually quite severe in young dogs. These findings also suggest that cicatricial focal lesions, being strategically located or of sufficient size, could cause functional disturbances in some patients. The manifestations of Chagas' disease in the digestive tract (mega-oesophagus, megacolon) may depend entirely on the destruction of ganglionic neurons in Auerbach's plexus during early infection, as suggested by Köberle (1974). Another obscure manifestation, such as skeletal muscle denervation (Cica et al 1979) may also result from the same mechanism. However, similar lesions in the heart would be devoid of a dynamic tendency and so would not have the grave prognosis of the chronic cardiac form of Chagas' disease.

Recently Chiale et al (1982) observed that ajmaline, a strong conduction-depressing drug, produced more changes (especially right-bundle branch block) in asymptomatic chagasic individuals than in normal controls. The authors concluded that their findings may indicate localized areas of injured myocardial tissue, not enough to alter the ECG by itself, but able to give rise to severe abnormalities after exposure to the drug.

Apical ventricular aneurysm, a peculiar gross finding in patients with Chagas' disease (Fig. 4), may also be found during the indeterminate (asymptomatic) phase of infection. Furthermore, this aneurysm can generate arrhythmias, some of them with fatal potential, which is probably an important cause of sudden death in previously asymptomatic chagasic patients. Thus, apical ventricular aneurysm may appear to the cardiologist as an unequivocal sign of progressive lesions in the myocardium. The pathogenesis of this aneurysm is not yet known. It probably results from interference with the conducting stimulus responsible for activation of the myocardium in the apical region. A delayed contraction at the apex may permit the blood within the heart to cause increased pressure and dilation at the apex during systole. The apex of the left ventricle is stimulated by the third division of the left bundle branch, the anteroseptal division, which originates from the 'bifurcation' of the right and left (anterior division) bundle branch (Durrer et al 1970), an area frequently damaged in Chagas' myocarditis (Andrade et al 1978). Such damage may also occur during the acute phase and be represented later on by a cicatricial lesion.

Chronic cardiac form of Chagas' disease

It is not known for how many people the indeterminate stage of Chagas' disease will evolve to the chronic cardiac form, nor which factors influence such a transformation.

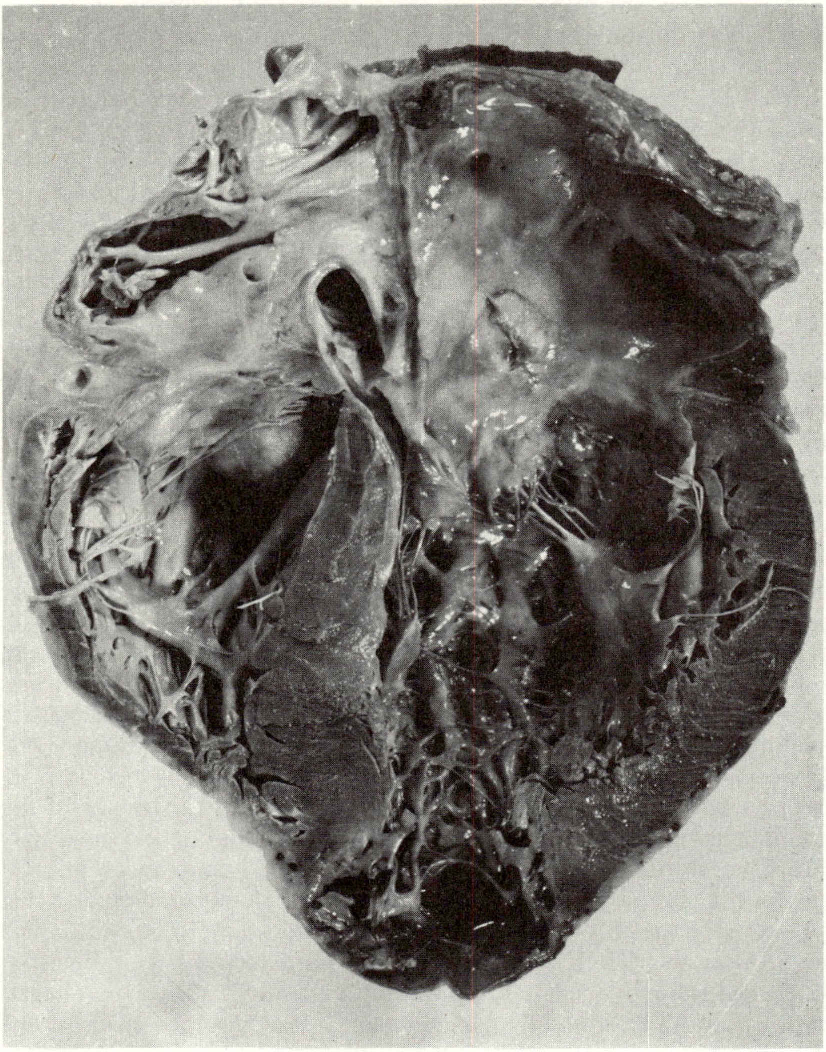

FIG. 4. A dilated and hypertrophied heart from a patient with chronic Chagas' myocarditis, showing an apical aneurysm in the left ventricle. Thinning and dilation of the apical region is seen without evident fibrosis of the surrounding myocardium.

The chronic form is characterized by a chronic, diffuse, active myocarditis, which has four main histological characteristics. (i) The cellular infiltrate, composed of macrophages and lymphoid cells, tends to accumulate focally in areas where the local myocardial fibres show varying degrees of degenerative change. (ii) Fibrosis appears as an outstanding feature, not only in focally dense areas but also in delicate and diffuse interstitial areas, sometimes involving each cardiac fibre (Fig. 5). (iii) Congestion and oedema are found throughout the myocardium. (iv) The parasites are difficult to find in histological sections (e.g. in only 30% of our material). All these findings indicate a progressive inflammatory process that is continually being reactivated, leading to diffuse myocardial destruction and fibrosis and not being directly related to the presence of parasites. This process appears in only a certain proportion (20–30% ?) of infected individuals, after a prolonged time from the initial infection, and is difficult to reproduce experimentally.

This chronic process is found only in the heart. No similar progressive type of chronic inflammatory lesion is found in the intestine, the brain or elsewhere. In the heart the active lesions may involve the conducting system (Andrade et al 1978) and the parasympathetic ganglia (Amorim & Olsen 1982), but some changes in these structures sometimes appear as old scars, the inflammation being scanty or absent (Fig. 6). The apical aneurism can be considered as an almost pathognomonic feature of Chagas' disease and from it some important thromboembolic manifestations may originate (Oliveira et al 1981).

Since the very earliest studies it has been suspected that immunological factors play a part in the pathogenesis of chronic Chagas' myocarditis. The histological findings are reminiscent of a cell-mediated chronic delayed-type hypersensitive reaction, but several obscure aspects need to be elucidated before one can explore further in this direction. The antigen or antigens involved are unknown. Besides *T. cruzi* antigens proper, there seem to be cross-reacting antigens in host cardiac and skeletal muscle tissues (Sadigursky et al 1982), which make autoimmune reactions a likely possibility. Moreover, neo-antigen(s) resulting from the host–parasite interactions may be important in a disease that is caused by an at least partially intracellular parasite. The reasons for the prolonged interval of the indeterminate stage are also unknown, as is why the lesions appear only in a small proportion of those infected. These difficulties stem mainly from the lack of an appropriate animal model for chronic Chagas' myocarditis. So far only the dog has presented some indications of being a suitable animal model (Andrade & Andrade 1980), and even this has not yet been widely recognized.

The immunological background is similar for the chronic cardiac form and the indeterminate form. In fact, towards the end of the acute phase all the indicators of immunity and hypersensitivity found in the late phases are already present. Besides the presence of serum antibodies that can agglutinate and lyse the parasites (with complement) *in vitro*, there are also sensitized lymphocytes that in the presence of parasite antigen can stimulate macro-

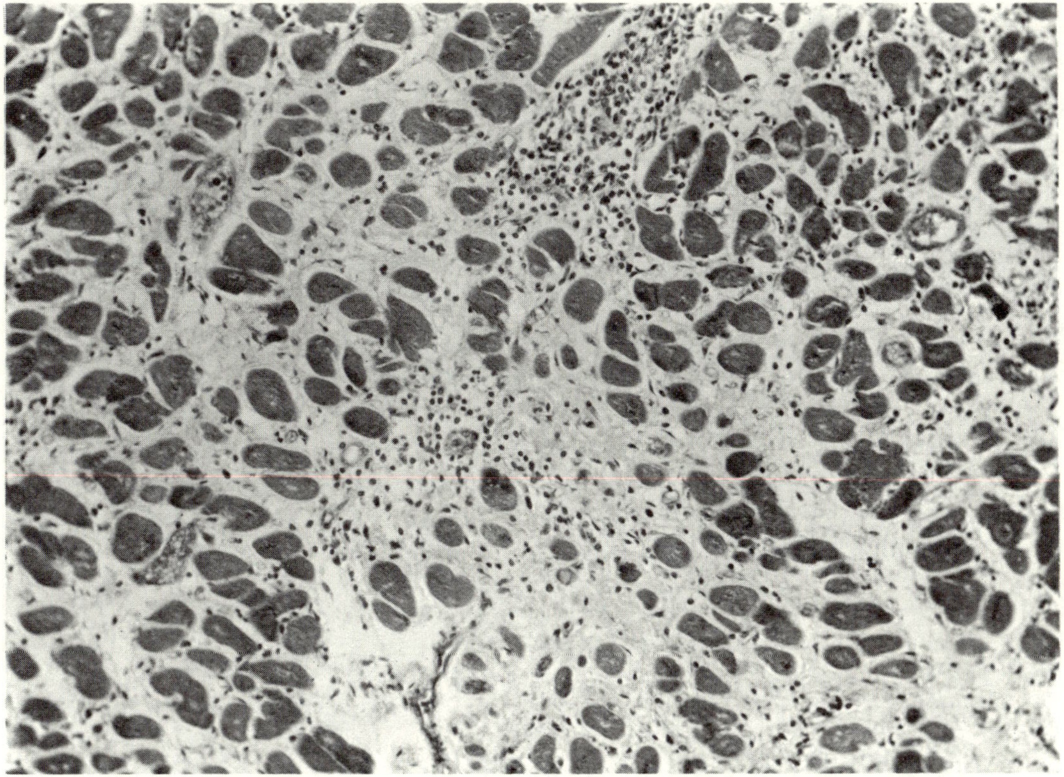

FIG. 5. A typical histological appearance of chronic Chagas' myocarditis. There is a diffuse and focal mononuclear cell infiltration with diffuse interstitial fibrosis. Myocardial fibres vary from states of atrophy to hypertrophy. Haematoxylin and eosin staining; magnification × 120.

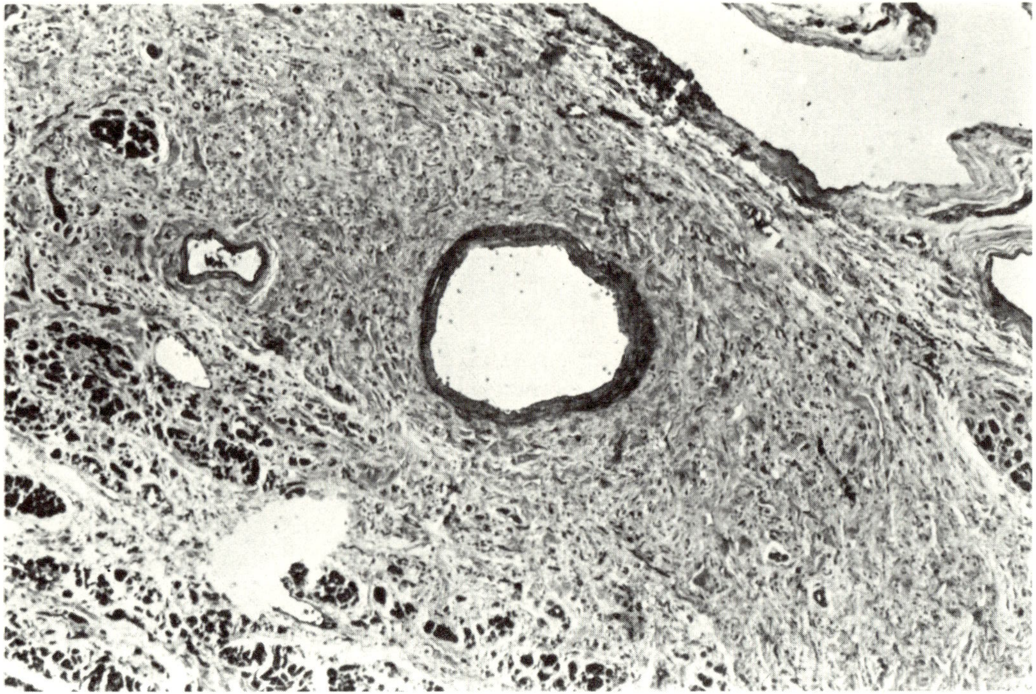

FIG. 6. Sinus node in a 32-year-old male with chronic Chagas' myocarditis. The node tissue is represented by a condensed fibrous stroma. The small dark dots resembling lymphocytes actually represent atrophic node cells. The fibrotic node appears as an old scar. Masson trichrome staining; magnification $\times 50$.

TABLE 1 Summary of the main characteristics of *T. cruzi* infection during the different clinical stages of Chagas' disease

Clinical stages	*Parasite*	*Host*	*Main lesions*	*Outcome*
Acute 2–4 months	Rapid multiplication	Inflammation	Generalized infection Myocarditis Meningo-encephalitis	Clinical cure (95%)
↓				
Indeterminate 5–10 years or more (30–20%)	Evasion Latency (?)	Immunity Humoral Cellular	Fibrous sequelae Conduction tissue Nervous tissue (autonomic)	Asymptomatic infection
↓				
Chronic	Antigens Neo-antigens Cross-reacting antigens	Delayed-type hypersensitivity	Chronic diffuse, progressive, fibrosing myocarditis	Death

phages to ingest and destroy the parasites (Brener 1980). At the same time several types of auto-antibody can be demonstrated, such as those against cardiac and skeletal muscles (Szarfman et al 1981), nerve fibres (Khoury et al 1979), neurons (Ribeiro dos Santos & Hudson 1981) and laminin (Szarfman et al 1982). On the other hand, lymphoid cells from infected hosts can be shown to adhere to and destroy allogeneic cardiac cells, but not kidney cells *in vitro* (Santos Buch & Teixeira 1974). Other evidence of delayed-type hypersensitivity to *T. cruzi* antigens, such as lymphocyte blastogenesis and cutaneous reactions, can also be observed in infected hosts (Brener 1980).

In conclusion, all the markers of hypersensitivity are found in hosts that present with either chronic asymptomatic infection or the cardiac form of Chagas' disease. One is therefore tempted to suggest that differences in the two conditions may lie in the state of the immunological suppressive factors which, while they seem to be successful during the indeterminate stage, appear to have been overcome to allow for the development of chronic progressive myocarditis (Table 1). Scott (1981) has recently shown in the mouse with chronic *T. cruzi* infection a specific suppression of delayed hypersensitivity to *T. cruzi* antigens but not to an unrelated antigen. Further studies have demonstrated a persistent suppression of responses by immunoglobulin G antibody, in mice with chronic *T. cruzi* infection, which is mediated by suppressor T lymphocytes (S. Reed, personal communication). More studies are needed to define better the nature of specific and non-specific suppression occurring during chronic Chagas' disease.

Acknowledgement

Thanks are due to the Brazilian Research Council (CNPq) and Rockefeller Foundation (CEDRE) for financial support, and to Dr Steven Reed for help with the English text.

REFERENCES

Acquatella H, Schiller NB, Puigbó JJ et al 1980 M-mode and two-dimensional echocardiography in chronic Chagas' heart disease. A clinical and pathologic study. Circulation 62:787-799

Amorim DS, Olsen EGJ 1982 Assessment of heart neurons in dilated (congestive) cardiomyopathy. Br Heart J 47:11-18

Amorim DS, Mançо JC, Gallo L Jr, Marin Neto JA 1979 Clinica: forma crônica cardíaca. In: Brener Z, Andrade ZA (eds) *Trypanosoma cruzi* e doença de Chagas. Editora Guanabar-Koogan, Rio de Janeiro, p 265-311

Andrade ZA, Andrade SG 1980 A patologia da doença de Chagas experimental no cão. Mem Inst Oswaldo Cruz Rio de J 75:77-95

Andrade ZA, Andrade SG, Oliveira GB, Alonso DR 1978 Histopathology of the conducting tissue of the heart in Chagas' myocarditis. Am Heart J 93:316-324

Andrade ZA, Andrade SG, Sadigursky M, Maguire JH 1981 Experimental Chagas' disease in dogs. A pathologic and ECG study of the chronic indeterminate phase of the infection. Arch Pathol Lab Med 105:460-464

Brener Z 1980 Immunity to *Trypanosoma cruzi*. Adv Parasitol 18:247-292

Chiale PA, Przybylski J, Laiño RA et al 1982 Electrocardiographic changes evoked by ajmaline in chronic Chagas' disease without manifest myocarditis. Am J Cardiol 49:14-20

Cica REP, Sanz OP, Aristimuño GG et al 1979 Muscle denervation in chronic Chagas' disease. Medicina (B Aires) 39:579-588

Durrer D, Van Dam RT, Freud GE, Janse MY, Meijler FL, Arzbaecher RC 1970 Total excitation of the isolated human heart. Circulation 41:899-912

Khoury EL, Ritacco V, Cossio PM et al 1979 Circulating antibodies to peripheral nerve in American trypanosomiasis (Chagas' disease). Clin Exp Immunol 36:8-15

Köberle F 1974 Pathogenesis of Chagas' disease. In: Trypanosomiasis and leishmaniasis with special reference to Chagas' disease. Associated Scientific Publishers, Amsterdam (Ciba Found Symp 20) p 137-158

Oliveira JSM, Oliveira JAM, Frederique V Jr, Lima Filho EC 1981 Apical aneurysm of Chagas' heart disease. Br Heart J 46:432-437

Ribeiro dos Santos R, Hudson L 1980 *Trypanosoma cruzi*: immunological consequences of parasite modification of host cells. Clin Exp Immunol 40:36-41

Ribeiro dos Santos R, Hudson L 1981 Denervation and the immune response in mice infected with *Trypanosoma cruzi*. Clin Exp Immunol 44:349-354

Sadigursky M, Acosta AM, Santos Buch CA 1982 Muscle sarcoplasmic reticulum antigen shared by a *Trypanosoma cruzi* clone. Am J Trop Med Hyg 31:934-941

Santos Buch CA, Teixeira ARL 1974 The immunology of experimental Chagas' disease. III: Rejection of allogeneic heart cells in vitro. J Exp Med 140:38-53

Scott MT 1981 Delayed hypersensitivity to *Trypanosoma cruzi* in mice: specific suppressor cells in chronic infection. Immunology 44:409-417

Szarfman A, Luqquetti A, Rassi A, Rezende JM, Schmuñis GA 1981 Tissue reacting immunoglobulins in patients with different clinical forms of Chagas' disease. Am J Trop Med Hyg 30:43-46

Szarfman A, Terranova VP, Rennard SI et al 1982 Antibodies to laminin in Chagas' disease. J Exp Med 155:1161-1171
Vianna G 1911 Contribuição para o estudo da anatomia patológica da 'Moléstia de Carlos Chagas'. Mem Inst Oswaldo Cruz Rio de J 3:276-293

DISCUSSION

Warren: Quite often with parasitic diseases, by the time a pathologist decides to do a biopsy—an invasive procedure that it would be unethical to do in the absence of symptoms—the patient has already reached an advanced stage of disease. It is difficult, therefore, to study the early, immunologically mediated events that are probably responsible for initiating the lesions in humans. Dr Andrade has made great advances in looking at this indeterminate stage, even though by that time the conduction system in the heart is already destroyed. Modern concepts of immunoregulation and modulation are now revealing that by the time the indeterminate phase is reached—two or three months after infection—the measurable immunological parameters may not indicate the mechanisms that initiated the pathological condition, although they may highlight mechanisms that modulate the condition. Yet the complexities of finding a decent animal model that allows the disease to be studied throughout its time course are also great, and Dr Andrade has mentioned that although the dog is a good model for some things it is not for others.

Nogueira: Perhaps all the damage done in the acute phase could explain most of the pathology that we see. Have you tried to immune-suppress the dogs in the so-called indeterminate phase, when you can show the parasite by xenodiagnosis? If the dog becomes immune-suppressed for a while, parasites would start multiplying, the whole inflammatory process would resume, and more damage would ensue. Scar tissue is left by the acute infection, and this summation of lesions may lead to heart decompensation. Have you studied that?

Andrade: We have no evidence to indicate that acute recurrent inflammation occurs in dogs with *Trypanosoma cruzi* infection. We are in the process of studying more dogs in the chronic indeterminate stage. Your suggestion is a good one, and if we could successfully produce the chronic disease in dogs we would better understand what is going on in humans with Chagas' disease.

Nogueira: Epidemiological and experimental data from the work of the Harvard School of Public Health and others are now suggesting that the so-called indeterminate phase is not a silent or pseudo-cure phase before the development of the so-called autoimmune disease. All the patients in the indeterminate phase have lesions, as you have shown, and they may show alterations in the electrocardiogram. One can prove that parasites are present if one does xenodiagnosis frequently enough. Thus, the indeterminate phase is not necessarily totally new and different from the chronic phase. It is more like a continuum; the state of immunity of the host and a disturbance in the host–parasite balance may influence the outcome of infection.

Andrade: The particular concept, definition and pathological characterization of the indeterminate phase of Chagas' disease that I am using are as I presented in my paper.

Hudson: You described a severe reduction in neurons in an interatrial ganglion, and you saw fibrosis but few lymphocytes. Could your examination of the tissues have been *after* the initial inflammatory event, which had been precipitated by an infiltration of mononuclear cells and replaced, in the distant past, by fibrosis?

Andrade: In humans we can say only that we see a late lesion, but we are not sure what has happened before. The dogs, however, do develop an acute disease, during which neuronal destruction occurs. Later on, fibrosis appears in the autonomic nervous tissue, which we can attribute fairly confidently to a previous acute inflammation.

Hudson: When speaking about the pathogenesis of Chagas' disease one has to try to explain why neuronal destruction may occur early in the acute phase whereas gross pathology may often not be seen until late in the chronic stage. What happens in the intervening period?

Andrade: Neuronal destruction does not always follow the same pattern. One can see a few or a thousand cardiac neurons destroyed in the chronic indeterminate stage of Chagas' disease (Andrade & Andrade 1979). It seems that even when all the neurons are missing, the 'denervated' heart can function automatically without much of a problem. But in the intestine and the oesophagus if the destruction is too extensive there will probably be adverse effects later on. It seems that throughout life the neurons are being destroyed and disappear, so a young person will have many more neurons in the oesophagus than an older person (Koeberle 1961). Older people sometimes present with dysphagia, which is considered to result from this progressive loss. If a person's oesophageal neurons are destroyed by the disease to a certain degree, but not sufficient to produce megaoesophagus, the later physiological loss of neurons may cause megaoesophagus to develop subsequently.

Nussenzweig: It is obvious that a thorough description and characterization of the lesions in humans is very important for a subsequent understanding of the dynamics of the process. But the necessary information can be obtained only with great difficulty in humans. One needs an experimental host to manipulate this system and to define the various causes and effects. Dogs have been used in a number of experimental studies but, from what you showed, this model presents considerable difficulties. What is your view on the suitability of the rabbit model for reproducing the chronic phase of Chagas' disease? I understand that Teixeira et al (1975) have produced chronic lesions in rabbits and that attempts to reproduce these experiments have been made in several other laboratories. On the other hand, some investigators have used certain strains of mice and different strains of *T. cruzi*, and have claimed that these provide valid experimental models for chronic infections. From the point of view of investigation of the pathology of the disease, how worthwhile do you think it is to pursue these models?

Andrade: First of all, I should define what I think is a suitable model of Chagas' disease. It should show an acute infection when inoculated for the first time, with patent parasitaemia and parasites in the tissues, followed by recovery in a significant number of the infected animals, with evidence of immunity (sometimes hypersensitivity) and no symptoms. This should be followed, after a prolonged period, by the appearance of chronic disease in a few of the animals. The canine model seems to be like that. If 100 mice are inoculated, we might recover from acute infection, say, 50 mice, and find chronic inflammation and some fibrosis in the atria of all these mice, 400 days afterwards. If the animals are killed at any time in between, we will find myocarditis and parasites. This means that mice develop persistent infection, with the production of persistent inflammation due to periodic rupture of parasitized myocardial fibres. So this is not like the human model or the canine model. We have tried to infect rabbits and we obtained a short acute phase, but we didn't see much in the myocardium. Later on we did not see lesions. So, in our hands, the rabbit is a very difficult animal to work with as a host of Chagas' disease (Andrade & Andrade 1979).

Warren: I believe that an animal model need not mimic exactly each stage of a disease. If we had listened to all the people who told us that the mouse doesn't develop gross clay-pipe stem fibrosis, we would never have done any work on schistosomiasis in mice. Nevertheless we have learned something about the disease from our work in mice. Chimpanzees can develop clay-pipe stem fibrosis when infected with *Schistosoma mansoni* or *Schistosoma japonicum*. Yet these animals do not develop portal hypertension or oesophageal varices, which are the fatal manifestions for the patient. The mouse does develop oesophageal varices. If one wants to study granulomas (egg lesions), there are some experimental animal species that do not support the entire life-cycle of the parasite; i.e. they do not develop adult worms that produce eggs. However, if eggs are isolated and injected into these animals, they will produce typical granulomas. So one can study granulomas by looking just at that specific phase of the pathology in a variety of experimental animals. In our studies of filariasis, David Grove and I developed a model that involved the intravenous injection of microfilaria of *Brugia malayi* into mice. The mouse will not support the whole cycle and develop adult worms that produce microfilaria. But intravenous injection of microfilaria from gerbils into mice leads to prolonged circulation of the microfilaria. These eventually disappear, and the mice are immune to re-infection. Kazura & Davis (1982), using that model, have not only learned an enormous amount about the mechanism of that reaction but have actually developed an effective vaccine. Injection of a tiny amount of antigen subcutaneously into mice will immunize them against the microfilaria stage of the disease. So the mouse is a useful model, even though the whole life cycle cannot be recreated in it, because it has been so well characterized immunologically.

Andrade: The usefulness of a model depends on what you want to ask. Even experiments on cultured cells can reveal many fundamental answers. But for the interpretations about the pathogenesis of chronic Chagas' disease in humans, the wrong animal may give wrong results. One needs a good model that will give information about the mechanisms of cardiac damage in chronic human disease. On the other hand, if one wants to study chemotherapy, or the acute phase of the disease and the immunoresponse, there seems to be no better animal than the mouse.

Gutteridge: For the acute stage of Chagas' disease you seem to believe that chemotherapy is possible. Is this true also for the indeterminate and chronic stages, or is it then too late to improve the clinical condition of the patient with chemotherapeutic agents?

Andrade: During acute infection one can kill the parasite with the chemotherapeutic drugs now available (Andrade et al 1980). The rate of multiplication renders the parasite quite sensitive to drugs. In the later chronic indeterminate or chronic progressive stages of the disease most attempts at chemotherapy do not achieve a cure. We still need better drugs that can eliminate the parasite at any time during infection.

Warren: Are any available drugs guaranteed to cure the patient?

Andrade: Not as far as I know.

Gutteridge: Even if one had a drug that could successfully eliminate all amastigotes from patients in the chronic phase, would that drug also improve the survival and well-being of the patient, or would it be too late to intervene with chemotherapy?

Andrade: What happens later seems to be the result of the persistence of the parasite which overcomes the immunological equilibrium of the host.

Gutteridge: Would the lesions self-heal if you could actually eradicate the total parasite burden, or would you simply expect no further development of the disease?

Andrade: I think you're implying that an autoimmune process may already have started. In that case I don't know what would happen if the parasite was eradicated. If autoimmunity is present then there would be no reason for taking out the parasite, because this would not interfere with the evolution of the disease. But one would need first to prove that autoimmunity was already present.

Martinez-Palomo: You mentioned that some of the dogs may go from the acute to the silent phase. Will any of them also go to the chronic stage which, judging from the outcome, is really the significant phase? Is the last (chronic) stage in humans really a reactivation or could it sometimes be a reinfection or an association with another pathological process such as viral myocarditis or atherosclerosis?

Andrade: In Venezuela, Anselmi et al (1965, 1967) studied the canine model and produced chronic progressive disease in dogs. They infected 25 dogs and found progressive lesions in three of them. In Brazil, Pellegrino (1946) and Laranja & Andrade (1980) obtained dogs in the chronic progressive phase, and the ones we saw had first developed the acute disease and then gone through an indeterminate phase. Sixteen months later chronic myocardial inflammation and fibrosis developed, without parasites in the myocardial fibres; we assumed that the animal had then developed the chronic progressive stage. I cannot tell whether viral myocarditis was present. In humans, chronic Chagas' myocarditis had no relationship to atherosclerosis and also does not seem related to viruses.

Warren: The dogs that you described ranged, in their initial weights, from 1.2 to 8.0 kg, so they are likely to be an assortment of mongrels. Has any work been done on laboratory-bred dogs under standardized conditions?

Andrade: Kramer (1972) did some acute studies on Beagle dogs. We have tried to use a group of litters, containing 5–9 dogs at one time. They should be inoculated when they are two to three months old. If an adult dog is inoculated it will probably not show acute manifestations of disease.

Pulido: The results that Dr Andrade mentioned from the Venezuelan group (Anselmi et al 1965, 1966, 1967) were also subject to this problem of a variety of breeds and weights being used, and so the infection was also variable.

Wyler: One might anticipate that patients who have subclinical disease but already have fibrosis in the conduction system might be particularly sensitive to certain cardiotropic drugs that would decrease conduction, such as digitalis. Is there any clinical evidence that this occurs?

Andrade: Yes. Chiale et al (1982) used ajmaline, a conduction depressor drug, which has barely any effect on normal people. But when it was given to people with asymptomatic Chagas' disease several of them developed conduction disturbances, especially right-bundle branch block. The normal control group, on the other hand, in the few instances in which they presented abnormalities, developed left-bundle branch block.

REFERENCES

Andrade ZA, Andrade SG 1979 Patologia. In: Brener Z, Andrade ZA (eds) *Trypanosoma cruzi* e doença de Chagas. Editora Guanabara-Koogan, Rio de Janeiro

Andrade SG, Andrade ZA, Sadigursky M 1980 Combined treatment with a nitrofuranic and a corticoid in experimental Chagas' disease in the dog. Am J Trop Med Hyg 29:766-773

Anselmi A, Pifano FC, Suarez JA, Domingues A, Vasquez AD, Anselmi G 1965 Experimental *Schizotrypanum cruzi* myocarditis. Am Heart J 70:638-656

Anselmi A, Pifano F, Suarez JA, Gurdiel O 1966 Myocardiopathy in Chagas' disease: comparative study of pathologic findings in chronic human and experimental Chagas' myocarditis. Am Heart J 72:469-481

Anselmi A, Gurdiel O, Suarez JA, Anselmi G 1967 Disturbances in the AV conduction system in Chagas' myocarditis in the dog. Circ Res 20:56-64

Chiale PA, Przybylski J, Laiño RA et al 1982 Electrocardiographic changes evoked by ajmaline in chronic Chagas' disease without manifest myocarditis. Am J Cardiol 49:14-20

Kazura JW, Davis RS 1982 Soluble *Brugia malayi* microfilarial antigens protect mice against challenge by an antibody-dependent mechanism. J Immunol 128:1792-1796

Koeberle F 1961 Patologia y anatomia patologica de la enfermedad de Chagas. Bol Of Sanit Panam 51:404-428

Kramer AW Jr 1972 Experimental Chagas' disease in purebred beagle dog acutely infected with *Trypanosoma cruzi* (B strain). Rev Inst Med Trop Sao Paulo 14:291-300

Laranja FS, Andrade ZA 1980 Forma crônica cardiaca da doença de Chagas no cão. Arq Bras Cardiol 35:377-380

Pellegrino J 1946 O electrocardiograma na fase crônica da doença de Chagas experimental no cão. Mem Inst Oswaldo Cruz Rio de J 44:615

Teixeira ARL, Teixeria ML, Santos Buch CA 1975 The immunology of experimental Chagas' disease. IV: Production of lesions in rabbit similar to those of chronic Chagas' disease in man. Am J Pathol 80:163-180

Immunopathogenesis of experimental Chagas' disease in mice: damage to the autonomic nervous system

LESLIE HUDSON

Department of Immunology, Jenner Wing, St George's Hospital Medical School, London SW17 0RE, UK

Abstract Infection of mice with *Trypanosoma cruzi* produces pathological change which in many ways parallels the evolution of Chagas' disease in human patients. An essential element in this experimental pathology is the intense denervation observed during the resolution of acute-stage parasitaemia. Host cells, from a variety of tissues, have been shown to absorb parasite antigens and thus to become targets for the host's own anti-parasite immune response. The definition of common antigenic determinants, shared by *T. cruzi* and human neuronal cells, might explain why the electrical conduction systems and the autonomic nervous system are especially vulnerable to the postulated autoimmune process. We have the models, the tools and the hypotheses, and now we await the proof.

1983 Cytopathology of parasitic disease. Pitman Books, London (Ciba Foundation symposium 99), p 234-251

Given the difficulties of diagnosis and clinical management of disease, the pathologist is frequently the last person to see the patient. Often, however, he or she may have the meagre consolation of the final word and is in a position not only to describe the disease pathology but also to uncover the chain of events leading to its production.

Pathologists have yet to attain this desirable state with regard to Chagas' disease, in either human infection or animal models. Even so we have reason for optimism in that we now have the tools and technologies with which to sift the various hypotheses advanced to explain the pathogenesis of Chagas' disease, several of which were advanced by contemporaries of Carlos Chagas himself (1879–1934).

What can the experimental scientist, working far from the endemic area and rarely, if ever, seeing the human disease, add to the study of this problem? In essence, the scientist may offer the same assets that have been intimately involved in the steady advance of biomedical research in other areas over the past few decades—the standardization and definition of model systems in which the supposed pathogenic mechanisms can be tested. For the immunologist Chagas' disease provides a panacea of research possibilities, among which must be counted the real possibility of an 'autoimmune disease' precipitated by an already defined aetiologic agent—*Trypanosoma cruzi*.

Disease pathogenesis

It is impossible, and at present unhelpful, to attempt a unifying hypothesis that would embrace all aspects of *T. cruzi* infection and Chagas' disease. Although a variety of host and parasite factors have been invoked to explain the wide diversity of observed pathology, research groups are only now approaching the problem of identifying and assessing these factors. A model that reproduces the great variability seen in the response to human infection would be of little value to the experimental scientist. Animal models that produce cardiopathy with or without megaformations of the digestive tract are thus more likely to be of interest than those reproducing the most frequent outcome of human infection with *T. cruzi*, the so-called inapparent infection.

Similarly, one must attempt to apply Occam's razor—the principle that entities are not to be multiplied beyond necessity—to the multitude of possible aetiological events and their interrelations. There seems little doubt that during the *acute* phase the parasite can exert a direct pathogenic effect which results in acute myocarditis produced by the non-specific inflammatory response that is provoked by disintegrating parasites. If the inflammatory response is severe, then cardiac structure and function may be modified, but at the end of the acute phase, when the cellular infiltration decreases, normal structure and function usually return.

The major paradox of this disease is illustrated by the *chronic* stage, in which parasite numbers decline to virtual insignificance and yet the disease symptoms become most apparent. If this paradox can be explained by the emergence of a parasite-triggered autoimmunity then it would be reasonable to suggest that there might also be a connection between acute-stage events and chronic-phase symptoms. An attractive working hypothesis was advanced by Köberle (1974). He suggested that Chagas' disease might be a neuropathy resulting from the destruction of ganglion cells and nerve fibres in distinct parts of the body. Compelling evidence was presented in support of this notion. Data have been published from Köberle's and other laboratories to show that denervation is well advanced before the end of the acute phase and is complete long before the so-called chronic chagasic syndromes of cardiopathy and megaformations become apparent. Although there is little doubt that the acute-stage pathology must be directly related to parasite load, this key point has yet to be verified for the chronic stage. The implications are as important as they are obvious. If parasite-initiated, acute-stage events mediate or influence the pathology of the chronic stage then there is real hope that any immunotherapy or immunoprophylaxis which significantly lessens acute-stage parasitaemia might also ameliorate or prevent the chronic-stage pathology. This notion should be validated because current attempts at immunoprophylaxis are at present unlikely to produce sterile immunity.

Model systems of host and parasite

Populations of *T. cruzi* show considerable genetic heterogeneity, as demonstrated by variation between strains in morphology, drug resistance, pathogenicity and isoenzyme analysis. Indeed, even in a single strain one may find as much heterogeneity between stable parasite clones as between wild populations. Individual clones of the Sylvio (Postan et al 1982), or Y, strain of *T. cruzi* (Fig. 1) may be selected to produce either an acute, uniformly lethal infection at 6–10 days or a chronic infection with the mice surviving indefinitely and with a low level of parasitaemia. Although this degree of intraspecies variation may be unimportant for some studies, it is likely to explain the discrepant immunological findings reported by different groups working with the same parasite strain (reviewed by Hudson 1981). The recent application of *restriction endonuclease fingerprinting* to this problem (Goncalves et al 1983) is likely to provide a definitive means of typing existing clones and strains to ensure a uniformity of parasite material between research groups.

The mouse has been the most frequently used species for the study of *T. cruzi* infection. Consequently, the accumulating evidence that this species is also a good model for human Chagas' disease has been greeted with a feeling of relief in many laboratories, including our own. Implicit in this relief was the realization that the pathology does not crucially depend on a single mouse strain, parasite clone or infection regimen. For example, Laguens and co-workers (1980) have reported chagasic pathology in both inbred and outbred mice infected with 25–50 Tulahuen strain parasites. Conversely, Cover & Gutteridge (1982) induced pathology in Ajax mice treated with Bayer 7602Ac and infected with 2×10^5 Sonya-strain blood trypomastigotes.

As patent parasitaemia develops in mice, histological examination shows occasional nests of amastigotes in skeletal and cardiac muscle as well as in the sub-serosal muscles lining the large intestine and bladder. Inflammatory infiltrates of mononuclear cells produce cytolytic and necrotic lesions, which

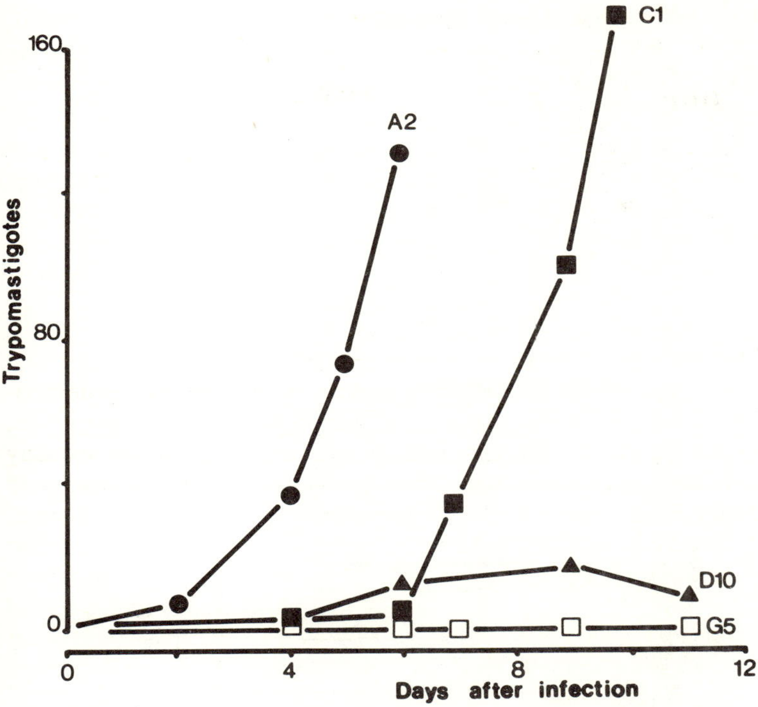

FIG. 1. Blood parasitaemia in (C3H × C5B1) mice infected with 5×10^7 cloned trypomastigotes derived by limiting the dilution culture of the Y strain of *T. cruzi*. Vertical axis depicts trypomastigote numbers in a standard volume of heparinized blood.

eventually fibrose, in regions remote from parasite foci. Neuronal degeneration is strikingly similar to that predicted by Köberle (1974) (Fig. 2) and is associated with profound electrocardiographic (ECG) abnormalities (Fig. 3). *Post mortem* examination reveals a generalized muscular atrophy associated with dilation of the colon and bladder.

With the exception of its obvious logistical and immunological attractions, it is difficult to assess the value of the mouse model in relation to the rabbit model originally described by Teixeira et al (1975) and the dog model described by Andrade (this volume). The mouse model is known to show specific anomalies; for example, the myenteric plexus is not involved in mice but is a significant feature in some forms of the human disease, and the bradycardia seen on murine ECG examination (Fig. 3) is not a significant feature of the human disease. Caution demands that we await further developments in each model system.

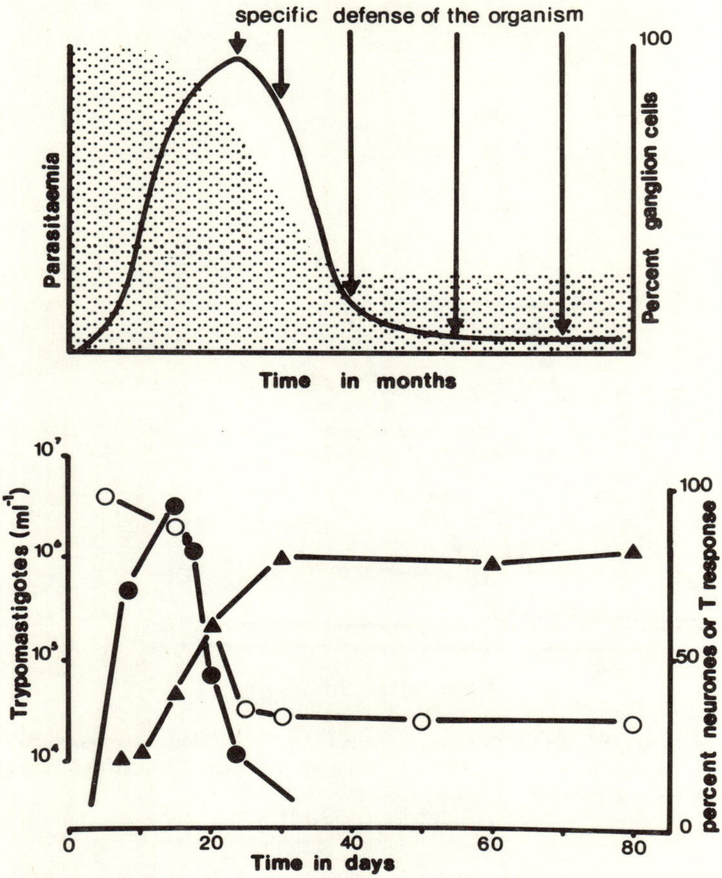

FIG. 2. Denervation as a function of time in *T. cruzi* infection. The upper figure (based on Köberle 1974) shows the course of ganglion cell destruction (stippled area) in relation to parasitaemia and the emergence of the immune response. Although this time course was deducted from *post mortem* material from Chagasic patients, it is strikingly similar to the accelerated kinetics shown by data from infected mice (lower figure). Numbers of cardiac neurons (open circles) were found to decline as parasitaemia resolved (filled circles) in response to the emergence of the anti-parasite immune response (filled triangles), measured as the response of lymphocytes producing migration inhibition factor in response to *T. cruzi* antigen *in vitro*. Antibody kinetics show a similar relationship to parasitaemia.

Evidence for immunological involvement

The initial immune response provoked by *T. cruzi* infection is directed against the parasite itself. The parasite burden is rapidly reduced to a level where

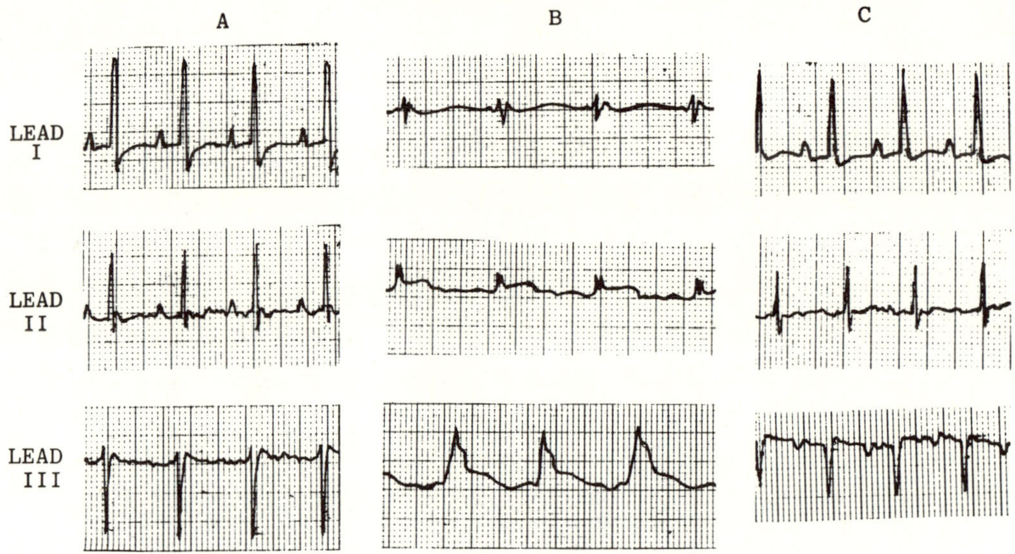

FIG. 3. Electrocardiogram (ECG) recordings in normal mice or mice infected with *T. cruzi*. (a) Normal A-strain control mice. (b) Mice infected with Sonya-strain trypomastigotes following treatment with Bayer 7602AC (courtesy of B. Cover). The trace from lead II shows a raised ST wave, suggestive of myocardial infarction, with a widening of the QRS complex (lead III). The bradycardia shown by this mouse is a consistent, but mouse-specific, ECG alteration following *T. cruzi* infection. Treatment with the drug alone produced no ECG alteration. (c) Mice infected with Y-strain trypomastigotes and treated with three doses of 0.5 ml of CE5 monoclonal antibody. The ECG trace is within the variation shown by normal mice.

pathology mediated by direct effects of the parasite, via mechanical destruction or toxin production, must be insignificant. Chronic-stage pathology is thought to arise as an aberration of this anti-parasite response; the host itself becomes the target. Evidence that the parasite is not involved in chronic-stage pathology comes from studies in infected patients undergoing immunosuppressive therapy for a concomitant illness: the parasitaemia breaks out again but the pathological effects are not reactivated or exacerbated (Barousse et al 1980).

Auto-antibodies against muscle and nerve cells are a consistent feature of chagasic serology in humans and animals, but present evidence shows no correlation with the development of the disease (Peralta et al 1982). Similarly, auto-aggressive T lymphocytes, which are reactive with heart muscle cells *in vitro*, have been demonstrated in infected patients, mice and rabbits but at present can provide only circumstantial evidence of aberrent immunological reactivity.

The first compelling evidence for the immunopathogenesis of chagasic lesions came from studies by Teixeira et al (1975) using rabbits. These investigators immunized rabbits weekly for nine months with subcellular fractions of *T. cruzi* and found that the rabbits developed pathological features similar to those in rabbits with chronic *T. cruzi* infection. However, the most direct demonstration of immune involvement comes from transfer of lymphocytes from infected to normal mice (Laguens et al 1981). Recipient mice were given 10^6 lymphocytes from *T. cruzi*-infected donors and, in the absence of transferred infection, half of them developed definite ECG alterations and lymphocytic infiltration of the myocardium within an astoundingly short period of 1–4 days. Although these findings are consistent with disease transfer, their rapid evolution is unexpected when one considers the time course of other lymphocyte-induced autoimmune processes that use homogenous antigen-specific T-cell lines (Ben-Nun & Cohen 1982).

Mechanisms of cell destruction

In an association as complex as that between *T. cruzi* and its mammalian host it is unlikely that a single mechanism will account for the widespread and varied cell destruction that results in Chagas' disease. Even when limited to the present context of nerve cell destruction, the evidence still suggests that the postulated mechanisms might change in their relative importance at different stages of the disease.

Parasite modification of host cells

Our initial observations on the destruction of parasitized host cells emerged from experiments done for quite different reasons. On the assumption that the destruction of the intracellular amastigote stage was likely to be the most rewarding target for immunoprophylactic regimens, we pulsed cultures of muscle and neuron cells with *T. cruzi* trypomastigotes and then we examined them at serial time points for the appearance of cell-surface antigens induced by intracellular infection.

Up to 72 h after infection, and before the appearance of the first round of extracellular parasites, no parasite antigens were detected, even though about 30% of the cells were heavily infected. After parasite release, however, *T. cruzi* antigen was found on the surface of both the infected and the uninfected cells (Ribeiro dos Santos & Hudson 1980a). Subsequent experiments showed that parasite antigens, derived either naturally from tissue-culture supernatants or after disruption of amastigotes by freezing and thawing, could be used to sensitize the host cells passively. Parasite-sensitized cells thus became susceptible to lysis by cytotoxic T lymphocytes and by antibodies either with complement or in combination with K cells, derived from *T. cruzi*-infected mice. Significantly, T cells from mice infected for 30 days lysed the cells treated with parasite antigen but had no effect on untreated, normal cells. After 90 days of infection, T cells were isolated that could lyse muscle and neuronal cell lines in the absence of prior treatment with parasite antigens, indicating that auto-aggressive T-cell reactivity had developed. The specificity of this T-cell reaction was shown by the observation that HeLa cells acted as targets for these '90 day' lymphocytes only after treatment with parasite antigens (Ribeiro dos Santos & Hudson 1980b).

Neuronal cell destruction was quantitated in the hearts of infected mice by microscopic examination of serial heart sections, and was found to occur before the appearance of neuron-specific T lymphocytes. The temporal relationship of these findings suggests that neuron-specific T lymphocytes resulted from the neuronal destruction and so could not have initiated it.

It is worth noting that the original aim of these experiments, to identify infection-induced host-cell membrane modification, was not lost; in a study analogous to that described above, it was shown that chemical inhibitors of the nuclear enzyme ADP-ribosyl transferase can be used to block DNA ligation which has been postulated as an obligatory event in amastigote-to-trypomastigote differentiation but these inhibitors do not affect cell proliferation (Johnstone & Williams 1982, Williams 1982). It is thus possible to maintain an intracellular infection with cell proliferation and to circumvent the problem of antigen release and adsorption (Fig. 4).

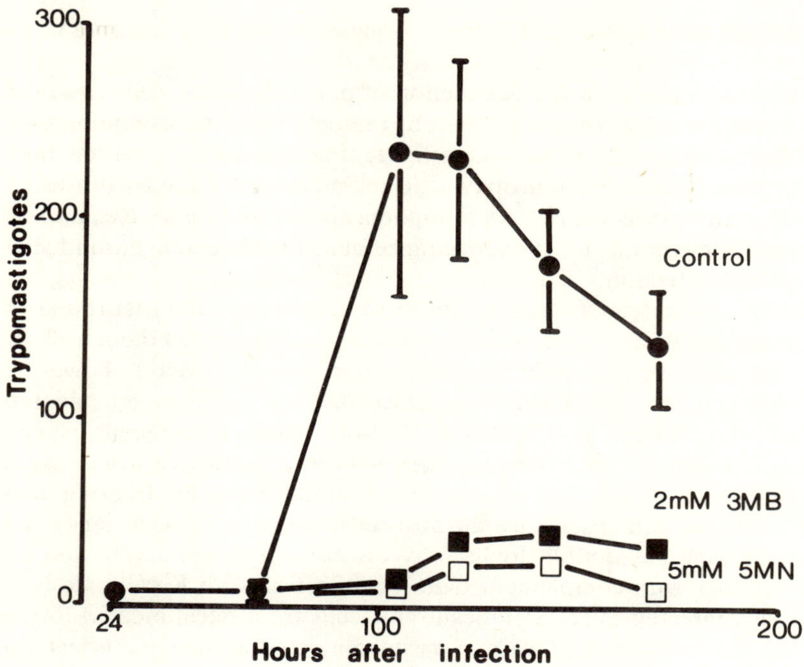

FIG. 4. Release of trypomastigotes from a muscle cell line heavily infected with intracellular *T. cruzi* amastigotes. Vertical axis shows parasite numbers per microscope field. Filled circles, control cultures; filled squares, infected cells cultured in the presence of 2 mM-3-methoxybenzamide (3MB); open squares, 5 mM-5-methylnicotinamide (5MN) (unpublished data of G. T. Williams). These specific inhibitors of the nuclear enzyme ADP-ribosyltransferase have been shown to prevent the DNA ligation essential for eukaryotic cell differentiation (Johnstone & Williams 1982). Although amastigote-to-trypomastigote differentiation was inhibited, host-cell and amastigote proliferation were unaffected. Differentiation was resumed when inhibitors were replaced by fresh medium at any of the time points shown on the horizontal axis (Williams 1982).

Host–parasite cross-reactive antigens

Serological studies in humans and animals have shown that some components of anti-*T. cruzi* sera may be absorbed by muscle or neuronal cells. Conversely, serum titres of EVI (endocardium, vessels and interstitium) and NP (peripheral nerve) antibody may be reduced by cross-absorption with *T. cruzi*. Given the problems of interpretation associated with these conventional serological manoeuvres, it was an obvious step to attempt to define these putative cross-reactive antigens by the use of monoclonal antibodies.

In brief, reciprocal screening of anti-parasite and anti-neuronal hybridoma supernatants detected an immunoglobulin M (IgM) λ monoclonal antibody,

CE5, which reacted with viable *T. cruzi* organisms and with human and rat central and peripheral subpopulations of neurons known to degenerate in Chagas' disease (Wood et al 1982). CE5 antibody from ascitic fluid has been shown to immunoprecipitate a polypeptide of relative molecular mass (M_r) 87 500 from the *in vitro* translation products of poly A+ RNA isolated from *T. cruzi* epimastigotes (L. Hudson & H. Eisen, unpublished observations). This demonstrates that CE5 reacts with an epitope specified by the parasite genome and is not a passively acquired host-cell component.

Administration of CE5 ascitic fluid to *T. cruzi*-infected mice results in a reduction in parasitaemia (Fig. 5). However, whereas other anti-*T. cruzi*

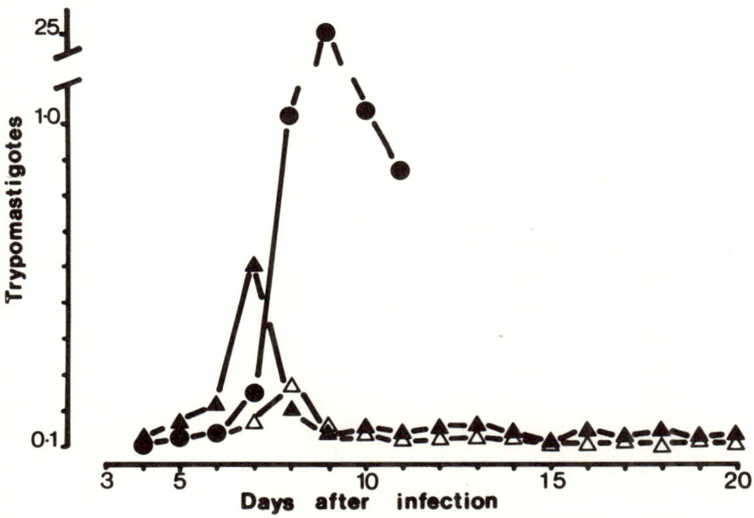

Antibody Treatment	Survivors at 80 days*	Mean time to death	Range
MOPC 104E	0/10	12	12-13
CE5	0/10	23	17-33
4G10	8/10	24+	22-25

* Termination of experiment   + Of two non-survivors

FIG. 5. Effect of monoclonal antibodies on the course of *T. cruzi* infection in mice. Mice were treated with 0.5 ml of ascitic fluid containing monoclonal antibody (as below) six hours before infection with 2×10^5 Y-strain blood trypomastigotes. Antibody treatment was repeated at five days after the infection. Upper figure shows the course of blood parasitaemia in infected mice following treatment with: MOPC 104E (filled circles), an IgM anti-dextran myeloma protein; CE5 (filled triangles), an IgM anti-rat dorsal root ganglion monoclonal known to cross react with *T. cruzi* (Wood et al 1982); and 4G10 (open triangles), an IgM monoclonal antibody reactive with surface components of viable *T. cruzi* parasites, but without any known anti-host cross-reactivity. The lower table shows survival of mice depicted in the graph.

monoclonals (for example 4G10, Fig. 5) allow the mice to survive indefinitely after a transient parasitaemia, all mice treated with CE5 showed a recrudescence of slender-form trypomastigotes and died by the 33rd day after infection (see lower table in Fig. 5). No evidence of ECG abnormalities were detected (Fig. 3). Two of the five mice, observed close to death, showed an inability to regain their normal position when rolled onto their backs, but instead rolled along the bench. Although no pathological examinations were done, this alteration of behaviour indicates that Purkinje cell destruction may have occurred. Mice treated with CE5 antibody alone showed no alteration in behaviour.

Recent findings indicate that the CE5-defined antigen is by no means unique. Two further monoclonal antibodies raised against *T. cruzi* have been shown to bind to neural antigens blotted onto nitrocellulose sheets (J. Wood, personal communication).

Conclusions

The role of parasite modification of host cells in *T. cruzi*-infected mice has recently been reviewed (Hudson & Ribeiro dos Santos 1981). However, it is valuable to consider these findings in relation to our more recent work with monoclonal antibodies, even with the present incomplete evidence. One may speculate that cross-reactive antigens are available on viable parasites in sufficient amounts to stimulate B and T lymphocytes *in vivo*. However, the CE5-defined antigen (as a representative of these cross-reactive antigens) is present on the surface of viable neurons in very limited amounts (Wood et al 1982) but can be detected easily when the cell is permeabilized. The adsorption of parasite antigens, and a consequential attack by the host's own anti-parasite immune response, may be sufficient to begin this 'permeabilization' process *in vivo*, thus exposing a leaky neuron to an already existing autoimmune response. The chronic release of neuronal antigens would serve, in turn, to amplify the cycle of self-destruction. This mechanism could account for the relative selectivity of neuronal destruction following infection with a parasite which may potentially invade any cell in the body, and yet rarely chooses neurons.

Prognosis

At present we have few criteria on which to judge the likely evolution of Chagas' disease in an infected patient. Within a single locality, one patient may present with an inapparent infection and another may die with cardiopathy and/or intestinal manifestations. If autoimmune involvement in Chagas' disease stands the test of time and experiment, then the answers to these problems must be implicit in the antigenic nature of the particular invading organisms and the quality of the immune response they provoke.

A direct measurement of EVI and NP antibody titres have been shown to have no correlation with disease classification and so we must look for more refined criteria. These criteria might involve the identification of particular antigens or their relevant antibodies, and cross-reactive epitopes would be obvious candidates. Similarly, although T cells have been shown to be involved in Chagas' disease, we have yet to investigate the quality of this response in detail. Immense possibilities are offered by the potential isolation and characterization of T cell clones specific for *T. cruzi* and for neurons. A useful analogy may be made with the outstanding studies of Cohen (see Ben-Nun & Cohen 1982) on experimental autoimmune encephalomyelitis. These workers established clones specific for myelin basic protein and showed that not only could these T-cell lines produce disease when injected into normal rats but also that they could be used as immunogens and so could provoke a population of suppressor cells capable of preventing evolution of the disease.

In Chagas' disease, similar T-cell clones would certainly aid our understanding of the pathogenic mechanisms and, in addition, might allow us to halt the disease process in a host that already harbours the parasite.

In such a brief presentation it is impossible to do justice to the immense research effort—much of it within Latin America itself—that has recently established definable parasite clones, workable animal models and the exciting possibilites of T-cell cloning, and hybridoma and recombinant DNA technologies. With such powerful weapons in our armoury who, but the most dedicated pessimist, would dare to predict anything but eventual success?

Acknowledgements

I am very grateful to Brian Cover and Gwyn Williams for permission to reproduce their unpublished data in this article, and to Kay Dorelli for typing the manuscript. Unpublished findings from this laboratory are from research work supported by grants from the UNDP/World Bank/WHO Special Programme for Research and Training in Tropical Diseases and from the Medical Research Council of Great Britain.

REFERENCES

Barousse AP, Costa JA, Epasto U, La Plume H, Segura EL 1980 Enfermedad de Chagas' e inmunosupresion. Medicina (B Aires) 40:17-26

Ben-Nun A, Cohen I 1982 Spontaneous remission and acquired resistance to autoimmune encephalomyelitis (EAE) are associated with suppression of T cell reactivity: suppressed EAE effector T cells recovered as T cell lines. J Immunol 128:1450-1457

Cover B, Gutteridge WE 1982 A putative mouse model for chronic Chagas' disease in man. Mol Biochem Parasitol (Suppl): 367-368

Goncalves AM, Chiari E, Deane MP, Carneiro M, Romanha AJ, Morel CM 1983 Schizodeme characterisation of natural and artificial populations of *Trypanosoma cruzi* as a tool in the study of Chagas' disease. In: Newton B (ed) Application of biochemical and molecular biology techniques to problems of parasite and vector identification. UNDP/World Bank/WHO Schwabs and Co. Ag., Basel (Trop Dis Res Ser), in press

Hudson L 1981 Immunobiology of *Trypanosoma cruzi* infection and Chagas' disease. Trans R Soc Trop Med Hyg 75:493-498

Hudson L, Ribeiro dos Santos R 1981 Immunological aspects of chagasic cardiopathy. In: Lessof MH (ed) Immunology of cardiovascular disease. Marcel Dekker Inc, NY, p 141-155

Johnstone AP, Williams GT 1982 Role of DNA breaks and ADP-ribosyl transferase activity in eukaryotic differentiation demonstrated in human lymphocytes. Nature (Lond) 300:368-370

Köberle F 1974 Pathogenesis of Chagas' disease. In: Trypanosomiasis and leishmaniasis with special reference to Chagas' disease. Associated Scientific Publishers, Amsterdam (Ciba Found Symp 20), p 137-158

Laguens RP, Meckert PC, Basombrio MA et al 1980 Infección crónica del ratón con *Trypanosoma cruzi*. Modelo experimental de enfermedad de Chagas. Medicina (B Aires) 40:33-39

Laguens RP, Meckert PC, Chambo G, Gelpi RJ 1981 Chronic Chagas' disease in the mouse. II: Transfer of the heart disease by means of immunocompetent cells. Medicina (B Aires) 41:40-43

Peralta JM, Manigot DA, Muscelli EOA, Magalhães TCR, Almeida EA, Bastos A 1982 Anticorpos EVI e NP na infecção chagásica crónica estudo em pacientes con diferentes formas clínicas. Rev Inst Med Trop São Paulo 24:6-10

Postan M, McDaniel JP, Dvorak JA 1982 Differences in the susceptibility of C3H/HEN$^-$ mice to two clones of *Trypanosoma cruzi* isolated from a common source. Mol Biochem Parasitol (Suppl):374-375

Ribeiro dos Santos R, Hudson L 1980a *Trypanosoma cruzi*: binding of parasite antigens to mammalian cell membranes. Parasite Immunol (Oxf) 2:1-10

Ribeiro dos Santos R, Hudson L 1980b *Trypanosoma cruzi*: immunological consequences of parasite modification of host cells. Clin Exp Immunol 49:36-41

Teixeira ARL, Teixeira ML, Santos-Buch CA 1975 The immunology of experimental Chagas' disease. IV: Production of lesions in rabbits, similar to those of chronic Chagas' disease in man. Am J Pathol 80:163-178

Williams GT 1983 Specific inhibition of intracellular and extracellular differentiation in *Trypanosoma cruzi* using inhibitors of ADP-ribosyl transferase. Science (Wash DC), in press

Wood J, Hudson L, Jessel T, Yamamoto M 1982 A monoclonal antibody defining antigenic determinants on subpopulations of mammalian neurones and *Trypanosoma cruzi* parasites. Nature (Lond) 296:34-38

DISCUSSION

Nogueira: The immunofluorescence that you described was with fixed organisms. Does your anti-CE5 monoclonal antibody also stain live organisms?

Hudson: It will stain live amastigotes but will stain epimastigotes only when they are fixed; it will stain fixed but not live trypomastigotes.

Nogueira: These features suggest that the antigen is not a surface component.

Hudson: It is a surface component on amastigotes.

Nogueira: But you also described immunofluorescence with *Trypanosoma cruzi* trypomastigotes. Was this with the same anti-CE5 antibody that you used to produce passive protection in mice (Fig. 5 in your paper)?

Hudson: Yes.

Nogueira: So how can you explain the decrease in parasitaemia when the anti-CE5 antibody was administered passively?

Hudson: I don't know. This antibody might react with an antigen on the surface of amastigote-infected cells, and this is something that we have not investigated. (**See note on p 251.*)

Nogueira: Do you know the molecular nature of the component in the neurons and in *T. cruzi*, by cell labelling and immunoprecipitation experiments?

Hudson: Yes. We have studied this quite extensively and a series of components of different relative molecular mass has been described (Wood et al 1982).

Nogueira: Is the component in trypomastigotes the same as that in amastigotes?

Hudson: Immunoprecipitation from [^{35}S]methionine-labelled parasites revealed bands of similar molecular mass on sodium dodecyl sulphate–polyacrylamide gel electrophoresis (L. Hudson, unpublished observations.)

Piras: Is there any difference in the staining with the monoclonal antibody against the neurons, depending on whether the *T. cruzi* strain that you use is neurotropic or not?

Hudson: I don't know. We have only looked at the Y strain, and we don't ever see infected neurons in our mice. This would be worth testing.

Andrade: I would like to emphasize that involvement of the myenteric plexus does occur in the mouse with *T. cruzi* infection. Some time ago we showed that if the animals were treated with corticoid, destruction of the neurons could be avoided. At that time there was a controversy about whether the amastigote was releasing a neural toxin, and we wanted to abolish inflammation. The destruction of neurons took place only when inflammation was present (Andrade & Andrade 1966). Alencar (1964) in Brazil counted Purkinje cells in the central nervous system, selecting these cells by chance because they are actually easier to count. He found that humans with chronic Chagas' disease had a decreased number of Purkinje cells. However, he used, as controls, patients with chronic cardiac failure and, using the same technique, he found a similar number of neurons in both groups. He concluded that the neuronal loss was due to anoxic or ischaemic damage to the Purkinje cells.

Hudson: Amastigotes do not produce a neural toxin (Ribeiro dos Santos & Hudson 1980). However, we were excited to find that, in the human disease, Purkinje cells were affected (Brandão & Zulian 1966, Köberle 1974). The problem is always in trying to relate experimental findings to observations in human pathology. In London I have little opportunity to observe patients with Chagas' disease!

Sharma: I was wondering if the mRNA product that you have seen on the gels is the protein part of the glycoprotein; therefore the low M_r of the translated product would not be surprising. Is this antigen-specific mRNA? Did you isolate total mRNA from trypomastigotes?

Hudson: Yes. We took total mRNA from *T. cruzi* trypomastigotes, then did immunoprecipitation on the translation products. Harvey Eisen is doing sucrose-density fractionation at the moment to try to get the specific mRNA out. The CE5-defined antigen is about 1% of the total translated products, so we may have a chance of getting its mRNA out.

Sher: You said that cytolytic T cells are involved in the pathogenesis of these lesions, and you described damage to infected cells. Do you have any system for measuring cytotoxic T-cell activity against non-infected cells that express the CE5 antigen, and can you block that activity with the monoclonal antibody?

Hudson: We really need to develop T-cell lines to look at these antigens. Ben Nun & Cohen (1982) were able to obtain T-cell lines that were antigen-specific. More importantly, for Chagas' disease, they were able to immunize with these T-cell lines and were able to stop the disease-causing potential of the T-cells. This is relevant to our discussion after Dr Andrade's paper when we were considering whether anything can be done for patients once they have developed Chagas' disease. This approach is perhaps equivalent to an anti-idiotype immunization, which may halt the pathogenic process. If this is an autoimmune process, once established it might become self-perpetuating, and getting rid of the parasite would therefore be unhelpful.

Sher: Is the T-cell-mediated killing that you observe restricted by the major histocompatibility complex?

Hudson: No. The killing of the cells was not H2-restricted, which is odd. But Louis et al (1981) showed, when using whole spleen cells from mice that had been infected with one of the *Leishmania* species, that there was no H2-restriction. When they started making T-cell lines from these mice they then saw H2-restriction. This is a further reason why we need T-cell lines.

Sher: To go back to my first point, I believe that people have been able to block cytolytic activity, using antibodies to block the target determinant. That approach might be useful to you if you do detect T-cells that will kill cells expressing the antigen.

Hudson: Yes, but the problem is that such an approach is not open-ended. The results can be interpreted only if the antibody produces inhibition of T-cell killing.

Butterworth: There is another possible interpretation of this direct killing by lymphocytes. We heard previously about the neuraminidase that is released from the trypomastigotes (see Nogueira, this volume), and this neuraminidase may presumably remove sialic acid residues from the target cells in your tissue-culture system. I believe that the removal of sialic acid residues from some normal cells renders them susceptible to natural-killer (NK)-cell killing. So you may be seeing the effect of an increased NK-cell activity after removal of sialic acid residues from both the infected and the uninfected target cells.

Hudson: A whole series of studies have looked at that phenomenon. As I mentioned in my paper one could reproduce host-cell sensitization passively with *T. cruzi* antigens *in vitro*. When T cells from mice infected for 30 days are used, killing is mediated entirely via parasite antigens. When T cells from mice infected for 90 days are used, parasite-antigen-coated muscle cells and also uncoated syngeneic muscle cells will be killed. However, HeLa cells will not be killed with these same T cells, unless they are sensitized with antigen. So even at the 90-day stage, a degree of specificity is retained. This would argue against the involvement of NK cells.

Warren: Can you explain why the antigen adheres so readily to so many different cell types? What is the mechanism?

Hudson: The antigen seems to prefer to stick to cells that are adherent during their normal growth pattern, and it is probably binding to something like a fibronectin structure on the surface.

Sher: Szarfman et al (1982) have shown that patients and experimental animals develop antibodies to laminin, which is a component of connective tissue. This antigen can also be detected on the surface of trypomastigotes. Could the anti-CE5 monoclonal antibody be recognizing laminin?

Hudson: I don't know.

Butterworth: You prepared clones by limiting dilution. Are they stable, and do they all, regardless of their virulence, express the antigen recognized by the monoclonal antibody?

Hudson: In both James Dvorak's work (Postan et al 1982) and our own, the parasite clones were stable. So the A2 clone, which was very virulent, has remained virulent. With regard to antigen expression, we have looked at only three of the 35 clones that we have made, and they all expressed the antigen. At least one of them was very poorly infectious, and the other one was A2. So from these limited observations antigen expression does not correlate with infectivity or virulence.

Gutteridge: Presumably your Y strain is a fairly old laboratory strain that has been passaged rapidly in mice at seven-day intervals for years and years. By now one might have expected to have selected, from that original uncloned population, the genotype that was best adapted to such passage. It is amazing that apparently you still have a highly mixed population, as measured by kinetics of growth. This must serve as a warning to all who work on such uncloned parasite lines.

Pereira: Is there any evidence that neuronal destruction is complement-mediated? I ask this because neuraminidase treatment of certain mammalian cells activates the complement pathway.

Hudson: We do know that, *in vitro*, anti-CE5 antibody plus complement is able to kill viable neuronal cells, and complement-mediated lysis is thus possible when the antibody is administered *in vivo*. I don't know whether infection *alone* could induce neuronal destruction by complement fixation. Do you have any information on this yourself?

Pereira: No.

Gutteridge: The inhibitors of differentiation that you studied were interesting. The concentrations that you had to use were relatively high; have you done any experiments to see if they affect development of parasitaemia *in vivo*?

Hudson: We have not used these inhibitors with parasites, but we do know that in mice treated with the inhibitors and then immunized with hapten carrier conjugates, one can specifically suppress the immune response. This happens if the inhibitors are given up to 12 h before the antigen, *with* the antigen, or up to 12 h *after* antigen administration (C. Broomhead & L. Hudson, unpublished observations). So inhibition occurs only during the phase when the cells are differentiating. Perhaps one could therefore suppress the initiation of an immune response, and yet leave an existing immune response untouched. For the control of parasite infection, it might not be helpful to use an inhibitor that would suppress the immune response, so one would need a specific inhibitor for parasite ADP-ribosyl transferase. Our present inhibitors are probably the worst ones to use with parasite infections because they were originally identified by their effects in mammalian cell systems.

REFERENCES

Alencar A 1964 Atrofia cortical na cardiopatia chagasica crônica. Hospital (Rio de J) 66:808-815

Andrade SG, Andrade ZA 1966 Doença de Chagas e alteracoes neuronais do plexo de Auerbach. Rev Inst Med Trop Sao Paulo 8:219-224

Ben-Nun A, Cohen I 1982 Spontaneous remission and acquired resistance to autoimmune encephalomyelitis (EAE) are associated with suppression of T cell reactivity: suppressed EAE effector T cells recovered as T cell lines. J Immunol 128:1450-1457

Brandão HJS, Zulian R 1966 Nerve cell depopulation in chronic Chagas' disease. A quantitative study in the cerebellum. Rev Inst Med Trop Sao Paulo 8:281-286

Köberle F 1974 Pathogenesis of Chagas' disease. In: Trypanosomiasis and leishmaniasis with special reference to Chagas' disease. Associated Scientific Publishers, Amsterdam (Ciba Found Symp 20) p 137-158

Louis JA, Moedder E, MacDonald HR, Engers HD 1981 Recognition of protozoan parasites by murine T lymphocytes. II: Role of the H-2 gene complex in interactions between antigen-presenting macrophages and *Leishmania*-immune T lymphocytes. J Immunol 126:1661-1666

Postan M, McDaniel JP, Dvorak JA 1982 Differences in the susceptibility of C3H/HEN mice to two clones of *Trypanosoma cruzi* isolated from a common source. Mol Biochem Parasitol (Suppl) p 374-375

Ribeiro dos Santos R, Hudson L 1980 *Trypanosoma cruzi*: immunological consequences of parasite modification of host cells. Clin Exp Immunol 49:36-41

Szarfman A, Terranova V, Rennard SI et al 1982 Antibodies to laminin in Chagas' disease. J Exp Med 155:1161-1171

Wood J, Hudson L, Jessel T, Yamamoto M 1982 A monoclonal antibody defining antigenic determinants on subpopulations of mammalian neurones and *Trypanosoma cruzi* parasites. Nature (Lond) 296:34-38

**Note added in proof* (see p 247)*

Using immunofluorescence we have now shown that CE5 antibody will bind to the surface of a BALB/c muscle tumour (S2) infected with *T. cruzi*. Uninfected S2 cultures showed no reaction (L. Hudson & S. J. Morgan, unpublished results).

Final general discussion

Problems of working with different parasitic strains

Warren: It is heartening that at the beginning of our symposium there was a considerable area of agreement about protozoan organisms between Dr Piras and Dr Nogueira, even though they are working with fibroblasts and macrophages, respectively, and possibly with different strains of *Trypanosoma cruzi*. In early work on *T. cruzi* confusion arose because people worked with different stages of the organisms but the field is now becoming more sophisticated. The development of research on leishmaniasis, by comparison, has now reached the confusing stage. Immunopathology of leishmaniasis, for example, is a difficult issue because it is so bound up with mechanisms of immunity; one is never sure whether one is dealing with host or parasite mechanisms (Warren 1982). Dr Chang has talked about *Leishmania donovani* and *Leishmania mexicana amazonensis* in mice macrophages. Dr Hernández has talked about *Leishmania braziliensis* in culture, and has also looked at the effect on mouse macrophages. Dr Pérez has talked about work on mice with *L. mexicana* from a patient and *L. mexicana amazonensis* that came from a wild reservoir. Dr Sher has talked about *L. mexicana* and *Leishmania tropica* in similar inbred strains of mice, using mouse macrophages. The various experimental conditions are, thus, very different. The picture can be even more confused when the authors of review articles draw conclusions about mechanisms while mixing up all these different factors. Strains of parasites are now being defined more carefully, and people are now using similar mouse strains and cell lines. The source of parasite strains is certainly important, as is the need to deal with relatively fresh strains so that observations can be related to the state of the patient from which the strain is taken.

Sher: I would like to emphasize my own view that research on leishmaniasis has been making good progress and that there is a consistent pattern of results emerging, particularly on the immunology of the infection in inbred mouse strains. Many of the data on the cell biology and biochemistry of the parasite are also quite consistent from laboratory to laboratory.

Pérez: There once was a lot of confusion but if we compare, for example, the

1983 Cytopathology of parasitic disease. Pitman Books, London (Ciba Foundation symposium 99) p 252-255

results of Behin et al (1979), Bradley (1974), Handman et al (1979), Howard et al (1980), Dr Sher's group and our group, we can see that the same strains of mice are resistant to *L. tropica*, *L. donovani* and to *L. mexicana* parasites. With American *Leishmania* species, perhaps we are forgetting that the genus is in the process of speciation. The American *Leishmania* species are more complex than we originally thought. We have a biological reactor represented by the vectors and the reservoir. The definition of differences between leishmanial parasites is going to be even more difficult than we realise. I am really against the idea of using parasites, as we all do, that have been kept for many years in cultures. We should begin to isolate parasites from vectors, reservoirs and human beings, and to use cryopreservation and cloning to look for a different experimental system for analysing them.

Hernández: We have been working with Dr J.V. Scorza (unpublished work) and we found profound differences in the isolates even in a small endemic region. Furthermore, the NR strain of *L. braziliensis* that we are working with didn't follow the classification reported in mosquitoes for *L. mexicana* and *L. braziliensis*. We have more clues than before, and the problem now is how to organize it all.

Urbina: We have been studying metabolic differences between different leishmanial strains, one of which is non-pathogenic (which, as Dr Pérez pointed out, could be just an artifact of selection after so many years of passage), and another strain that is very infective. Typically, clear-cut growth patterns differentiate the two strains, and relate to an important difference in their aerobic metabolism capacity. The infective strain has a poor capacity to metabolize carbohydrates. Markers of aerobic metabolism, such as the enzymes of the TCA cycle, have very low activities compared with those in the non-pathogenic strain which are very active *in vitro*. Although these results are not clearly related to a pathogenic property, the infective strain thus has a low capacity for classical carbohydrate metabolism and its aerobic metabolism is slow compared with the laboratory-adapted strains.

Chang: Although different workers use different culture systems for studying *Leishmania* species, there is some general agreement about results on aspects of host–parasite interactions. In at least three or four different host–parasite combinations, phagosome–lysosome fusion has been demonstrated, for example. The entry of the parasite into the macrophage has been shown, also in several systems, to be due largely to the phagocytic activity of the macrophages. It is important, nevertheless, to differentiate the different strains at the same time as other work is going on. It may not be fair to compare progress in studying *Leishmania* species with that in studying *T. cruzi* because Chagas' disease is geographically limited to South America, whereas leishmaniasis is caused by different strains and species in different parts of the world and will take more time to be fully understood.

Hernández: The key factor in the survival of the leishmanial parasite is the transformation at the first step from promastigote to amastigote. We should look at the factors that initiate differentiation as a means of understanding the whole issue (see also p 133-136). It has been shown that when promastigotes don't differentiate they are almost all killed by macrophages whereas the opposite happens with amastigotes (Lewis & Peters 1977, Hernández et al 1981). So differentiation is the key factor. The differences between promastigotes and amastigotes could resolve many of the problems arising from the particular strains that we are each working with. The ideal would be to describe as much as possible about each strain, in terms of isoenzymes, excretory factors, buoyant density of kinetoplasts, restriction enzymes, and so on. Ruth Nussenzweig mentioned earlier (p 172) the restriction enzyme patterns and the differentiation between strains. One can distinguish easily, for example, between different trypanosomes but not between different *Leishmania* species. There is a point at which one will find small differences but we don't know if these are significant. Some major features certainly deserve more attention: definition of the strains being used in laboratories may be important from the epidemiological, immunological and biochemical points of view. The parasite need not always kill the cell but may sometimes simply modify the cell so that it can live there, as I showed in my paper (this volume).

Sher: There seems to be a general trend in parasitology research to study the behaviour of clones. It may not necessarily be a good idea to deal with cloned populations of parasites, particularly in immunopathological studies in experimental animals. Obviously one will learn much about the genetic diversity of different parasite populations but in dealing with cloned organisms there is the danger that we will overlook the properties of natural, mixed isolates and thus fail to see the wood for the trees.

Hudson: Peter Medawar (1982) in his book 'The art of the soluble' said, in essence, that nobody gets credit for doing heroic experiments which fail; people simply think that you have tackled the wrong experiment. If one only studies clones then this is unreal because clones rarely, if ever, exist in the real world. The ideal is to reduce the system under study to its most simple elements, then to describe the components of the system, and then to see how those components interact by step-wise addition. Ultimately one then returns to real life. The danger for people working outside endemic areas, as I do, is that study of the parasite itself can be so fascinating that one neglects the much more complex entity of the human patient with the disease.

Piras: In relation to this cloning versus non-cloning approach, I was struck by the comment of Win Gutteridge after Leslie Hudson's paper that after so many passages in mice one can still clone such different *T. cruzi*. There must have been a tremendous selective pressure throughout the years, and nevertheless it was possible to isolate different clones. This must mean something. It would also be worthwhile to look at what happens to a cloned parasite after a few months or a few years: would it, for example, show up just as a single clone?

Mirelman: We still don't know enough about host effectors and microenvironments and how are they controlled. Changes in the host could modulate the expression of the parasite's genome under conditions that are controlled by the host's general state—for example, bacterial flora, nutrition, secondary infections, and intake of other medications. These factors may facilitate the development, *in vivo* in the human host, of a parasitic virulence that would not otherwise have developed under normal conditions. We must try to understand how the parasite may be affected by these varying conditions.

Warren: The simple problem is that not enough people are working in this field. The World Health Organization in its Tropical Diseases Research Programme is now supporting studies on six diseases—malaria, trypanosomiasis, leishmaniasis, filariasis, schistosomiasis and leprosy (see also p 260). In addition, the Edna McConnell Clark Foundation devotes significant funds to the study of schistosomiasis alone. However, the study of amoebiasis caused by *Entamoeba histolytica* has received relatively little financial support, as have the infections of hundreds of millions of people with ascariasis, trichuriasis, hookworm or giardiasis.

REFERENCES

Behin R, Mauel J, Sordat B 1979 *Leishmania tropica*—pathogenicity and *in vitro* macrophage function in strains of inbred mice. Exp Parasitol 48:81-91

Bradley DJ 1974 Genetic control of natural resistance to *Leishmania donovani*. Nature (Lond) 250:353

Handman E, Ceredig R, Mitchell G 1979 Murine cutaneous leishmaniasis: disease patterns in intact and nude mice of various genotypes and examination of some differences between normal and immune macrophages. Aust J Exp Biol Med Sci 57:9-29

Hernández AG, Arguello C, Ayesta C et al 1981 The surface membrane of *Leishmania*. In: Slutzky G (ed) The biochemistry of parasites. Pergamon Press, Oxford, p 47-65

Howard JG, Hale C, Chan-Liew WL 1980 Immunological regulation of experimental cutaneous leishmaniasis. I: Immunogenetic aspects of susceptibility to *Leishmania tropica* in mice. Parasite Immunol (Oxf) 2:303-314

Lewis DH, Peters W 1977 The resistance of intracellular *Leishmania* parasites to digestion by lysosomal enzymes. Ann Trop Med Parasitol 71:295-312

Medawar P 1982 Pluto's republic: incorporating 'The art of the soluble' & 'Induction and intuition in scientific thought'. Oxford University Press, Oxford

Warren KS 1982 Mechanisms of immunopathology in parasitic infections. In: Cohen S, Warren KS (eds) Immunology of parasitic infections. Blackwell Scientific Publications, Oxford, p 116-137

Chairman's closing remarks

K.S. WARREN

Health Sciences Division, The Rockefeller Foundation, 1133 Avenue of the Americas, New York, NY 10036, USA

Since this symposium is concerned with parasitic diseases (classically, those caused by protozoa and helminths) I would like to end by mentioning some recent broad insights into parasites provided by the mathematical ecologists, Robert May and Roy Anderson (1979). They have emphasized the gross differences between helminths and other parasites. They call helminths *macroparasites* and all other infectious agents, including protozoa, bacteria, viruses and fungi, *microparasites*. The principal difference, apart from multicellularity as compared to unicellularity, is that macroparasites do not usually multiply within the definitive host; ingestion, say, of one egg will result in development of at most one worm. All microparasites, on the other hand, multiply within the human host unless they are controlled by natural resistance, acquired immunity or drugs. Most of the papers presented at this symposium have covered intracellular microparasites (four papers on *Trypanosoma cruzi*, four on *Leishmania* species, one on *Toxoplasma gondii*), with the exception of David Mirelman's paper (Mirelman et al, this volume) on *Entamoeba histolytica* and David Wyler's paper (this volume) on a helminth infection (*Schistosoma mansoni*).

Problems in research on parasitic diseases

Variation among parasites

Studies of *E. histolytica* largely assume that there is a single species which may either be non-virulent or have varying degrees of virulence. *T. cruzi* has many strains, but the strains and the techniques for studying them are now becoming more standardized from laboratory to laboratory. The study of leishmaniasis

1983 Cytopathology of parasitic disease. Pitman Books, London (Ciba Foundation symposium 99), p 256-262

presents a particular problem, as we have been discussing, because of the many species and the large number of different strains within these species. A continuing difficulty has been how to distinguish between the strains: attempts at morphological differentiation have now been largely abandoned; isoenzymes have been studied; the kinetoplast DNA molecules have been subjected to restriction enzymes and then to gel filtration analysis; hybridoma techniques have been used, and so too has DNA hybridization. When I came to this symposium I thought that the hybridoma technique described by McMahon Pratt & David (1981) and the DNA hybridization studies of Wirth & McMahon Pratt (1982) might solve most of these problems, but after our final discussion of the multitude of strains of *Leishmania* and the difficulties in distinguishing between them, I am not sure!

A particular problem with *T. cruzi*, and also with *Leishmania* species, is that people have been working with different stages of the organisms—promastigotes, epimastigotes, amastigotes and trypomastigotes. Indeed, not very long ago these stages themselves were not very well defined. Some stages develop in an insect vector, others in a variety of mammalian hosts, including humans, and some are grown in tissue culture. Increasingly, people in individual laboratories are studying several different stages of the parasite simultaneously to compare their different characteristics, and this is a most promising development.

The source of the different strains is also important. Some have been maintained in laboratories for generations. Some strains are relatively fresh, but may be of human or animal origin. In some cases the precise clinical status of the source patient is defined, but even the site at which the parasite was obtained from the patient may be important. Cloning has now become a major tool, as wide variations can be observed in different clones obtained from a single isolate of the parasite.

The *Schistosoma* species of *japonicum*, *mansoni* and *haematobium* also give rise to problems because of different strains. *S. mansoni* from the New World appears to be more susceptible to oxamnaquine than that from Africa, as approximately four times the dose is required in patients from Africa (Davis 1982). Furthermore, cercariae of schistosomes shed from different snails appear to differ in their infectivity. E. H. Bloch's recent studies (unpublished work), using cinemicrophotography in chambers inserted into the skin of mice and hamsters, have shown that there is marked variation among the individual infective organisms, with some being attacked vigorously by host cells and others remaining virtually untouched.

Despite all these problems, much progress has been made, and if strain variation is taken into account in the planning of experiments we can expect even greater progress. Anything that can pinpoint precise differences among the various *Leishmania* strains, for example, is of great importance.

Variations among hosts

We also have to deal with marked variations in the hosts as well as in the parasites. Different laboratory animals are used, as well as different tissues, cells and cell lines from these animals. For *in vitro* studies different media are used. Among the different animal hosts, small laboratory animals such as hamsters, guinea-pigs and mice are used most commonly. A major advantage of laboratory mice, in addition to their small size and ease of handling, has been that they are exceedingly well characterized immunologically. As well as outbred mice, many different strains of inbred mice are being used by more and more laboratories, and there are considerable differences in the observed host–parasite relationships among them. Mice with metabolic and immunological defects of genetic origin may be particularly useful.

Work on the human host can be done not only *in vivo*, which is difficult to control, or *post mortem*, but also with living tissues taken from the human. Anthony Butterworth (1974) developed a model for working with *S. mansoni* and human white cells *in vitro* which has greatly advanced our knowledge of possible immune mechanisms in schistosomiasis. Nadia Nogueira and her colleagues (1982) have been studying human macrophages from patients with Chagas' disease in Brazil.

Temporal variations in the host–parasite relationship

Virtually all the protozoan and helminth infections that we have discussed here are chronic diseases, which go through several phases and have different clinical manifestations at different periods of time. It is not always necessary, however, for a given animal model to mimic the entire range of disease manifestations, both acute and chronic. For instance, granuloma formation around *S. mansoni* eggs injected into the tissues of mice, guinea-pigs, rats and hamsters appears to be similar even though these animals vary in their susceptibility to the infectious agent (Akpom et al 1970). Grove et al (1979) have been able to study *Brugia malayi* microfilaraemia in mice, even though the mice do not become infected with the parasite and undergo the whole cycle of development. Animal models can sometimes reveal a great deal even when they do not mimic the disease at all, as illustrated by Leslie Hudson's paper (this volume).

We must, of course, consider the human disease itself as an experimental model, but we have the problem of defining the stage at which a chronic disease is being studied. Now that immunomodulation and immunoregulation are becoming better understood, the point at which we examine the pathogenesis of a lesion or a clinical syndrome is crucial. Studying various immunological parameters in the later stages of infection may reveal mechanisms that regulate or suppress the lesion or syndrome rather than mechanisms responsible for initiating it.

General summary of the symposium

I would like to consider the work presented at this meeting at three different levels—ultrastructural, chemical and immunological. The elegant electron micrographs of Don Fawcett (see this volume, p 207-213) revealed how *Theileria parva*, the causative agent of East Coast fever in African cattle, penetrates passively into lymphocytes. In contrast, Nadia Nogueira (this volume) described active phagocytosis of trypomastigotes of *T. cruzi* by mouse or human macrophages. Once the parasites are intracellular they use different mechanisms of multiplication, as revealed by electron microscopy. *T. gondii* enters phagosomes and multiplies because there is a mechanism preventing phagosome–lysosome fusion (Jones & Hirsch 1972). K.-P. Chang has shown that phagosomes containing *Leishmania* fuse with lysosomes, but that the organisms grow well in this presumably inimical environment (Chang & Dwyer 1976). Nogueira & Cohn (1976) have found that while *T. cruzi* is taken up in a phagosome, the organism soon leaves the organelle to multiply within the cytoplasm of the host cell. Adolfo Martinez-Palomo's superb electron micrographs (see this volume, p 26-29) have illustrated the way in which *E. histolytica* destroys host cells by direct contact without damaging surrounding cells.

Chemical studies have elucidated the mechanisms of parasite adhesion to host cells, penetration, the host–parasite relationship within cells, how the host cell destroys the parasitic cell and vice versa. Dr Mirelman and others (this volume) have described an adhesion mechanism of *E. histolytica* through sugar-binding proteins (lectins). The lectin can be on the parasite and the sugar on the host cell or vice versa. The lectin–sugar binding can be blocked experimentally. Romano Piras and his colleagues (this volume) have also shown the importance of 'lectin-like' proteins in adhesion of *T. cruzi* to fibroblasts. They also described the system, probably proteolytic, which activates or exposes a pre-existing protein, with resulting enhancement of adhesion. Dr Nogueira and colleagues noted that opsonization by immunoglobulin G-type antibodies enhances uptake of *T. cruzi* by macrophages. At the stage when the organisms are within the cells, Elmer Pfefferkorn's studies (Pfefferkorn et al, this volume) with mutants of both the parasite (e.g. *T. gondii*) and the host cell have demonstrated some of the metabolic pathways involved in the host–parasite relationship. Seymour Klebanoff and colleagues (this volume) have studied the oxidative response of phagocytic cells to parasite invasion, and his work reveals a major mechanism by which the host destroys parasites. Dr Nogueira has found that lymphokines enhance oxidative killing of *T. cruzi* within host cells. Interestingly, Angel Hernández (this volume) has shown that *Leishmania* species excrete factors that may suppress the handling of these parasites by macrophages.

We then extended our consideration of the role of immune mechanisms in the killing of intracellular parasites into describing investigations of the immunological mechanisms leading to the destruction of the parasite (immunity) or to the development of disease in the host (immunopathology). Hilda Pérez (this volume) has studied the mechanisms of immunity to *Leishmania mexicana* in inbred mice and Alan Sher and his colleagues (this volume) have studied the same parasite, as well as *L. tropica*, also in mice. In relation to immunopathology, Dr Wyler described an immunological mechanism of fibrosis as a major factor in the pathogenesis of schistosomiasis. Zilton Andrade (this volume), studying *T. cruzi* infections in dogs, revealed early destruction of cardiac muscle cells by the multiplying parasites and the subsequent inflammation. In late chronic progressive lesions few, if any, parasites are seen and the mechanisms of cell damage are presumed to be immunological. Dr Hudson then suggested two mechanisms by which *T. cruzi* damages the autonomic nervous system of the host: adsorption of parasite antigens onto host cells and sharing of common antigens by parasites and host cells.

The current status of parasitology

I will now conclude with some general remarks on the relative neglect of the science of parasitology by funding agencies, by the governments of the developing world (where these infections are rife) and by modern scientists. In fact the protozoa and helminths comprise the largest number of what the Rockefeller Foundation has called 'the great neglected diseases of mankind'. These diseases are 'great' with respect to the numbers of people that are infected; for instance, for *T. cruzi*, 12 million; for *Leishmania*, 12 million; for *E. histolytica*, 400 million; and for *Schistosoma*, 200 million; (Walsh & Warren 1979). In the developed world, by contrast, there is an enormous interest in relatively rare diseases, such as multiple sclerosis. The sheer numbers of people infected with the great neglected diseases should justify more work being done on them.

Neither are there enough scientists working on these problems, owing to a lack of direct interest by those in the developed world, a lack of infrastructure for science in the developing world, and a seemingly particular neglect of the science of parasitology. A survey conducted by the American Society of Parasitologists of all graduate training programmes of the United States and Canada has revealed a failure to 'keep up' with modern science. For instance, of the total courses in all parasitology training programmes only 5% covered immunology, 4% biochemistry, and 1% ultrastructure (Weinstein 1981). An examination of published work in parasitology has revealed that the amount published is quite small. In 19 major English-language journals, in general and specialty parasitology, tropical medicine, general and specialty medicine and general and specialty science, a total of 972 articles was published in 1979. A similar number of articles was published that year in the Journal of Immunology alone (Warren 1981).

With respect to funding, it is interesting to compare the cancer research programmes of the United States government and the American Cancer Society with the World Health Organization's Tropical Diseases Research Programme. The former provide, respectively, $1000 million and $40 million annually for research on a disease of 10 to 20 million people worldwide, and the latter provide only $25 million for research globally on six major diseases: malaria, trypanosomiasis, leishmaniasis, filariasis, schistosomiasis and leprosy. It is also noteworthy that in its first five years the WHO programme received $90 million from bilateral and multilateral agencies, of which 40% came from four small northern European countries and only 0.7% from all the developing countries.

Nevertheless, it appears that changes are beginning to occur. Outstanding scientists are starting to work on parasitic diseases and are producing exciting results that have important practical implications. This Ciba Foundation symposium has clearly revealed what can be accomplished by the application of sophisticated modern techniques of ultrastructure, chemistry and immunology in the elucidation of the mechanisms and potential means of control of parasitic diseases. I believe that these developments will continue to accelerate as scientists and funding agencies realize the enormous potential for the good of mankind offered by research on these great neglected diseases.

REFERENCES

Akpom CA, Abdel-Wahab MF, Warren KS 1970 Comparison of formation of granulomata around eggs of *Schistosoma mansoni* in the mouse, guinea pig, rat and hamster. Am J Trop Med Hyg 19:996-1000

Butterworth AE, Sturrock RF, Houba V, Rees PH 1974 Antibody-dependent cell-mediated damage to schistosomula *in vitro*. Nature (Lond) 252:503-505

Chang KP, Dwyer DM 1976 Multiplication of a human parasite (*Leishmania donovani*) in phago-lysosomes of hamster macrophages *in vitro*. Science (Wash DC) 193:678-680

Davis A 1982 Management of the patient with schistosomiasis. In: Jordan P, Webbe G (eds) Schistosomiasis; epidemiology, treatment and control. Heinemann, London, p 184-226

Grove DI, Davis RS, Warren KS 1979 *Brugia malayi* microfilaremia in mice; a model for the study of the host response to microfilariae. Parasitology 79:303-316

Jones TC, Hirsch JG 1972 The interaction between *Toxoplasma gondii* and mammalian cells. II: The absence of lysosomal fusion with phagocytic vacuoles containing living parasites. J Exp Med 136:1173-1194

May RM, Anderson RM 1979 Population biology of infectious diseases: part I. Nature (Lond) 280:361-367

McMahon Pratt D, David JR 1981 Monoclonal antibodies that distinguish between New World species of *Leishmania*. Nature (Lond) 291:581-583

Nogueria N, Cohn ZA 1976 *Trypanosoma cruzi*: mechanism of entry and intracellular fate in mammalian cells. J Exp Med 143:1402-1420

Nogueira N, Chaplan S, Reesink M, Typhings J, Cohn ZA 1982 *Trypanosoma cruzi*: induction of microbicidal activity in human mononuclear phagocytes. J Immunol 128:2142-2146

Walsh JA, Warren KS 1979 Selective primary health care. N Engl J Med 301:967-974

Warren KS 1981 The present status of the parasitology literature. In: Warren KS, Purcell EF(eds) The current status and future of parasitology. Josiah Macy Jr Foundation, New York, p 142-151

Weinstein PP 1981 Teaching parasitology. In: Warren KS, Purcell EF(eds) The current status and future of parasitology. Josiah Macy Jr Foundation, New York, p 51-62

Wirth DF, McMahon Pratt D 1982 Rapid identification of *Leishmania* species by specific hybridization of kinetoplast DNA in cutaneous lesions. Proc Natl Acad Sci USA 79:6999-7003

Index of contributors

Entries in **bold** *type indicate papers; other entries refer to discussion contributions*

Indexes compiled by John Rivers

Subject index